# Strategies for ECG Arrhythmia Diagnosis:

## Breaking Down Complexity

# Strategies for ECG Arrhythmia Diagnosis:

## Breaking Down Complexity

**George J. Klein, MD, FRCPC**
Professor of Medicine
Division of Cardiology
Western University
London, Ontario, Canada

cardiotext
PUBLISHING

First paperback edition, 2018

Cardiotext Publishing, LLC
750 2nd St NE Suite 102
Hopkins, MN 55343
USA

www.cardiotextpublishing.com

Any updates to this book may be found at: www.cardiotextpublishing.com/strategies-for-ecg-arrhythmia-diagnosis

Comments, inquiries, and requests for bulk sales can be directed to the publisher at: info@cardiotextpublishing.com.



Library of Congress Control Number: 2016936753

ISBN: 978-1-942909-11-8

eISBN: 978-1-942909-24-8

2 3 4 5 6 7

# Table of Contents

# Contributors

## Written and Edited By:

**George J. Klein,** MD, FRCPC; Professor of Medicine, Division of Cardiology, Western University, London, Ontario, Canada

## Contributors:

**Lorne J. Gula,** MD, MSc, FRCPC; Associate Professor of Medicine, Division of Cardiology, Western University, London, Ontario, Canada

**Peter Leong-Sit,** MD, MSc, FRCPC; Assistant Professor of Medicine, Division of Cardiology, Western University, London, Ontario, Canada

**Jaimie Manlucu,** MD, FRCPC; Assistant Professor of Medicine, Division of Cardiology, Western University, London, Ontario, Canada

**Paul D. Purves,** BSc, RCVT, CEPS; Senior Electrophysiology Technologist, Cardiac Investigation Unit, London Health Sciences Centre, London, Ontario, Canada

**Allan C. Skanes,** MD, FRCPC; Professor of Medicine, Division of Cardiology, Western University, London, Ontario, Canada

**Anthony S. L. Tang,** MD, FRCPC, FHRS; Professor of Medicine, Division of Cardiology, Western University, London, Ontario, Canada

**Raymond Yee,** MD, FRCPC; Professor of Medicine, Director of Arrhythmia Service, Division of Cardiology, Western University, London, Ontario, Canada

# Preface

The ECG remains the cornerstone of arrhythmia diagnosis, even after an explosion of technology and rapid expansion of our understanding of arrhythmia mechanisms. While many traditional textbooks emphasize cataloguing arrhythmias and pattern recognition, the current book aims to teach a universal approach based on known electrophysiological principles. There is fundamentally no difference in the principles and strategies behind understanding the ECG and intracardiac tracings—both are absolutely complementary. Cases are used virtually exclusively to highlight important principles, with each case meant to provide an important diagnostic "tip" or teaching point.

A multiple-choice question is provided with each tracing not only to "frame the problem" for the reader but to provide some practice and strategies for answering cardiology board examination-type questions.

The book is meant for serious students of arrhythmias, be they cardiology or electrophysiology trainees or established physicians.

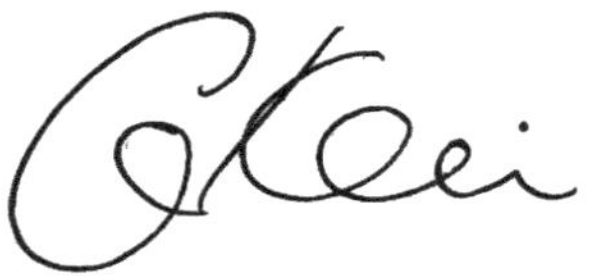

# Abbreviations

| | |
|---|---|
| **AF** | atrial fibrillation |
| **AFL** | atrial flutter |
| **AP** | accessory pathway |
| **AT** | atrial tachycardia |
| **AVCS** | atrioventricular conduction system |
| **AVN** | atrioventricular node |
| **AVNRT** | atrioventricular node reentrant tachycardia |
| **AVRT** | atrioventricular reentrant tachycardia |
| **BBB** | bundle branch block |
| **bpm** | beats per minute |
| **CL** | cycle length |
| **CSM** | carotid sinus massage |
| **ECG** | electrocardiogram |
| **EP** | electrophysiology |
| **ERP** | effective refractory period |
| **IVCD** | intraventricular conduction disturbance |
| **JT** | junctional tachycardia |
| **LAFB** | left anterior fascicular block |
| **LBBB** | left bundle branch block |
| **ms** | millisecond |
| **PAC** | premature atrial contraction |
| **PR interval** | interval from onset of P to onset of QRS |
| **PVC** | premature ventricular contraction |
| **RBBB** | right bundle branch block |
| **ST** | sinus tachycardia |
| **SVT** | supraventricular tachycardia |
| **VT** | ventricular tachycardia |
| **WC** | wide complex |
| **WCT** | wide complex tachycardia |
| **WPW** | Wolff-Parkinson-White |

# Explanatory Notes and Tables of Differential Diagnosis

## Cycle Length Variability ("Wobble")

Looking for CL variation during a tachycardia can be extremely productive. A simple but important principle is that *the cause of a CL change CANNOT be downstream from the observed change*. For example, if the P-P interval prolongs suddenly and prolongs the tachycardia CL, it cannot be VT!

## "Zone" Analysis of a Complex ECG

A complex ECG is often read from left to right, but it can be very useful to look at the recording and divide it into zones. For example, a tracing showing two different tachycardias can be divided into three zones: tachycardia 1, tachycardia 2, and a transition zone, each to be considered separately. It is often productive to start with the zone that is easiest or clearest to understand and then build from there.

It is also often productive to magnify zones of interest to clarify some subtle observations or make finer measurements.

## Regular Supraventricular Tachycardias

1. Atrial tachycardia
2. AVNRT
3. AVRT
4. JT
5. Atrial flutter
6. Sinus tachycardia
7. VT with narrow QRS

## Regular Supraventricular Tachycardia with VA Block (Fewer P's than QRS)

1. AVNRT
2. JT
3. Nodoventricular or nodofascicular reentry (uncommon)
4. VT with narrow QRS

## Wide QRS Tachycardia

1. Supraventricular tachycardia with aberrant conduction
2. Preexcited tachycardia
3. Ventricular tachycardia
4. Artifact
5. Paced rhythm
6. "Pseudo" tachycardia related to marked ST elevation . . . for example, sinus tachycardia with the elevated ST segment merging with the QRS giving appearance of a "wide" QRS

## Sudden Shortening of the PR Interval

1. Intermittent conduction over an accessory pathway ("intermittent preexcitation").
2. Junctional extrasystole
3. PAC
4. PVC
5. Shortening of the PR interval by resolution of delay in the AV node or His-Purkinje system, often after pause or rate slowing
6. Shift to a fast AVN pathway in a patient with dual AVN pathways

Of all these possibilities, the most common would be late-coupled PVCs, which interrupt the PR interval.

## Termination of a WCT with a Narrow QRS Complex at Same CL

1. SVT with spontaneous resolution of functional bundle branch block on the last cycle
2. Spontaneous termination of VT with a supraventricular (AV nodal or AV) echo beat after the last VT QRS
3. A capture beat terminating VT

This phenomenon is, with rare exceptions, related to spontaneous resolution of functional bundle branch block during SVT where the affected bundle branch is part of the circuit. For example, normalization of LBBB aberration in orthodromic AVRT over a left lateral AV pathway would result in shortening of the VA interval, which arrives prematurely in the AV node and may well block. A fortuitous atrial capture beat following the VT termination at the CL of VT is theoretically possible but very unlikely. This is because VT almost universally results in concealed retrograde penetration of the AV node even in the absence of VA conduction, and this would *delay* the arrival of the capture beat. Additionally, one would have to postulate that a relatively late-coupled capture beat at CL of VT would terminate VT without apparent fusion (essentially impossible) or that the VT terminated and a capture beat at the CL of VT fortuitously arrived at that time.

# Chapter 1

## The Electrophysiological Approach to ECG Diagnosis

The electrocardiogram (ECG) was introduced over 100 years ago and has been an integral part of cardiology diagnosis ever since, with ever-increasing understanding of the patterns observed and their relationship to physiology and pathophysiology. Virtually every cardiac assessment incorporates an ECG. Most students are taught a systematic approach to reading the ECG, with a heavy emphasis on pattern recognition. Arrhythmia analysis incorporates pattern recognition, of course, but is unique in requiring more than the ability to recognize patterns and to be systematic. The best arrhythmia electrocardiographers use their knowledge, overtly or not, of the physiology and pathophysiology of the conduction system and arrhythmogenesis to deduce the mechanism of complex arrhythmias.

Early electrocardiographers used deductive reasoning to predict the mechanisms of many arrhythmias, which were subsequently verified and amplified in the era of invasive electrophysiology and ablation. To this day, the ECG remains the pivotal diagnostic tool to bring attention to potentially important arrhythmias and focus the subsequent investigation and management. Indeed, electrograms recorded by intracardiac catheters are merely additional ECG leads that are "closer to the action" i.e., near-field.

Many outstanding cardiologists and electrophysiologists have diverse approaches to teaching arrhythmia diagnosis from the ECG. The intent of this brief text is to provide an approach with an emphasis on not only being systematic, but also using a conscious examination of the observations that one would expect given different arrhythmia mechanisms. ***You only see what you are looking for!***

Consider that a pure pattern reader might look at a wide complex tachycardia (WCT) and compare the findings to a long list of wide QRS ventricular tachycardia (VT) criteria found in the literature, often named after individuals who published them. In my experience, the average medical resident has no idea why, for example, an Rs complex in $V_1$ is a VT criterion. The electrophysiological approach teaches that the WCT, if it is aberration, should in general resemble RBBB or LBBB. Further, the more it is different from such, the higher the probability of VT. Of course, ventricular preexcitation essentially has "VT morphology" depending on where the accessory pathway inserts into the ventricle and must always be considered.

To take another example, a "northwest" axis is a "VT criterion" simply because it is generally not seen in the great majority of individuals with bundle branch block. It is simpler to ask oneself, "How similar is this ECG to a 'normal' bundle branch block pattern?" rather than attempt to memorize lists of seemingly unrelated "criteria" that essentially are derivatives of the above general principle.

Consider the WCT shown in **Figure 1-1A**. P waves are discernable in the ST segment (see lead 2) and there appears to be a one-to-one relationship between the P waves and QRS complexes. There are many possible discussion points for this tracing, but we can tell at a glance that this is likely to be VT, in all probability. The WCT is of LBBB type but $V_1$ is atypical in having a gradual (slow) downstroke of the S wave. There is a relatively big "jump" in the R wave between $V_2$ and $V_3$. The frontal axis is straight downward ("high to low" ventricular activation). There is a QS in lead 1, indicating ventricular activation predominately from left to right.

Going forward, pay attention to the QRS morphology when you encounter RBBB and LBBB and provide yourself with a mental range of reasonable variability, which you can then apply to WCT diagnosis.

*It is always worth examining previous ECGs* when these are available. In the example of WCT, I look especially for PVCs, which can be thought of as a 1-beat run of VT, allowing you to see an

Figure 1-1A

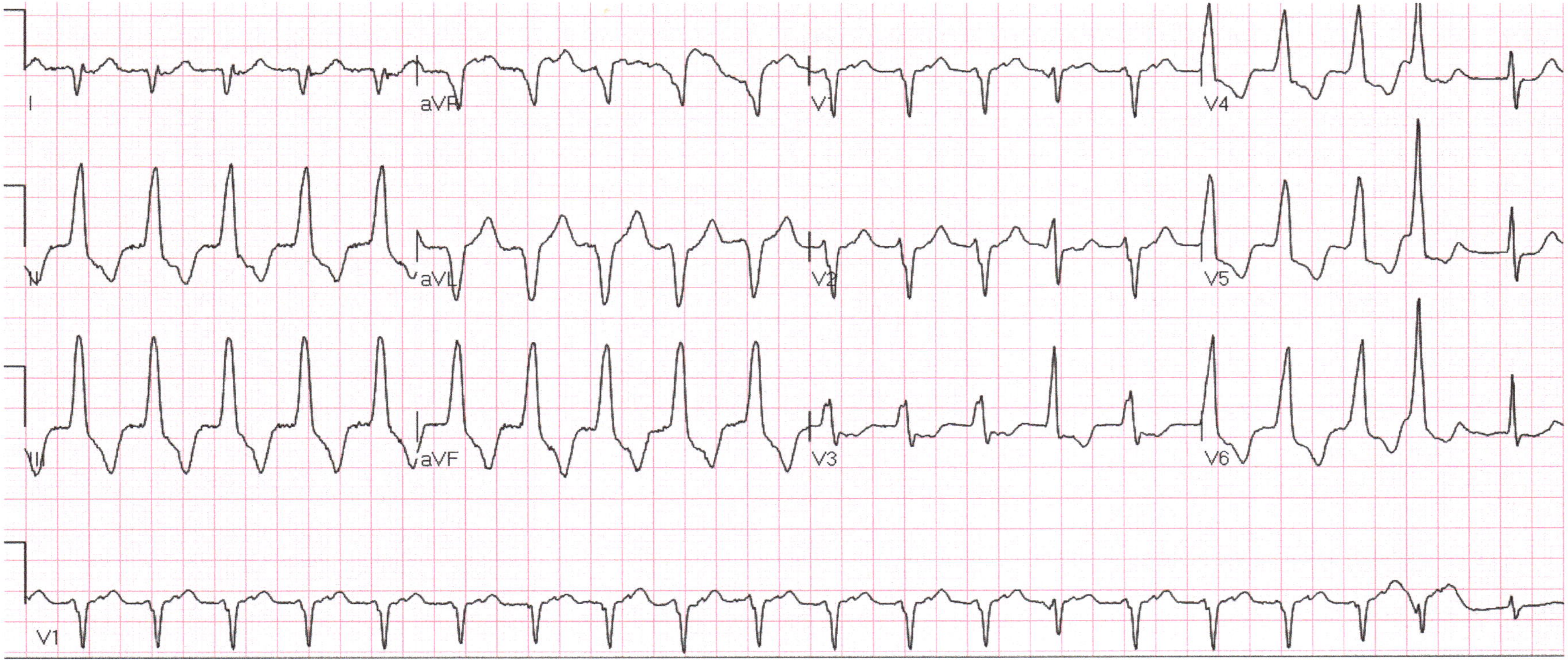


"onset" of tachycardia. In our example above, such a tracing (**Figure 1-1B**) was available. The diagnosis of the WC beats as PVCs is then quite straightforward, as they are not preceded by atrial activity and don't disturb ("reset") the ambient sinus rhythm. In this case, the obvious PVCs have an identical QRS to the WCT providing further support for the diagnosis of VT.

There is no intent in this text to provide an extensive catalogue of all possible arrhythmias. Rather, the emphasis is on the approach or "game plan" by which the electrocardiographer can prioritize a list of possible entities to explain the observations identified in the tracings. This is more important than arriving at a correct answer by a timely guess—the latter is not to be confused with a brilliant deduction.

In the analysis of ECGs, it is useful to think of evidence in terms of *probabilistic* versus *absolute* ("smoking gun"). For example, a supraventricular tachycardia showing any block to the atrium *absolutely and unequivocally* rules out atrial tachycardia. It also rules out any tachycardia where the atrium is a necessary link, such as atrioventricular

Figure 1-1B

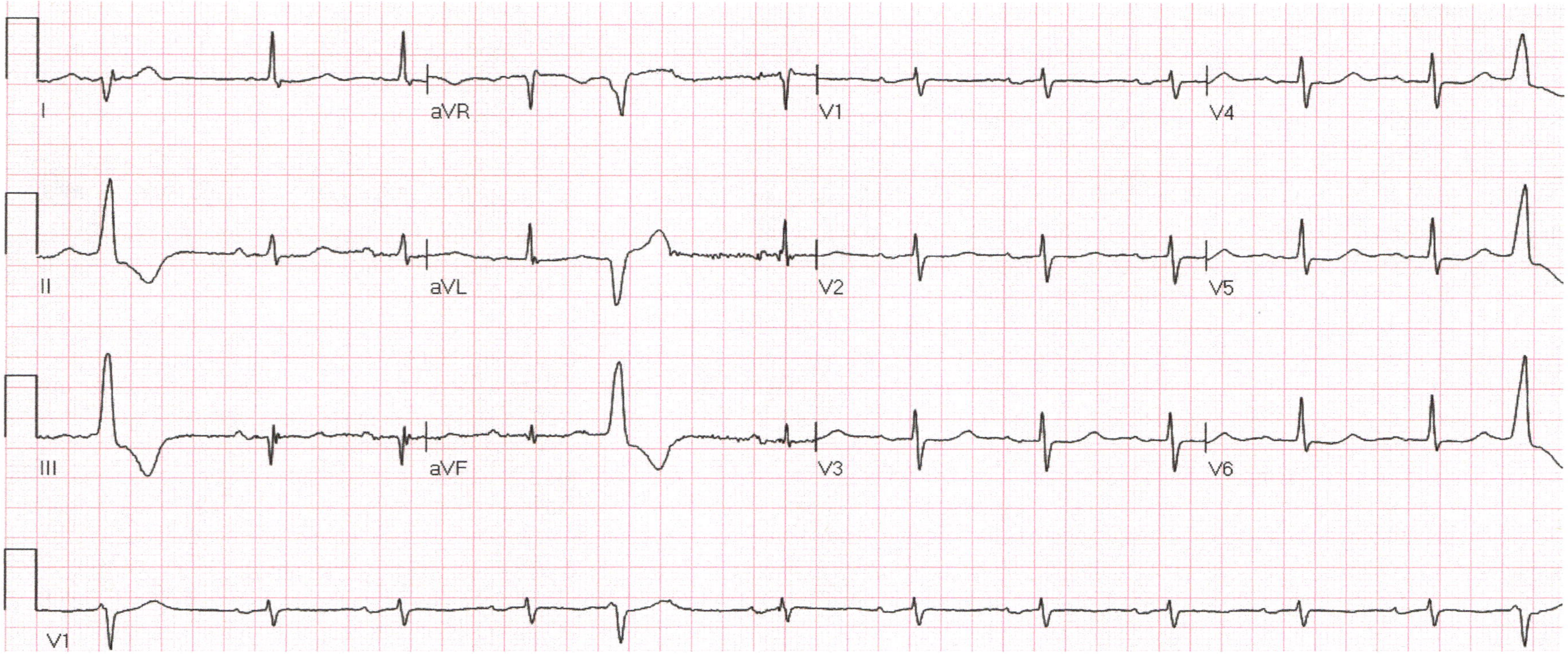


reentry. On the other hand, termination of a supraventricular tachycardia with a P wave (**Figure 1-2, arrow**) strongly militates against (does not *absolutely* disprove) atrial tachycardia, since it would be improbable for an atrial tachycardia to terminate entirely coincidentally with simultaneous AV block after the last tachycardia P wave. In the example presented here, the diagnosis was AVNRT. A diagnosis can frequently be made from one or more *probabilistic observations* that should be correct most of the time but are not infallible.

In this workbook, we frame the problem by providing a multiple-choice type of question for the reader. The question preamble or "stem" may put in the word "probably" or similar phrasing to indicate that the correct answer is based on the balance of probability. Outside of this format designed to help the readers with examination writing, readers need to frame their own problems for an unknown tracing to focus thinking. For example, if one frames the problem as a "wide QRS tachycardia," the differential diagnosis is limited (VT, SVT with aberration, preexcited tachycardia, paced rhythm, artifact). This allows one to test each possibility (that is, each hypothesis) for validity.

Figure 1-2

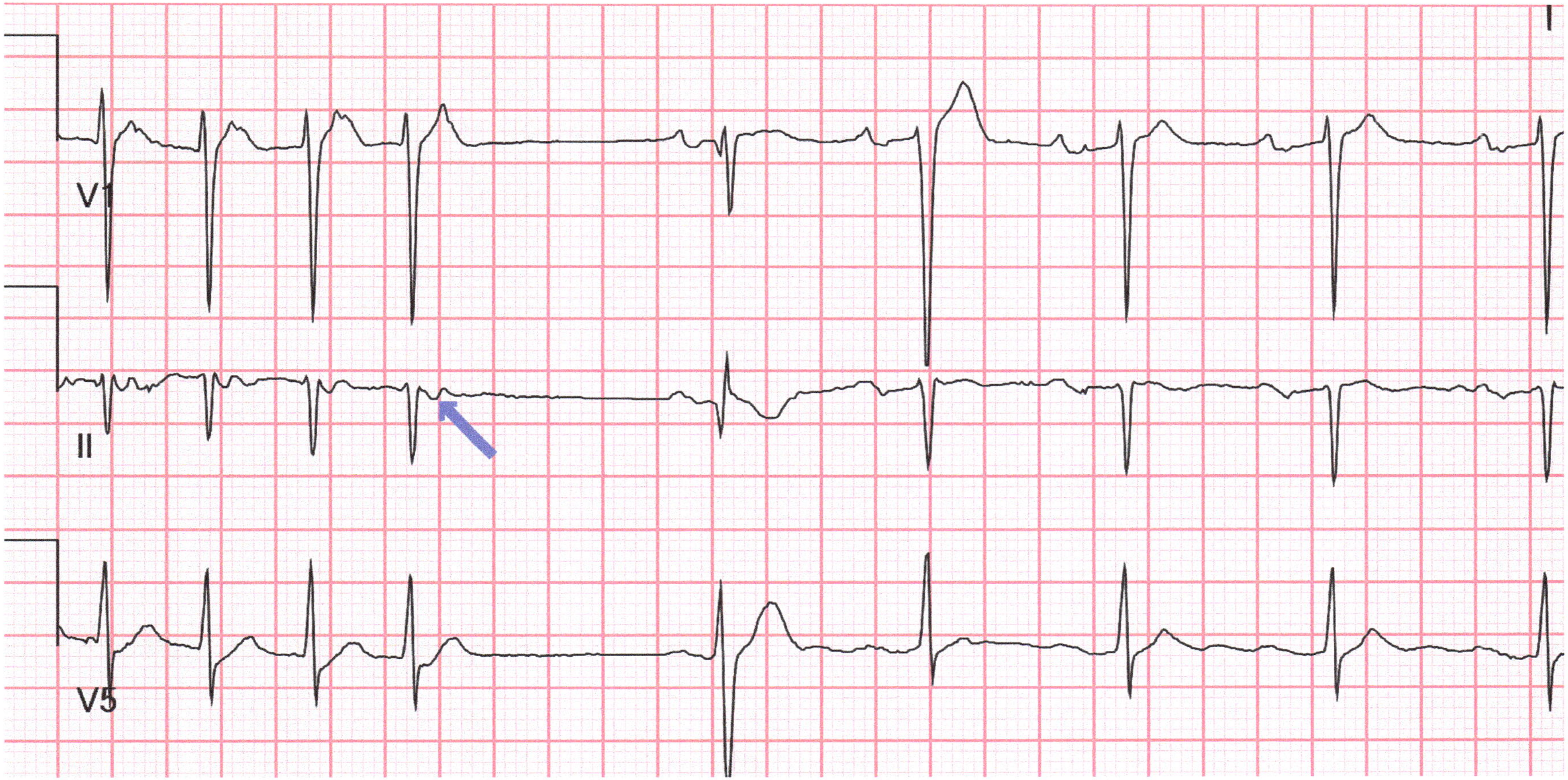


*Self-Check 1-1 and Self-Check 1-2* provide a starting framework that should be followed more or less with every single tracing. Pattern recognition is not discarded and is useful but needs to be supplemental to orderly observations that are put into a physiological framework. There are certain ways to look at the problem that may help that will be presented in the context of the cases. For example, dividing a complex tracing into segments, *focusing initially on a piece you can understand and building out from there,* as illustrated in **Question 6-13.**

Accurate measurement can be the key to interpreting arrhythmia. I find it useful to magnify the area of interest to better focus on the zone and make the appropriate measurements where the differences can be subtle as illustrated in **Question 2-3.**

The overall approach will become clearer with the exercises to follow. It might be worthwhile to reread this brief section periodically when going through the cases in the book.

## Self-Check 1-1

A systematic, electrophysiologic approach to ECG tachycardia diagnosis:

- Don't make up your mind too early. The "quick look" that depends on pattern recognition is done by all of us, but it can be risky to make up your mind too early. There is a tendency to rationalize subsequent observations to "fit" the original impression.
- Take the trouble to look at previous ECG tracings, when available.
- Describe what you see looking at the whole tracing. Examine zones away from the "action" of the tracing for clues.
- Avoid premature conclusions and "jargon" that suggest a mechanism prematurely.
- Consider the highlights: A to V relationship and P-wave and QRS morphologies. Recognition of atrial activity when possible is undoubtedly the single most useful diagnostic aid.
- Review the tracings. Tracings are frequently complex with changing features. It is not necessary to view it *temporally* from left to right, and it is frequently useful to focus initially on *any zone that is understandable* to you and then to build from there.
- Measure. Don't simply eyeball important intervals. Small changes in cycle length can be critical if consistent.
- Focus on ***zones of transition.*** These include onset and offset of tachycardia, change in cycle length and effect of ectopic beats. You will usually find the necessary diagnostic information in these zones.
- Center on a key observation and create a differential diagnosis; that is, "frame" the problem. For example, a tracing may have many interesting features, but if the QRS is wide, it is useful to just list the causes of wide complex tachycardia (WCT) consciously. We provide multiple-choice questions in this workbook that frame the problem for the reader, but in the real world, readers must frame their own problems prior to analyzing.
- Test each hypothesis for "goodness of fit." There may be a "smoking gun" or indisputable observation. Other observations, even if not indisputable, may allow meaningful prioritization of diagnoses by probability.

## Self-Check 1-2

If you got it wrong, did you. . .

- Make up your mind too early?
- Fall into the trap of using mechanistic jargon or labels rather than just observing initially with open mind?
- Just "eyeball" important intervals rather than measure carefully?
- Focus on a specific zone *without* considering the rest of the tracing?
- Miss a key observation?

# Chapter 2

## Diagnosis Through Physiology

Figure 2-1A

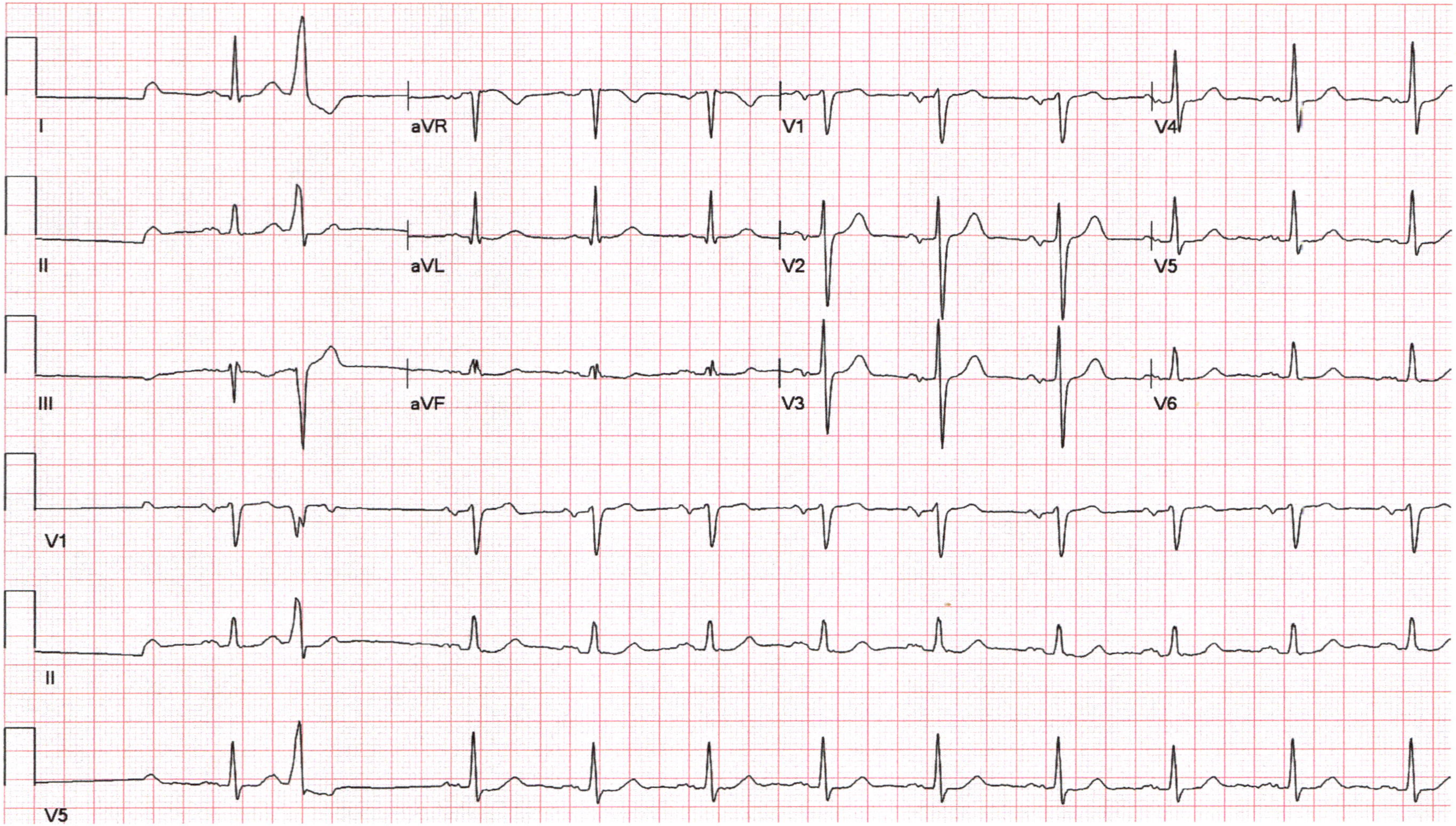

## Question 2-1

A 22-year-old woman has episodes of "rapid" heartbeats but other-wise is well. An ECG is obtained (**Figure 2-1A**). She is *most likely* to have which supraventricular tachycardia?

1. Atrial flutter
2. AVNRT
3. AVRT
4. Sinus tachycardia

## Answer

This question is "probabilistic" in that there is no absolute correct answer to such a question. We are told that the patient is a young woman, otherwise well—a patient in whom atrial flutter would be distinctly uncommon.

The ECG is normal, but we see a single PVC that provides the clue. $V_1$ is magnified in **Figure 2-1B**; P waves are highlighted by the black dots. The PVC is followed by a full compensatory pause and the sinus rhythm is not perturbed. The PVC does not conduct to the atrium even though it is early enough, suggesting at least a long retrograde ERP of the normal AV conduction system, and quite possibly no VA conduction at all. The next P wave is blocked, signaling concealed retrograde conduction into the AVN by the PVC. Orthodromic AV reentry is dependent on good retrograde conduction and AV node reentry is almost always, although not invariably, associated with retrograde conduction at baseline state, so that neither of these arrhythmias would be probable.

The best answer among our 4 options based on the information provided would be Option 4, sinus tachycardia.

Figure 2-1B

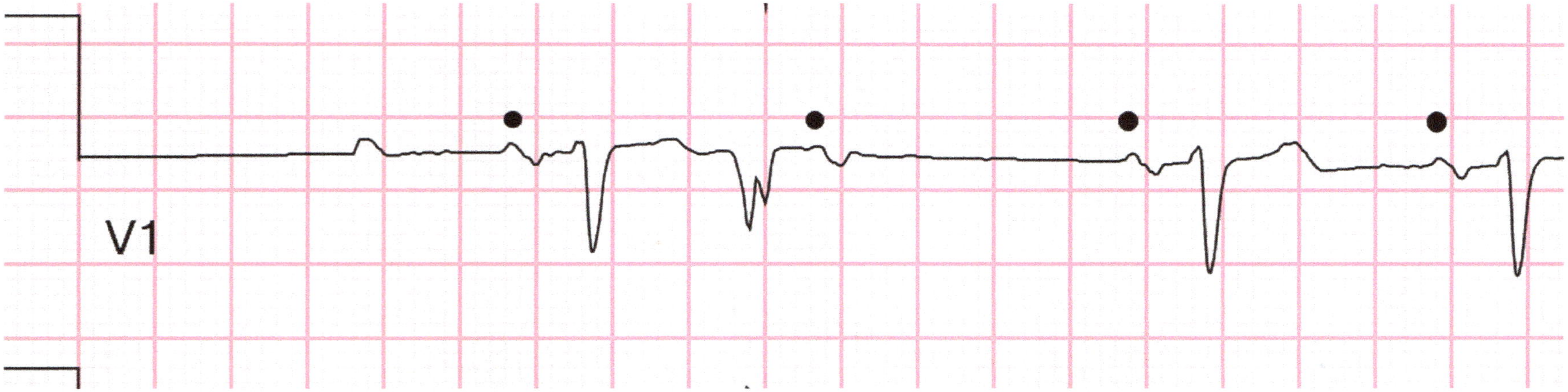

Figure 2-2A

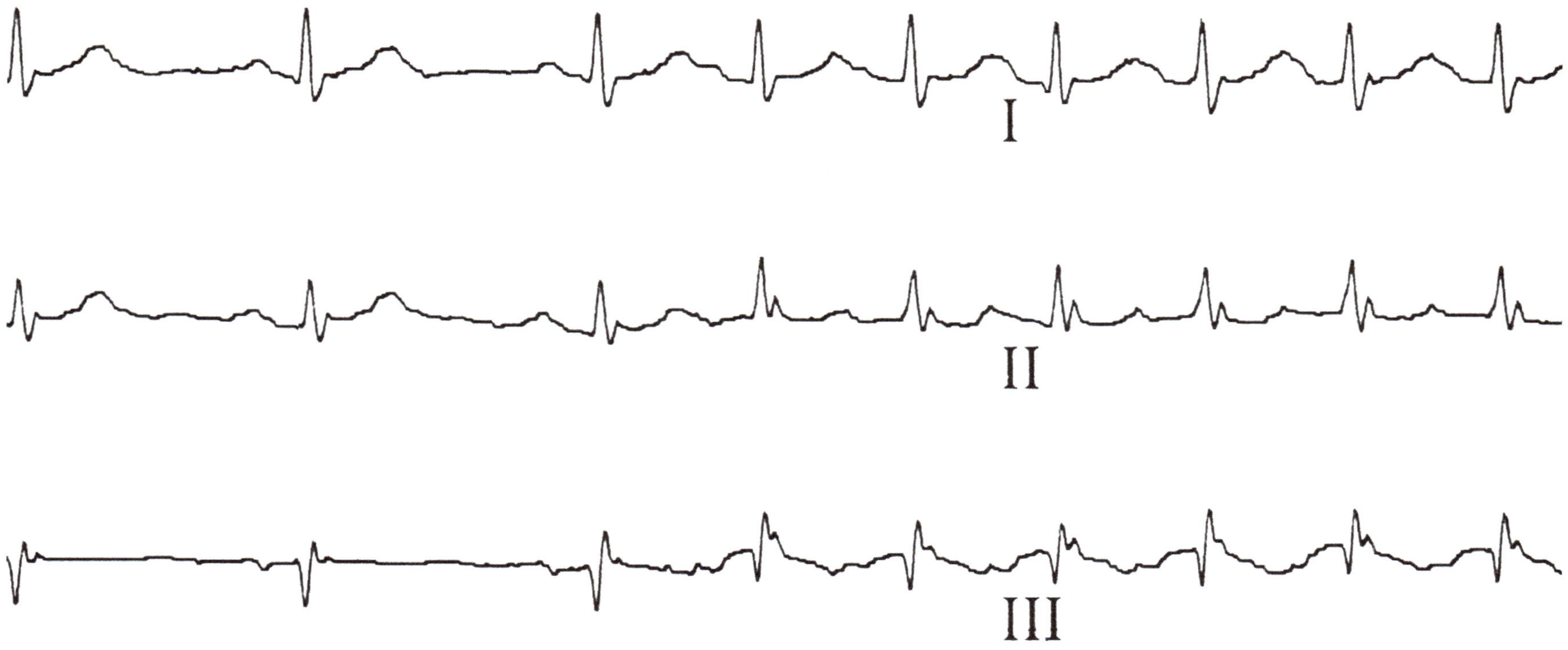


## Question 2-2

The SVT mechanism in **Figure 2-2A** is:

1. AT
2. AVNRT
3. AVRT
4. Need more data

## Answer

This tracing is meant to focus on the utility of the PR interval of the PAC initiating tachycardia in determining mechanism. We note (**Figure 2-2B**) that there is an initiating PAC and that P waves can be tracked superimposed on the T wave thereafter.

*The PR interval of the initiating PAC does not prolong.* This is useful information, since both AVN and AV reentry initiated by a PAC almost universally require some PR prolongation to allow the delayed arrival of the retrograde wave to initiate reentry. The example in Figure 2-2A therefore is clearly atrial tachycardia for this and other reasons (the P wave can be tracked through the tachycardia and remains upright in the monitored leads).

Does the contrary—i.e., PR prolongation of the initiating cycle—help narrow the diagnosis? Not really; PR prolongation is expected with a sufficiently premature PAC and, of course, is related to cycle-dependent prolongation ("decremental") of conduction in the AV node. Thus, the PR interval may prolong with the extrastimulus regardless of the mechanism of the subsequent tachycardia. However, a *marked* prolongation of the PR interval suggesting slow-pathway conduction will usually, although not universally, signal AVNRT. Consider that either AT or AVRT may involve a slow anterograde pathway even if the latter is not related to the SVT mechanism (see Question 6-8).

Figure 2-2B

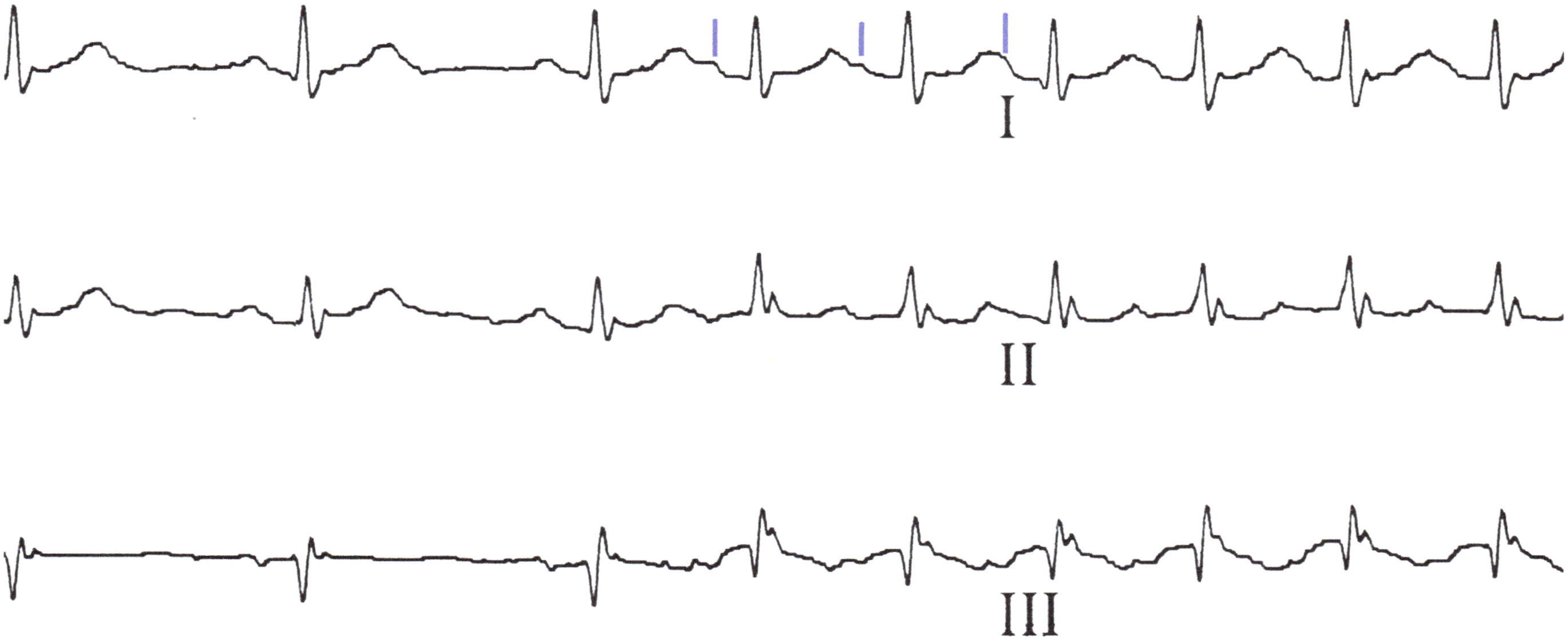

Figure 2-3A

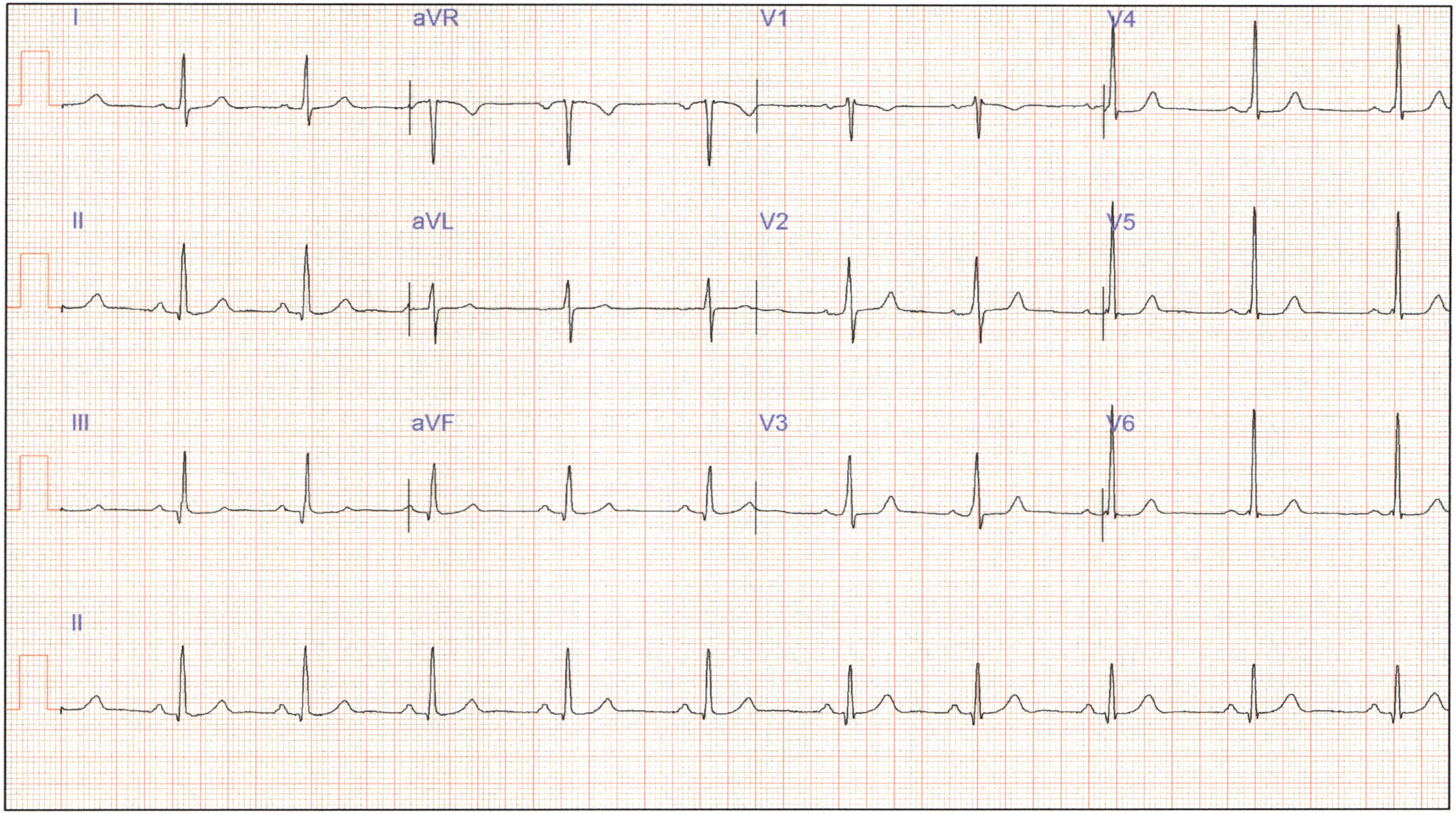

## Question 2-3

The tracing seen in **Figure 2-3A** illustrates:

1. QRS alternans
2. Intermittent preexcitation
3. Cycle length–dependent intraventricular conduction disturbance (IVCD)
4. Normal ECG

## Answer

The correct answer is *intermittent preexcitation*.

It is easy to dismiss this ECG as normal from a cursory look. Yet one should be struck by the difference in the frontal leads, which appear unremarkable, and the lateral precordial leads $V_4$ to $V_6$, which appear preexcited with a slurred upstroke and no PR segment. The lower rhythm strip also shows a change in QRS amplitude after the fifth cycle, along with a subtle change in QRS morphology.

It appears that the first of 5 cycles are normal and the last 5, with no apparent change in cycle length (CL), are preexcited. This observation can be made when the accessory pathway (AP) has a relatively long, anterograde ERP and conduction over the accessory pathway is "fragile" and lost with slight changes in heart rate, autonomic tone, or other undefined events. The former, of course, gives a strong clue that the accessory pathway would not allow rapid conduction in the event of atrial fibrillation (AF), a useful finding for noninvasive risk stratification.

How can one add another element of certainty to this observation? If visible preexcitation occurs in the rhythm strip, the PR interval should, of course, shorten. This difference is difficult to appreciate from the 12-lead ECG. **Figure 2-3B** is a magnification of the area of interest, and careful measurement makes it clear that this is indeed what happens. It is certainly difficult to make the observations by "eyeballing" the tracing. The difference of 16 ms would be very difficult to appreciate without doing this.

*This is not a complicated tracing per se, but highlights the use of magnification to make subtle points and measurements more clear.*

Figure 2-3B

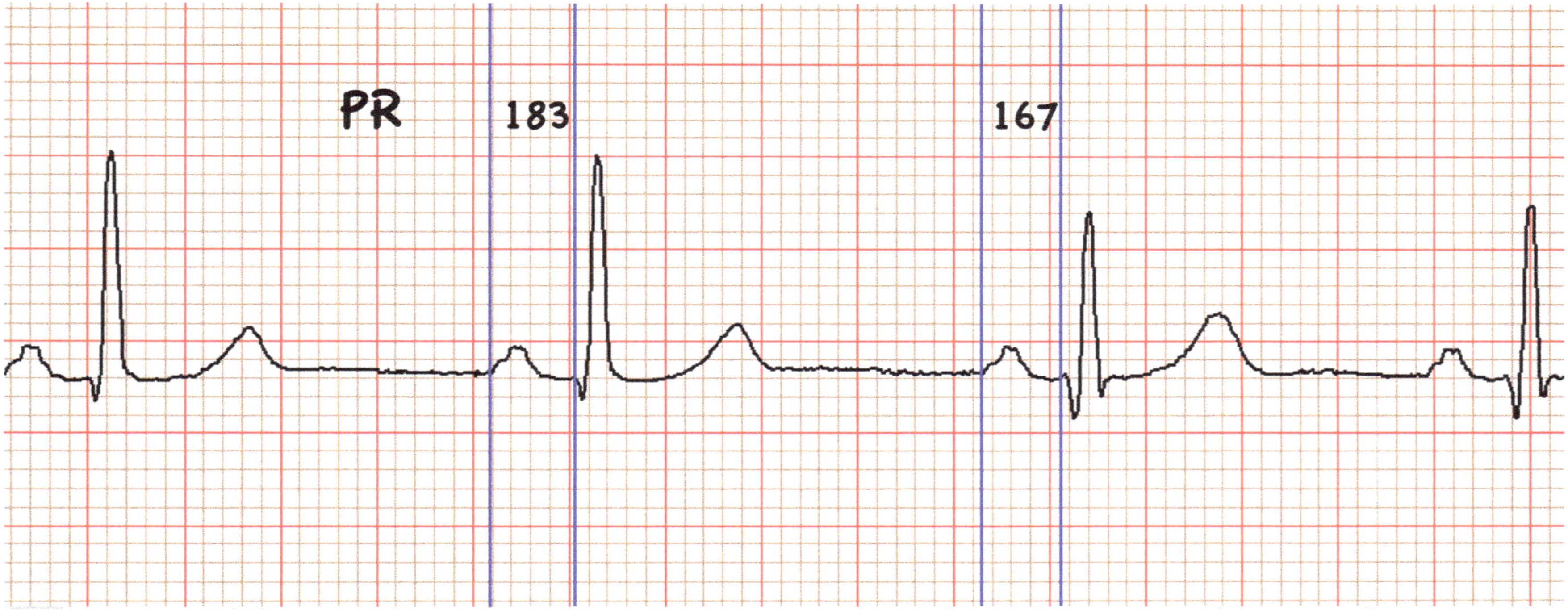

## Question 2-4

The following tracings (**Figures 2-4A** to **2-4D**) were extracted from a Holter monitor record of a 10-year-old boy referred for evaluation of the Wolff-Parkinson-White (WPW) pattern found in the course of a screening program at his school before a tryout for the soccer team. He is otherwise well. On the basis of this record, appropriate recommendations would be:

1. Electrophysiologic testing with a view to ablation if high-risk accessory pathway is found
2. β-blocker therapy for 1 year, after which the patient can be reevaluated
3. No therapy, but disallow competitive sports
4. Reassure with no further investigations

Figure 2-4A

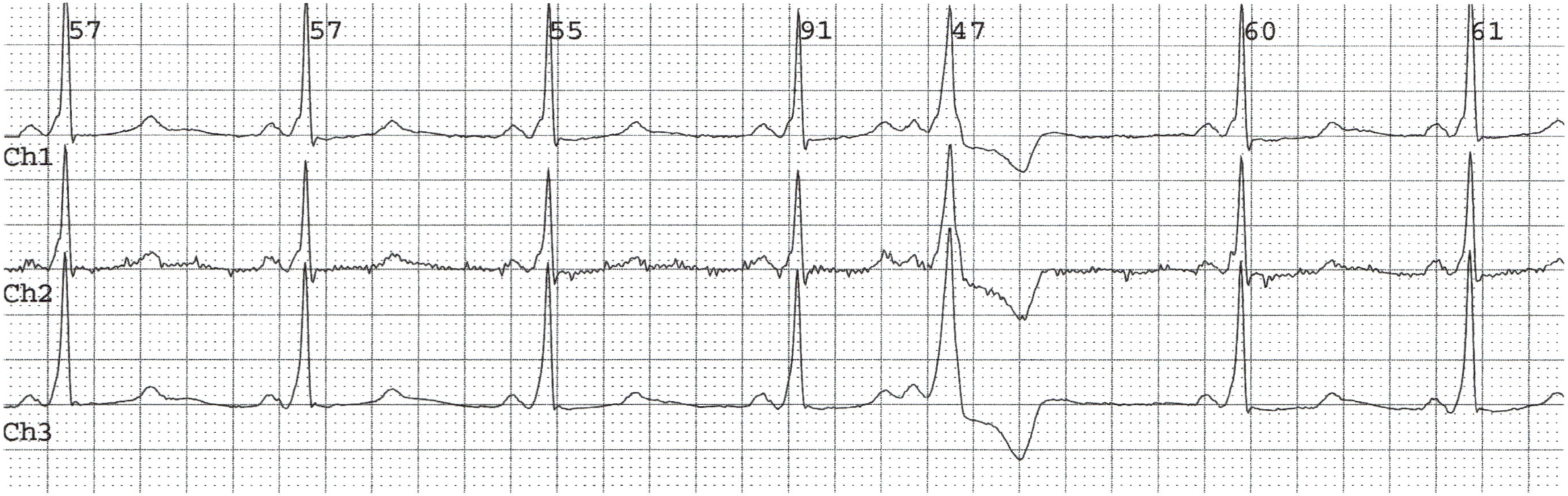


Figure 2-4B

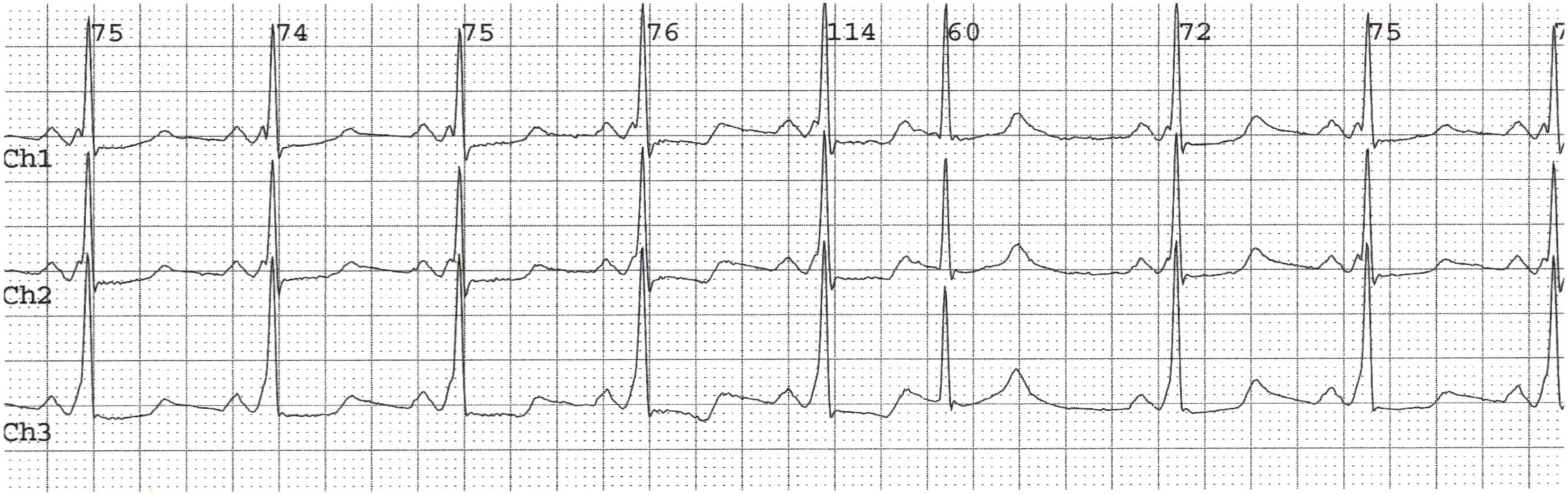


Question 2-4

Figure 2-4C

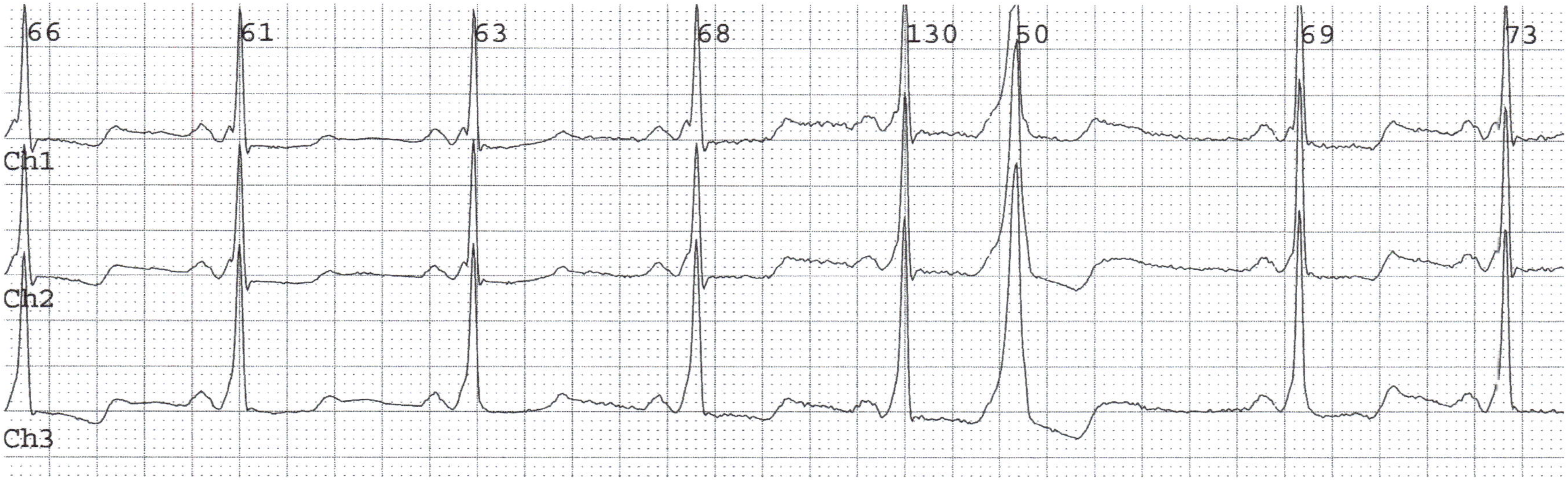


Figure 2-4D

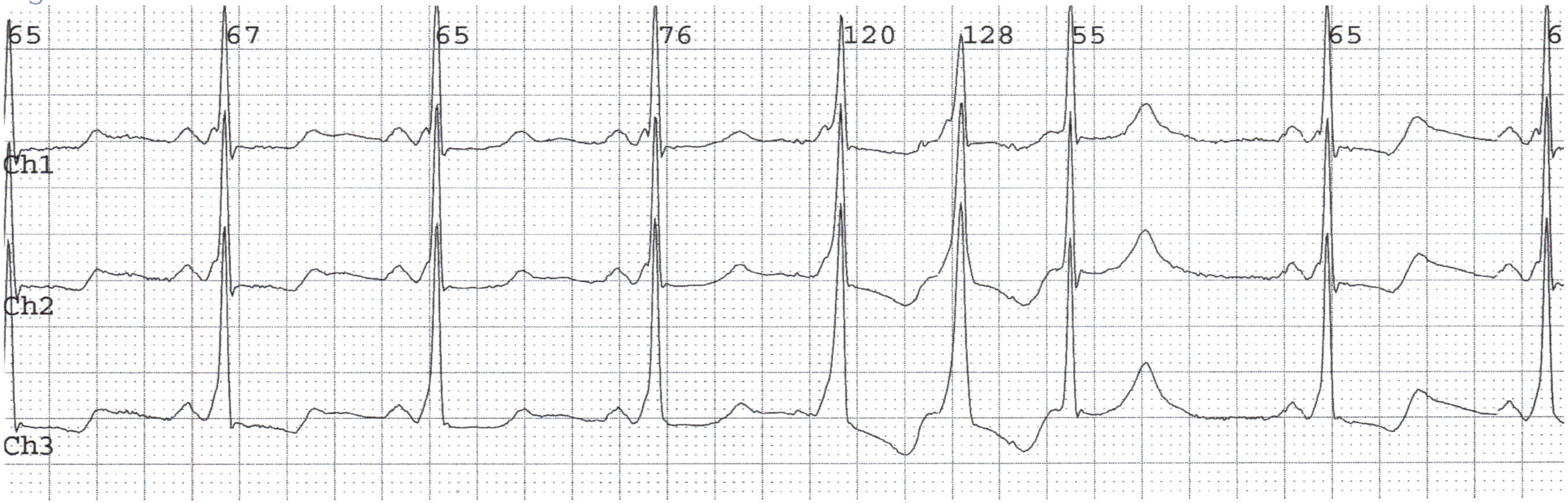

## Answer

Figure 2-4A shows a PAC that results in a more preexcited QRS complex. The PAC caused delay of AV node conduction, whereas conduction time over the AP did not prolong, resulting in more preexcitation. This is most compatible with a "typical" AV pathway.

A slightly earlier coupled PAC (Figure 2-4B) then reveals normalization of the QRS due to block in the AP. Block in the AP occurs with a relatively late-coupled PAC at least 500 ms after the preceding sinus cycle, and one might estimate the actual, measured anterograde refractory period of the AP to be in this range. This is clearly well above what would be expected to be associated with rapid anterograde conduction over the AP during atrial fibrillation (with a risk of VF).

Figure 2-4C shows a premature ventricular contraction (PVC) with no suggestion of retrograde VA conduction. The ST segment is smooth without an atrial deflection, and there is a full compensatory pause after the PVC. Intact retrograde conduction is of course necessary for orthodromic AV reentry.

Figure 2-4D shows 3 consecutive PACs. The last of these normalizes and exhibits a long PR interval, a perfect situation to start orthodromic SVT. Despite this, there is no retrograde conduction after the normalized QRS and hence no tachycardia. This patient would be most unlikely to experience clinical SVT.

One might consider the potential role of isoproterenol challenge during EP study, to ensure that conduction over the AP doesn't improve with catecholamines. However, all the risk parameters in this context were established during *baseline* studies without isoproterenol. The reader is challenged to find even a handful of cases in the medical literature where a patient with benign baseline parameters at EP study by published standards subsequently experienced VF!

This example illustrates the potential utility of a 24-hour Holter monitor in risk stratification of a WPW patient. As was apparent, the essential physiology was well defined, and little more could be gained by EP testing. This patient is essentially at no risk for developing life-threatening arrhythmia associated with the WPW pattern and can be safely reassured.

Figure 2-5A

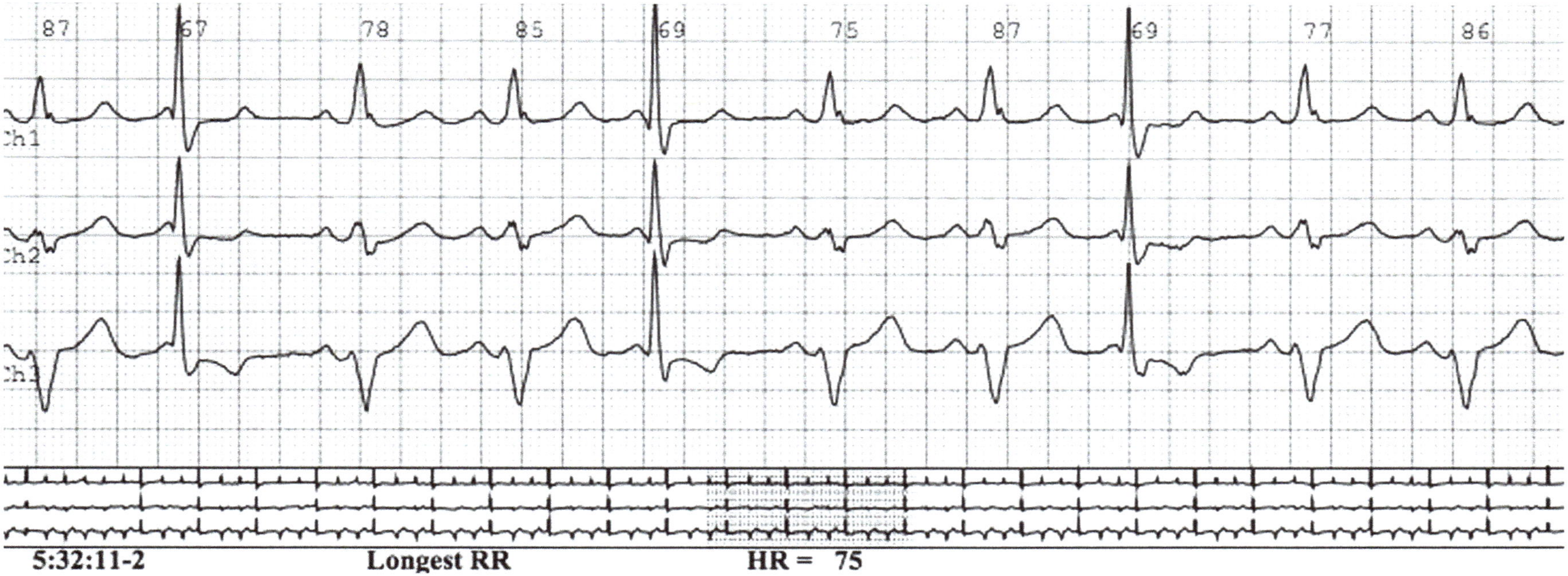


## Question 2-5

The narrow QRS cycles in **Figure 2-5A** are related to:

1. PACs
2. PVCs
3. Intermittent loss of preexcitation
4. Normalization of left bundle branch block (LBBB)

## Answer

Figure 2-5A shows sinus rhythm with a wide QRS as the baseline rhythm. The PR interval is approximately 160 ms, and there is a distinct flat PR segment. If we assume that channel 1 is in fact lead 1 (in this case, it was), this is most compatible with LBBB.

There are 3 narrow QRS cycles that are premature and are the subject of this exercise. The multiple-choice question includes the reasonable universal possibilities to explain these cycles. The sinus P waves are regular, and their timing is not affected by the ectopic activity, hence they can't be PACs. Similarly, there would be no reason to expect normalization of LBBB with prematurity of the QRS alone along with apparent shortening of the PR interval.

The apparent PR of these cycles is also slightly variable, and it is important to note that the QRS is also slightly variable in its morphology. Neither of these observations would be expected with preexcitation related to an AP where the degree of fusion between a normal and an accessory pathway (hence the QRS morphology) is generally constant at a constant sinus rate.

On the other hand, variable fusion *would* be expected with PVCs of slightly different coupling interval. The apparent normalization of the QRS may be related to the fact that the PVCs are occurring in the left ventricle. These PVCs "correct for" the intrinsic LBBB, a phenomenon called "pseudo normalization."

There is another way to look at this problem, which leads to a "rule" that the author has personally found useful over the years:

In the presence of baseline bundle branch block (i.e., "wide" QRS), any QRS that is narrower (or even just "different") is most probably of ventricular origin. This is true for single ectopic beats as well as VT.

This is intuitively reasonable, since a baseline bundle branch block would not be expected *in general* to transform into the alternate bundle branch block during an ectopic cycle or tachycardia. One might also consider that PVCs or VT of septal origin could be "narrow" because of cancellation of forces. PVCs originating in the His-fascicular network—or with good access to it—may also be quite "narrow."

The ventricular origin of the cycles fusing with sinus origin cycles in Figure 2-5A is even more obvious in **Figure 2-5B**. The ectopic QRS are enclosed by a full compensatory pause and, more important, the *ectopic narrow cycle is not preceded by any believable P wave.* (Carefully compare the diastolic interval preceding the PVC to the comparable interval in the preceding sinus rhythm cycle to see that no P wave is deforming it!)

Figure 2-5B

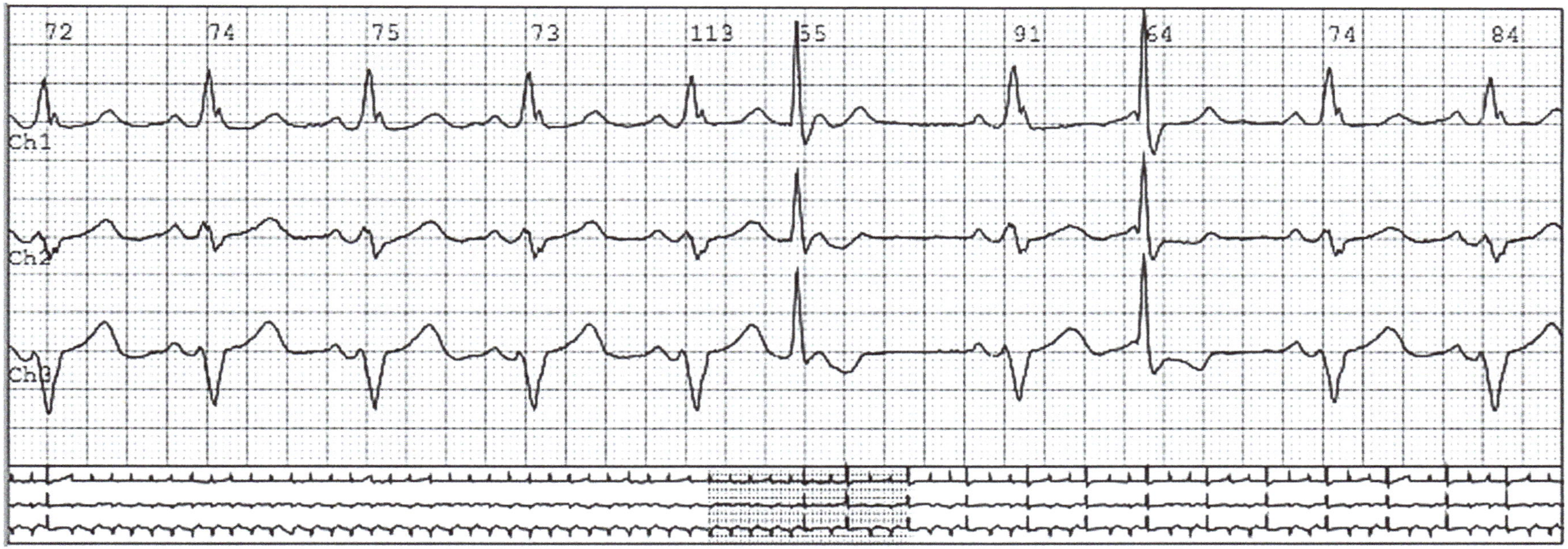

Figure 2-6A

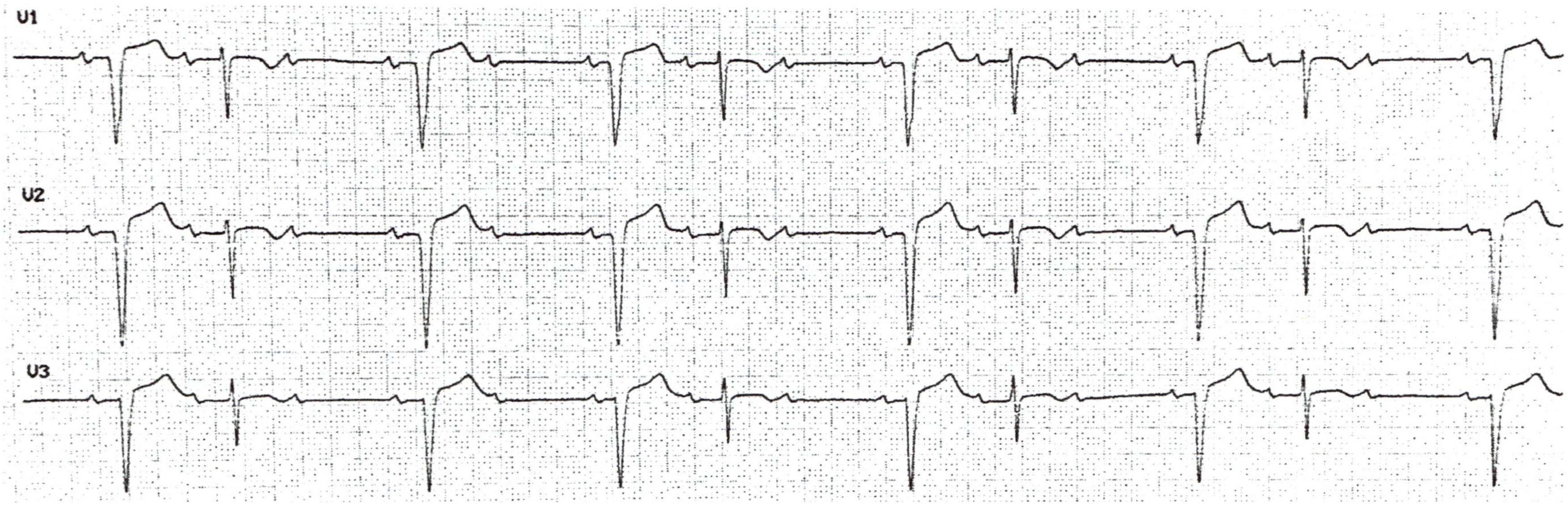

## Question 2-6

The blocked P wave in the middle of the tracing shown in **Figure 2-6A** is best related to block in:

1. AV node
2. His bundle
3. Right and left bundle branches
4. Need more data

## Answer

This tracing shows regular sinus rhythm with prolongation of the PR interval in the cycle prior to the blocked P wave, i.e., Wenckebach periodicity. There is one cycle with sudden block (beat 2). The validated correct answer is, of course, only obtainable with intracardiac recordings (not available), but a few observations can be made that are useful.

**Figure 2-6B** is a slightly magnified version of $V_1$ only. In beat 1, there is left bundle branch conduction delay, and conduction over the right bundle (RB) arrives at ventricular muscle in advance of that of the left bundle (LB)—hence a LBBB pattern.

In beat 2, the PR prolongs slightly, and there may be some delay in the AV node or the His bundle—but both the LB and RB *must* delay, the RB relatively more than the left, to equal the LB delay, and hence the QRS normalizes. Although other explanations are theoretically possible, it is difficult to otherwise explain this normalization credibly.

The phenomenon of normalization of LBBB due to development of delay in the RBB causing equal conduction delay suggests a low margin of safety of conduction over the bundle branches with prolongation of conduction time at modest resting rates for each bundle. It is therefore not a stretch to postulate a Mobitz 1 block pattern in the bundles, and that is our preferred answer to our question.

*Source:* Based on a tracing forwarded compliments of Drs. James Harrison and Mark O'Neill.

Figure 2-6B

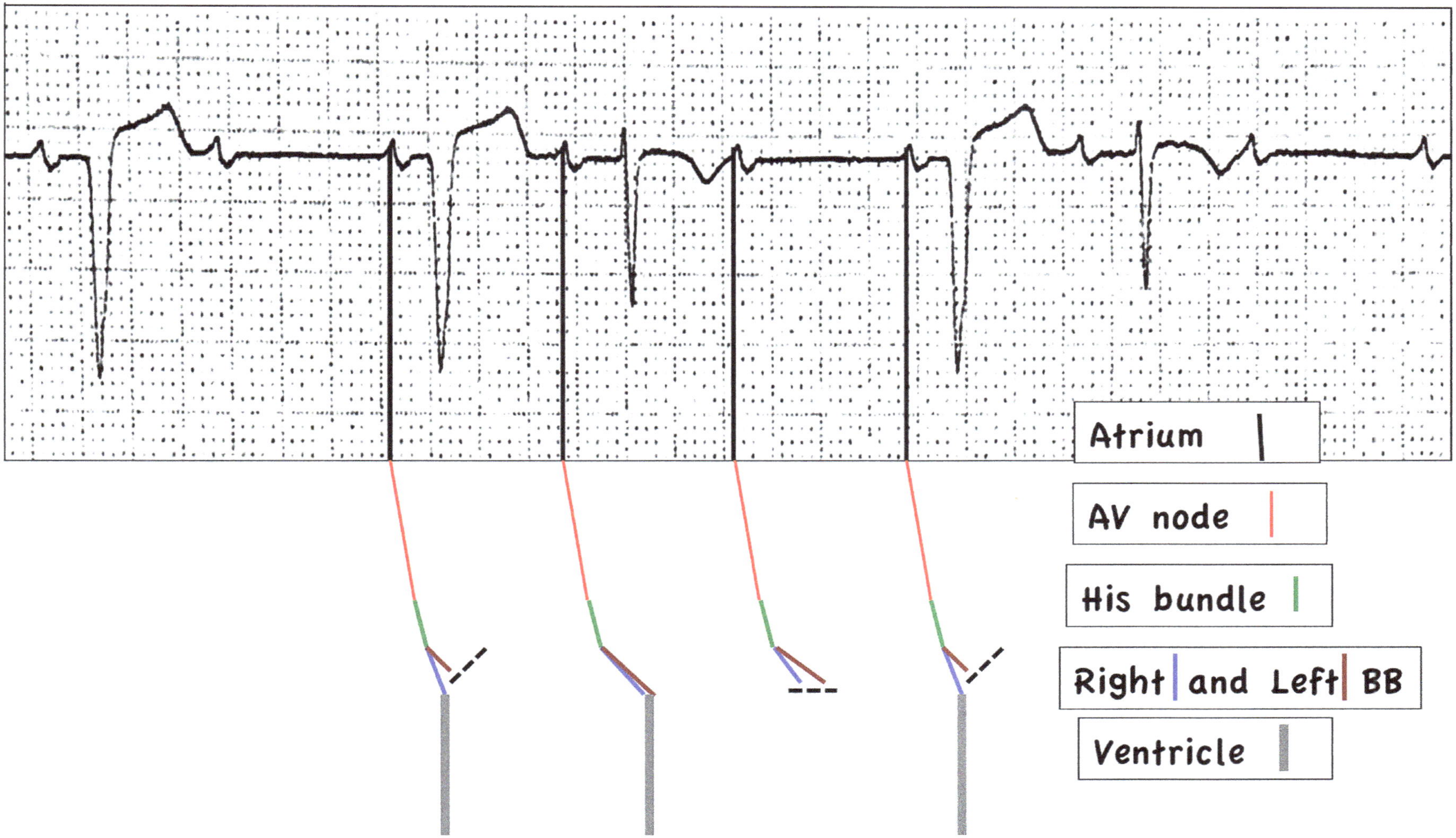
Atrium
AV node
His bundle
Right and Left BB
Ventricle

Figure 2-7

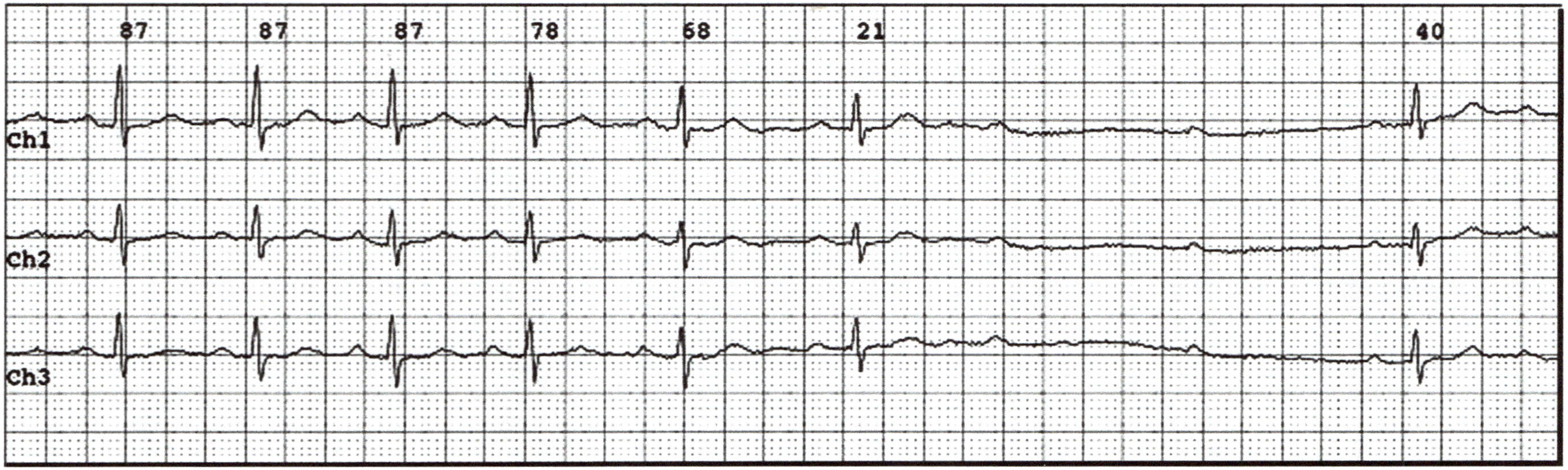

## Question 2-7

The tracing in **Figure 2-7** is recorded from an elderly gentleman previously well monitored after an episode of loss of consciousness. There were no symptoms noted on the patient log when the event shown in the tracing is logged at 12:38 AM.

The most appropriate next step would be:

1. Institute permanent pacing
2. Schedule electrophysiologic study
3. Continue monitoring
4. Arrange stress myocardial imaging

## Answer

This is a patient-management question that depends on correct ECG diagnosis—a “2-layered” question, if you will—of the kind popular in board-type examinations.

The first observation is that the event in question took place at 12:38 AM a time when this elderly man is probably sleeping. This raises the index of suspicion for vagally mediated events. The sinus rate slows gradually with minimal PR prolongation of the last conducted P wave. This is followed by 2 nonconducted P waves, and the pause is terminated by a sinus beat, also with a slightly longer PR interval.

*This is a “classical” example of a vagal pause with concurrent sinus bradycardia and AV block.* Consider that sinus bradycardia related to sinus node dysfunction would, if anything, result in improved AV conduction. Alternately, there would be no reason why primary AV conduction block should occur coincidently with sinus bradycardia.

Returning to our possible options, Option 1, initiating permanent pacing, is clearly wrong, since a satisfactory diagnosis for the patient's clinical loss of consciousness has not been made. One also needs to appreciate that electrophysiologic study (Option 2) in general has very low yield in patients with transient loss of consciousness in the absence of previous infarction. Finally, myocardial ischemia itself rarely causes isolated episodes of loss of consciousness, so Option 4 is unlikely to be helpful. The preferred answer is therefore Option 3—continue attempts at documenting an arrhythmia this is more convincingly related to the clinical loss of consciousness.

Question 2-8

Figure 2-8A

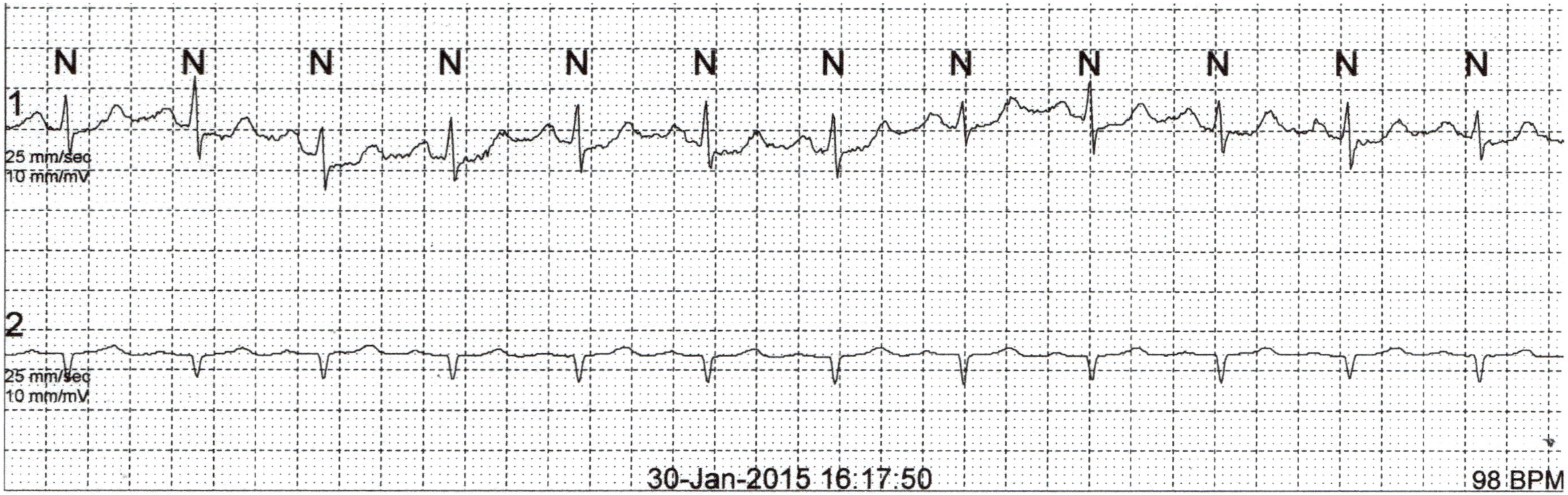


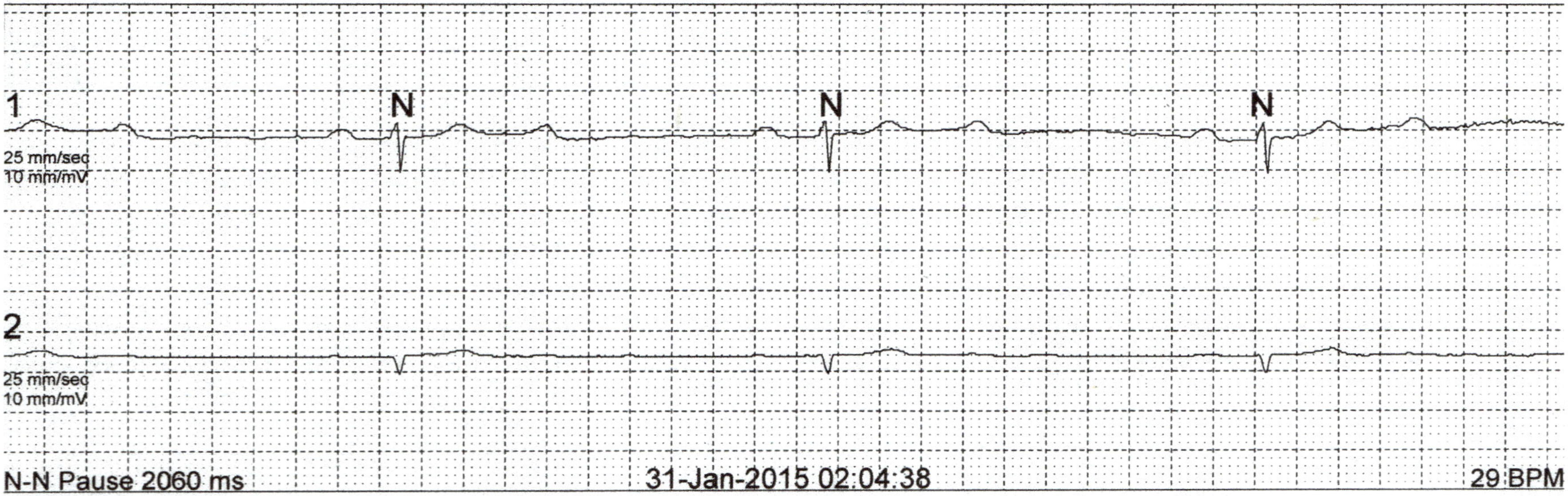

## Question 2-8

The patient whose tracing is shown in **Figure 2-8A** was referred for assessment of a prolonged episode of 2:1 AV block. There were no associated symptoms.
AV block is most consistent with:

1. AV node disease
2. His-Purkinje disease
3. High vagal tone
4. Need more data

## Answer

It is noted that the episode occurs at 2:04 AM, most probably during sleep. There is sinus bradycardia in conjunction with 2:1 AV block. The PR interval of the conducted beats is quite long, approximately 300 ms—considerably longer than that observed during waking hours as shown in the upper tracing. This is most compatible with vagal AV block, which should always be at least suspected for any significant bradycardia occurring during sleep.

By way of contrast to the above, the tracing in **Figure 2-8B** from a different individual shows a longer "mini" recording (lower trace) and a magnified portion of the beginning of a 5-second pause. It occurred at 9:55 AM and was not preceded by any substantive sinus slowing. One notes sinus irregularity with a normal PR interval after the pause. Finally, the 24-hour trend (not shown) was rather flat, with heart rate between 50 and 70 bpm.

This is all consistent with significant sinus node dysfunction that may require further investigation and probably permanent pacing.

Figure 2-8B

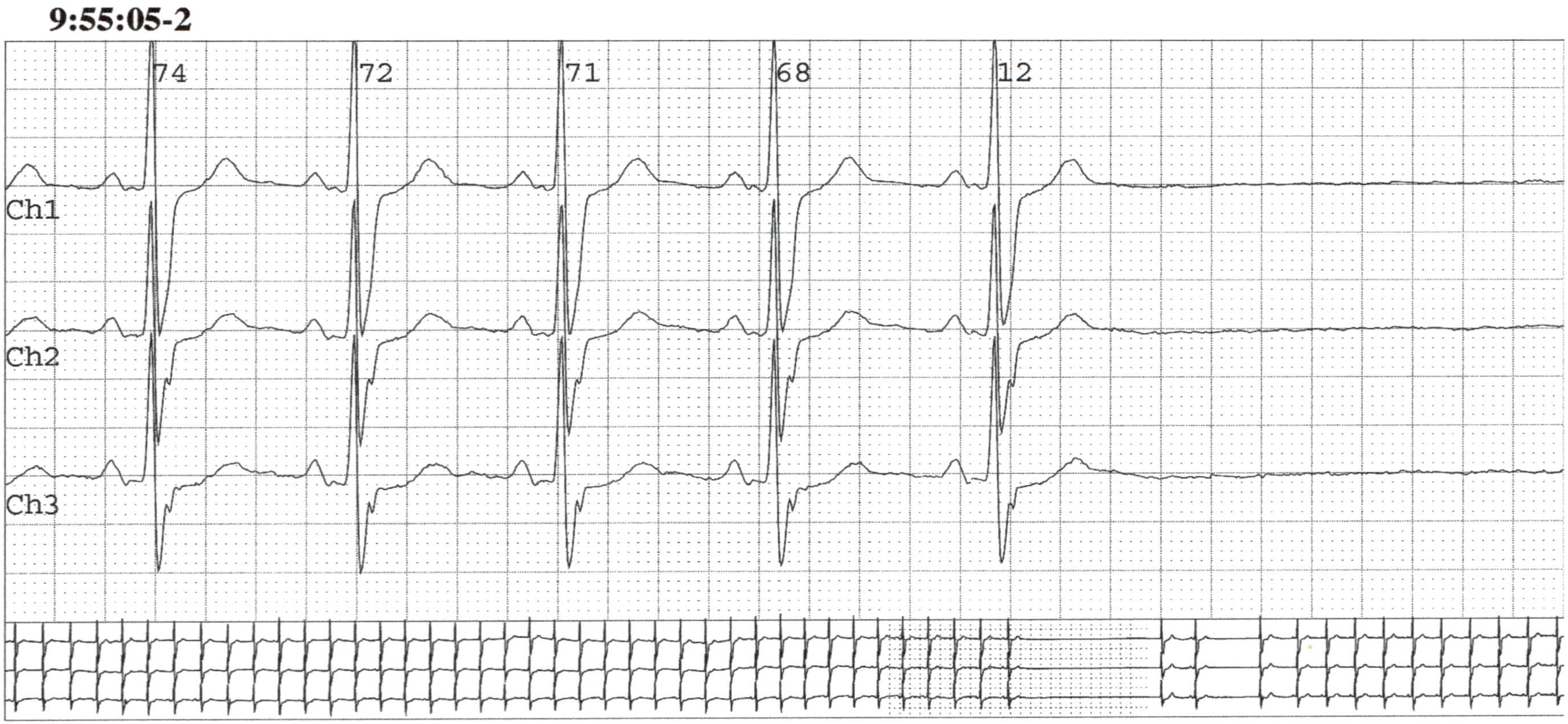

Figure 2-9A

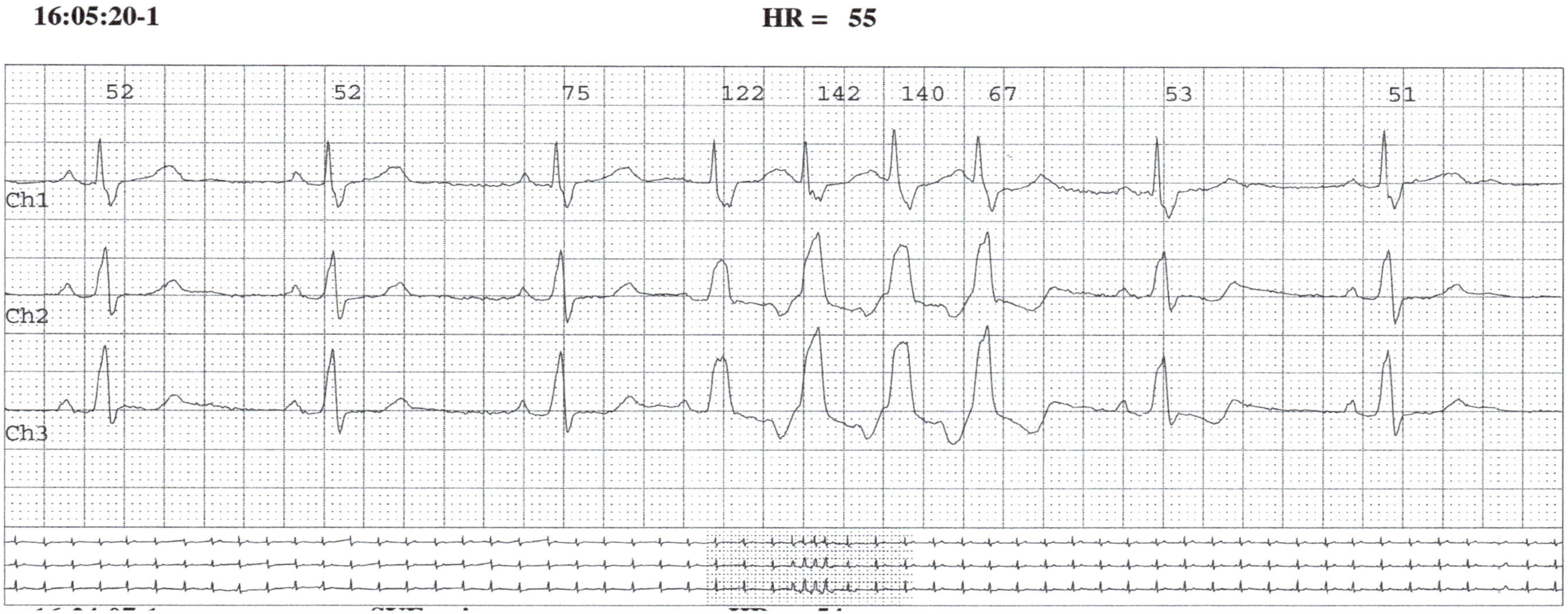


## Question 2-9

The patient whose tracing is seen in **Figure 2-9A** was referred for assessment of non-sustained wide complex tachycardia (WCT).

The mechanism of this WCT is:

1. VT
2. Atrial tachycardia (AT) with aberrancy
3. AVNRT with aberrancy
4. AVRT

Question 2-9

## Answer

We are fortunate to have a tracing free of artifact and have available the onset and termination of WCT as well as readily visible P waves (**blue dots** in **Figure 2-9B**).

Tachycardia begins with a PAC, making VT very unlikely. Furthermore, the tachycardia terminates without a P wave, making VT even more unlikely, since one would have to postulate that VT terminates coincidentally with VA block. Finally, we note the cycle length irregularity, which clearly shows that the change in the P-P interval (**blue letters**) *precedes* the change in the V-V interval, making VT absolutely untenable.

From the onset of this WCT, we observe that there is no PR prolongation associated with the initial PAC, making AVNRT unlikely.

It is a little more difficult to rule out antidromic AVRT absolutely. Recall that antidromic AVRT involves anterograde conduction over the accessory pathway. As such, the QRS during antidromic AVRT is fully preexcited on every cycle, and consequently *the QRS remains uniformly constant.* The slight variability of the QRS during WCT essentially rules out the antidromic AVRT option, leaving us firmly with the diagnosis of AT with aberrancy.

Figure 2-9B

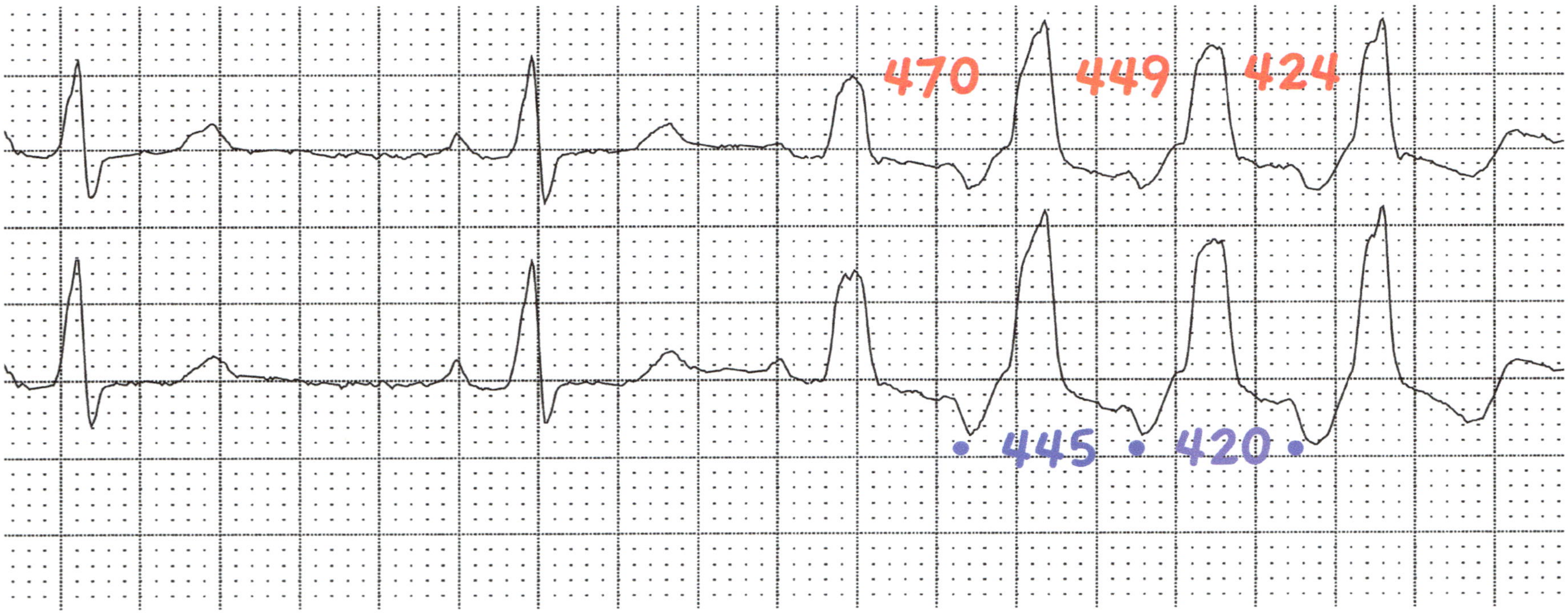

Figure 2-10A

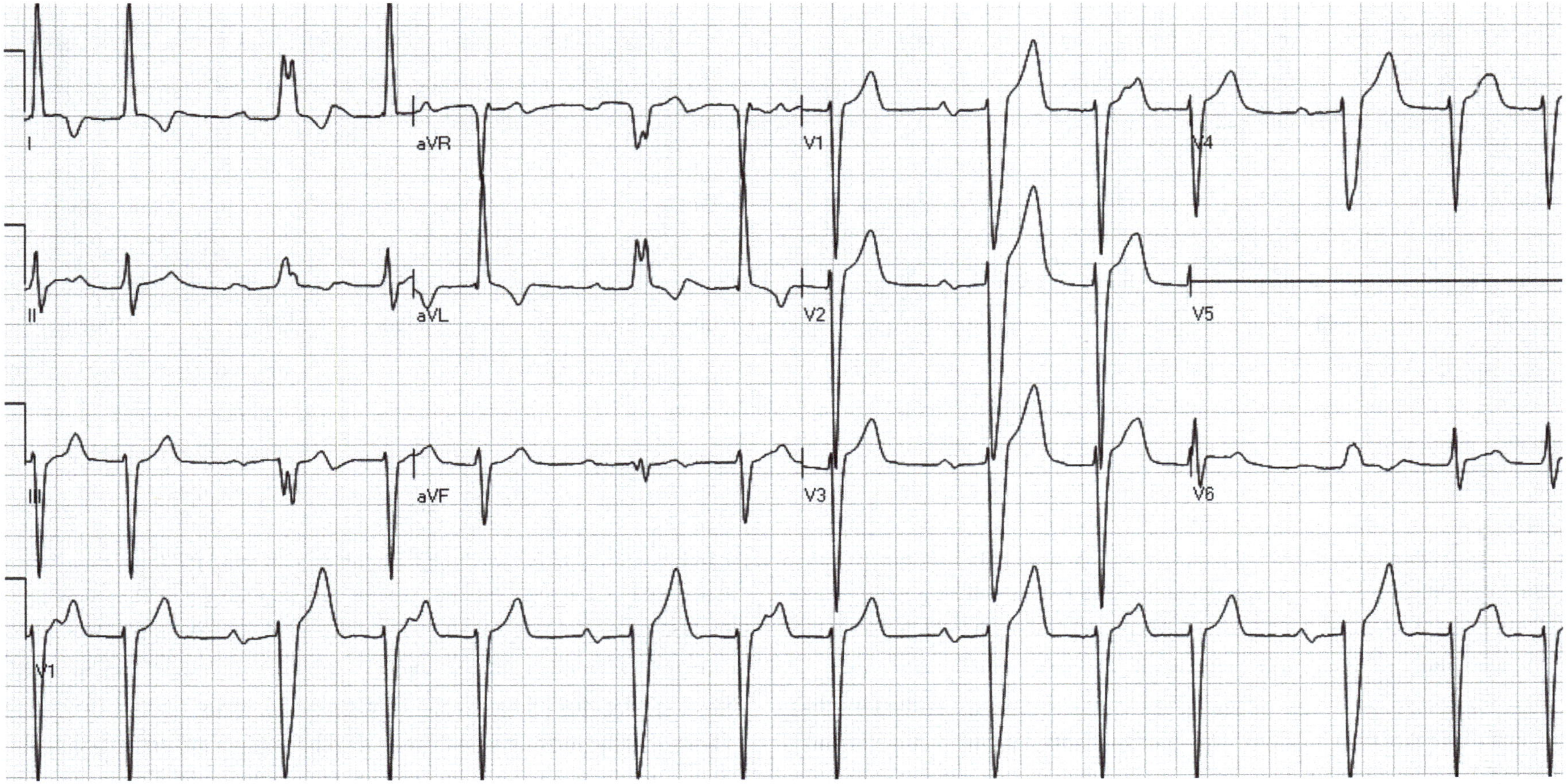


## Question 2-10

The changes in QRS morphology shown in **Figure 2-10A** are best related to:

1. CL dependent conduction over the LB
2. Ventricular ectopy
3. Longitudinal dissociation in the His bundle
4. Dual AV nodal pathways

## Answer

A global look at this 12-lead ECG shows a repetitive pattern ("group beating") of a wide QRS complex followed by 2 narrow, essentially normal QRS complexes followed by a pause. The wide QRS complex has a typical LBBB pattern and is preceded by a sinus P wave, so it is reasonable to begin here with the initial assumption that this indeed a sinus beat with LBBB (**arrow** in **Figure 2-10B**).

The ST segment of the first premature beat contains a "sharp" deflection most consistent with a P wave. Tracking the P waves (**blue dots**), it becomes readily apparent that the sinus rhythm is not perturbed by the 2 premature QRS complexes. Since there are no P waves preceding the premature beats, PACs are ruled out. *With a baseline LBBB in sinus rhythm, the narrow QRS cycles are in all probability ventricular* (see discussion in **Question 2-5**). The "normal" QRS can be explained by origin of the premature cycles in close relationship to the His–Purkinje system, perhaps bypassing the delay causing the LBBB.

Finally, we also note that the P wave buried in the ST segment fails to conduct to the ventricle, indicating concealed retrograde conduction to the AV node despite the absence of overt retrograde conduction to the atrium after the PVC.

The reader may propose additional potential mechanisms to explain the phenomena that may have validity. This is of little concern, as the main point of this exercise is to think systematically and physiologically and not necessarily to find a "right" answer.

Figure 2-10B

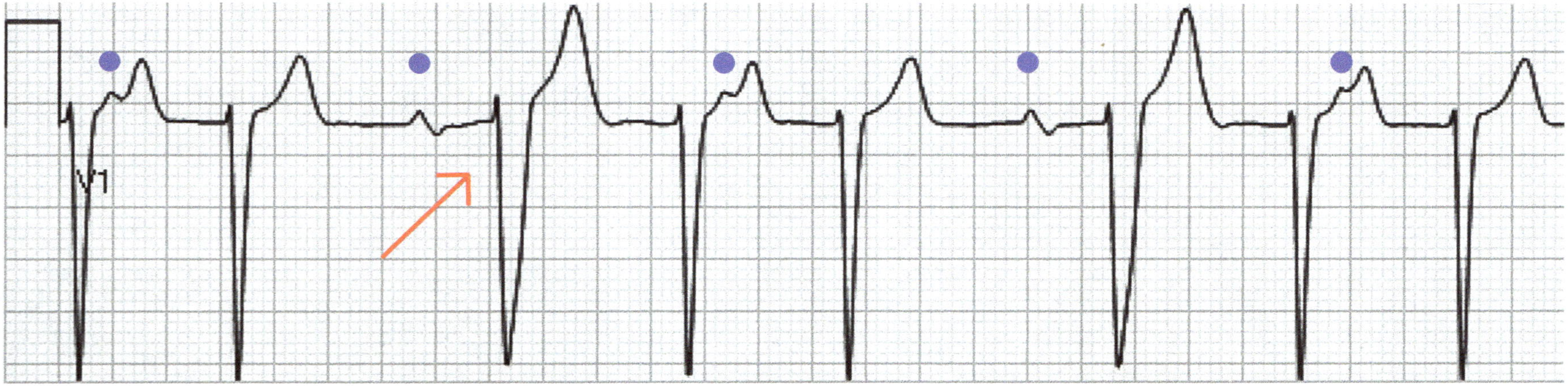

Figure 2-11A

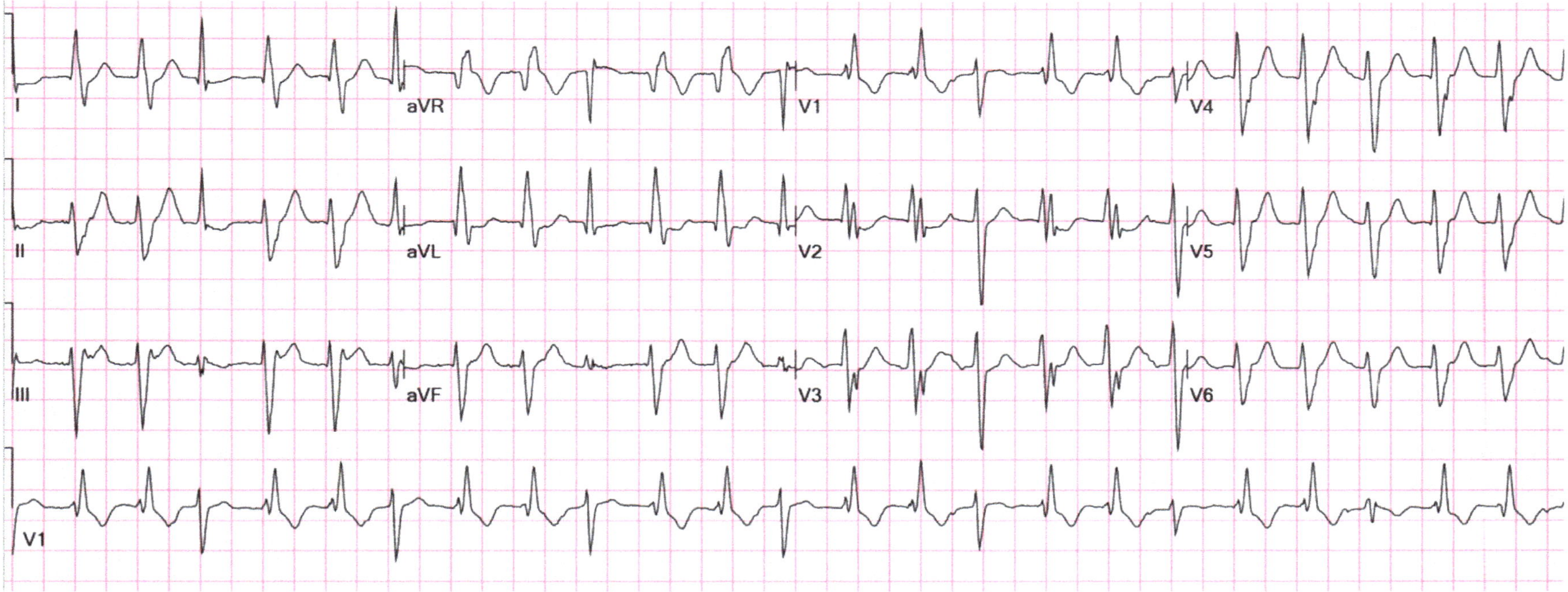




## Question 2-11

The arrhythmia mechanism on the tracing in **Figure 2-11A** is most probably related to:

1. Abnormal automaticity
2. Macroreentry (large circuit)
3. Microreentry (small circuit, focal)
4. Need more data

## Answer

This is admittedly an advanced tracing. Even though a definitive answer requires detailed electrophysiologic study, a cogent opinion can be arrived at deductively from the ECG alone.

We immediately note a repetitive pattern ("group beating") with 2 wide QRS complexes followed by a narrow one, the latter identical to the QRS seen in sinus rhythm in this individual (not shown). The wide complex cycles have a right bundle branch block (RBBB) pattern with left-axis deviation.

At this point, we search for P waves and do some detailed measuring to refine our observations (**Figure 2-11B**).

We now observe that the wide complexes are not preceded by P waves, but these are identified in the ST segment after every second cycle (**upright arrows**). Each P wave is subsequently followed by a normal QRS. Thus, we appear to have a dominant ventricular rhythm followed by a supraventricular complex at relatively fixed intervals.

Many will recognize this QRS morphology as typical of the "verapamil-sensitive" idiopathic left ventricular tachycardia. In the author's experience, presence of *both* RBBB and left anterior fascicular block (LAFB) is a very rare aberration pattern unless there is baseline LAFB. The narrow QRS are supraventricular capture beats, but the fixed coupling suggests they are not just random supraventricular captures fortuitously synced into a VT.

Ruling out the latter absolutely would require looking at longer strips but a reasonable explanation is that the capture beats are (atypical) AV nodal echo beats.

With that done, is there any hint to answer our question?

With the aid of our magnified strip, we see that the narrow QRS captures have a slightly variable QRS but generally *share the onset with the WC beats* (**blue rectangles**). This is best explained by postulating *fusion* between the next destined VT cycle and the capture beat.

The final bit of information comes from making a few measurements (**horizontal arrows**). We then note that the interval between 2 WC after a narrow QRS is *less than* twice the distance between 2 consecutive WC. That is, the capture-fusion beat has advanced or "reset" the tachycardia CL. This can only happen if the supraventricular capture beat has good access to a reentrant circuit with a large excitable gap! "Fusion plus reset" means macroreentry with very few exceptions!

This is compatible with known data on this type of ventricular tachycardia in which the circuit is closely related to the normal bundle branch system.

Although difficult, this question again highlights the importance of *magnification* of the tracing and careful *measurement* to make critical observations.

Figure 2-11B

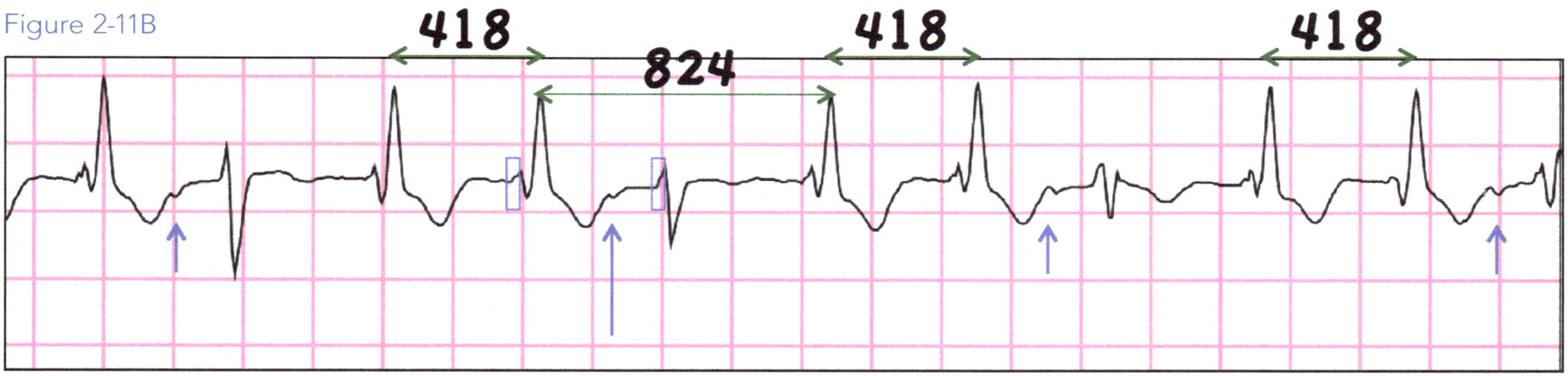

Question 2-12

Figure 2-12A

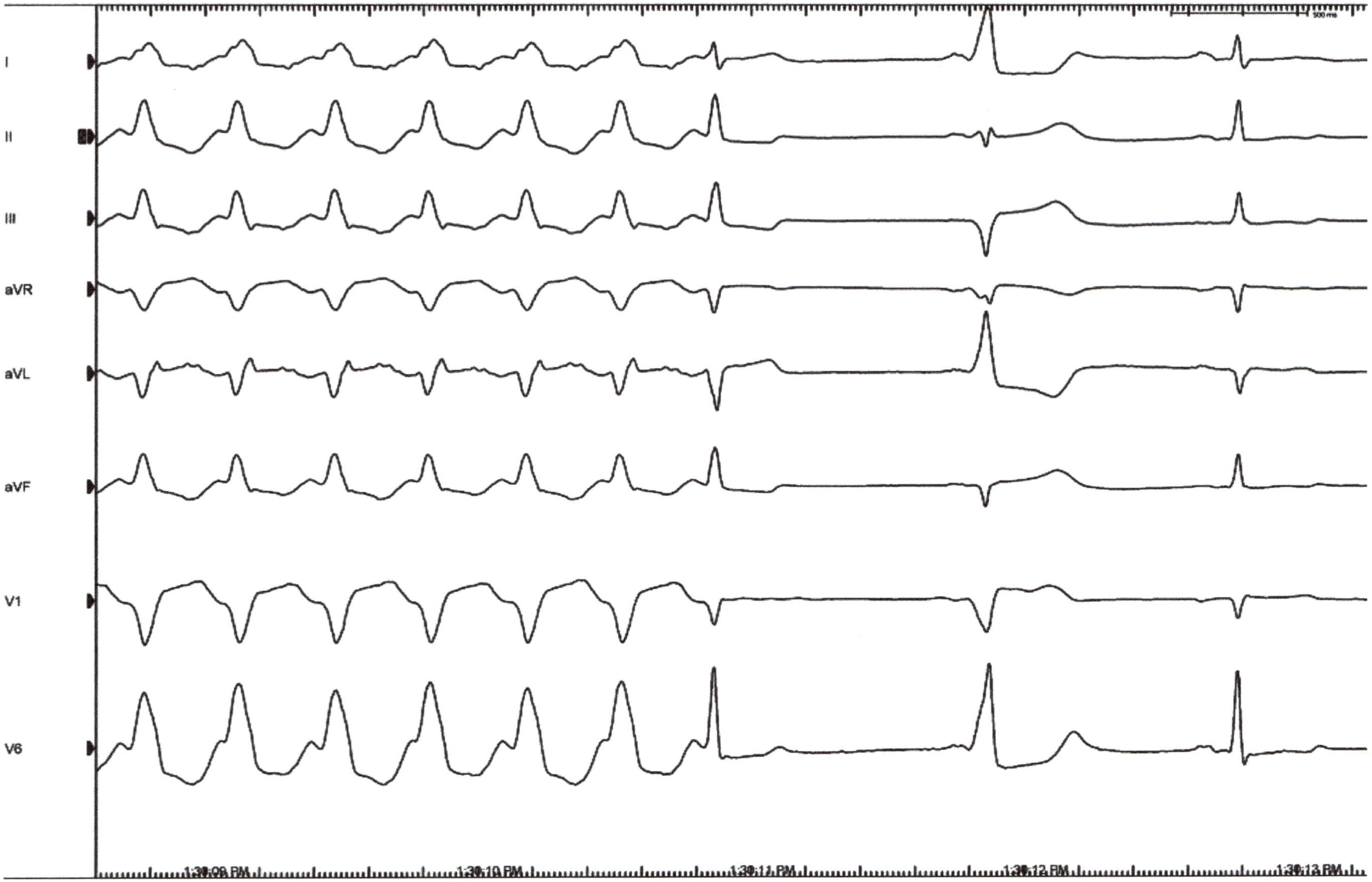

## Question 2-12

The mechanism of the WCT shown in **Figure 2-12A** is:

1. VT
2. Antidromic tachycardia
3. AVNRT
4. Orthodromic AVRT

## Answer

This WCT has LBBB morphology and terminates with a QRS that has an essentially normal QRS morphology (compare to sinus beat at end of the tracing). The key observations are highlighted in **Figure 2-12B**. The WCT is regular and the last QRS of tachycardia is not premature and in fact "on time." If this were VT, one would have to postulate a fortuitous capture beat, but it is virtually impossible for such a late capture beat to get into the VT circuit to terminate tachycardia, so this option is easily dismissed.

We next note the relatively sharp deflection in the ST-T wave, in all likelihood a P wave (**red dots**). The P wave is negative in lead 1 (activation left to right in the frontal plane) so that this can only be an atrial tachycardia (if it is an anterograde P wave) or a left AP if it is a retrograde P wave. Atrial tachycardia is not one of our options—and, furthermore, there would be no reason to expect an atrial tachycardia to stop coincidentally with normalization of QRS aberrancy or loss of bystander preexcitation. Similarly, there would be no reason for AVNRT to terminate coincidentally with normalization of LBBB aberrancy.

We now consider the option of antidromic tachycardia. Recall that antidromic tachycardia, by definition, involves an AP as the anterograde limb of the circuit and the normal AV conduction system as the retrograde limb. It is difficult to imagine this preexcited tachycardia terminating with a normal QRS beat at the exact CL of the tachycardia. The AP would have to block and the retrograde AV node would have to turn around and capture anterogradely—hardly feasible. If you think this through, an AV nodal echo could theoretically break an antidromic tachycardia but it would be difficult to see this happening with *no change* in the coupling of the last normal QRS to the previous one. Finally, the negative retrograde P wave in lead 1 would not be compatible with retrograde conduction over the normal AV conduction system, very rare potential exceptions notwithstanding.

The data are readily compatible with orthodromic AVRT over a left lateral AP, as was the case in this example. Spontaneous normalization of LBBB aberrancy and resumption of anterograde conduction over the LBB shortened the obligatory circuit (previously going via the RBB, transeptally, and then to the left AP). The shortened VA time encroached on the retrograde refractory period of the AP, and tachycardia stopped.

A very simple way to look at this is that only AVRT involves the bundle branches as part of a SVT mechanism and hence is the only arrhythmia potentially affected in some way by presence of absence of bundle branch conduction.

Figure 2-12B

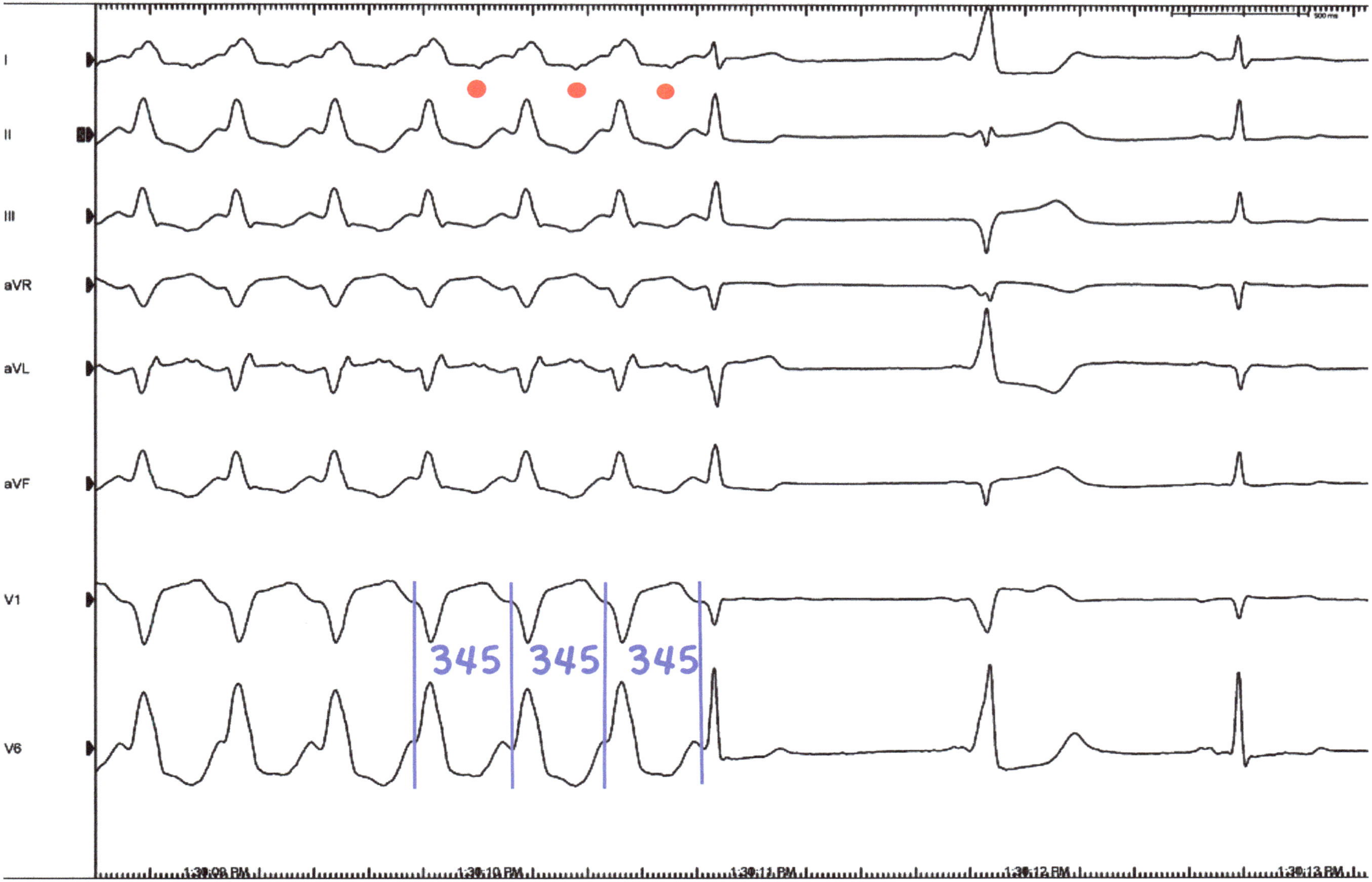
I
II
III
aVR
aVL
aVF
V1
V6
345
345
345
1:30:09 PM
1:30:10 PM
1:30:11 PM
1:30:12 PM
1:30:13 PM

Question 2-13

Figure 2-13A

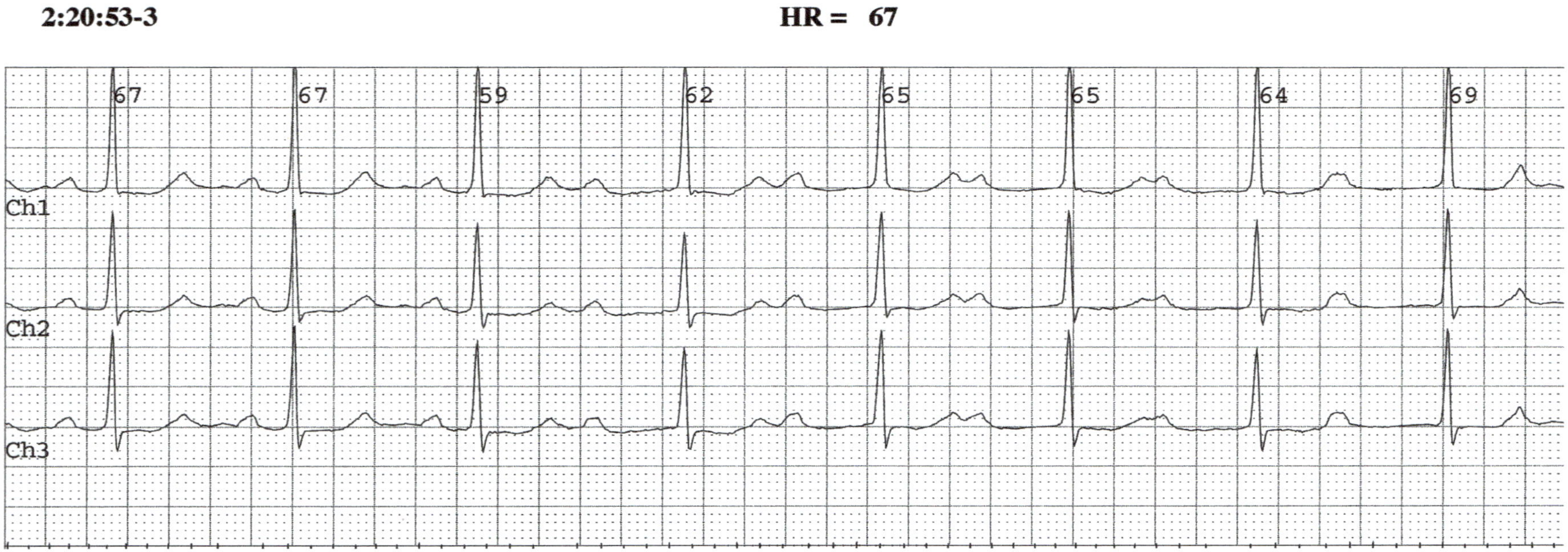

Figure 2-13B

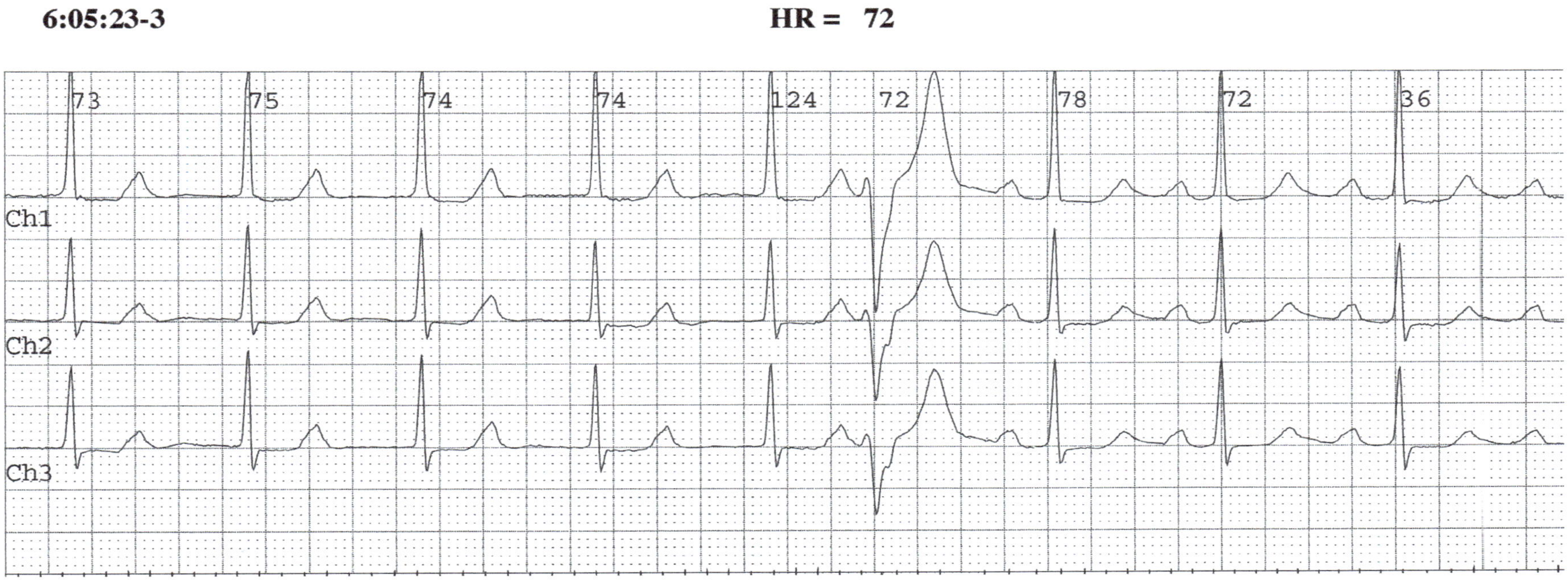




## Question 2-13

Based on the 2 tracings shown in **Figures 2-13A** and **2-13B**, the paroxysmal SVT occurring in this 77-year-old patient is most likely to be:

1. AT
2. AVNRT
3. AVRT
4. Junctional tachycardia (JT)

## Answer

This question is again "probabilistic" based on the physiology observed on the tracings, and the true answer is unknown. Further, it does not account for potential changes in autonomic tone that undoubtedly affects the physiology. This is nonetheless a useful exercise to speculate on what can be derived from the tracings through "physiological" thinking.

Figure 2-13A shows a sudden change from a normal PR interval to a long one after a slightly more premature sinus beat, best explained by the presence of dual pathway physiology and indicating block in a fast AV nodal and conduction over a slow one. This suggests a relatively long ERP over the fast pathway. Furthermore, there are no atrial echo beats even though the long PR would give ample opportunity for either a retrograde fast AV nodal pathway or a (concealed) unidirectional retrograde-only AP to return and initiate tachycardia. This suggests the absence of retrograde conduction.

The best answer would then be Option 1, AT. Recall that JT is a distinctly uncommon paroxysmal arrhythmia in adults.

In Figure 2-13B, we now see sinus rhythm starting with slow-pathway conduction (the P wave is superimposed on the preceding T wave). We see no retrograde conduction after the PVC, which we suspected from Figure 2-13A, and there has been no change in the sinus CL. Nonetheless, the PR interval abruptly *shortens*, and we revert to fast-pathway conduction.

This indicates that retrograde conduction must have at least reached the AV node, that is, *concealed retrograde conduction into* the AV node. Although the underlying anatomical physiology can at best be speculated upon, one can say that anterograde conduction over the pathway was facilitated by some degree of penetration of the PVC in the AV node.

This patient was asymptomatic, and of course no intervention is indicated solely on the basis of these observations.

Figure 2-14A

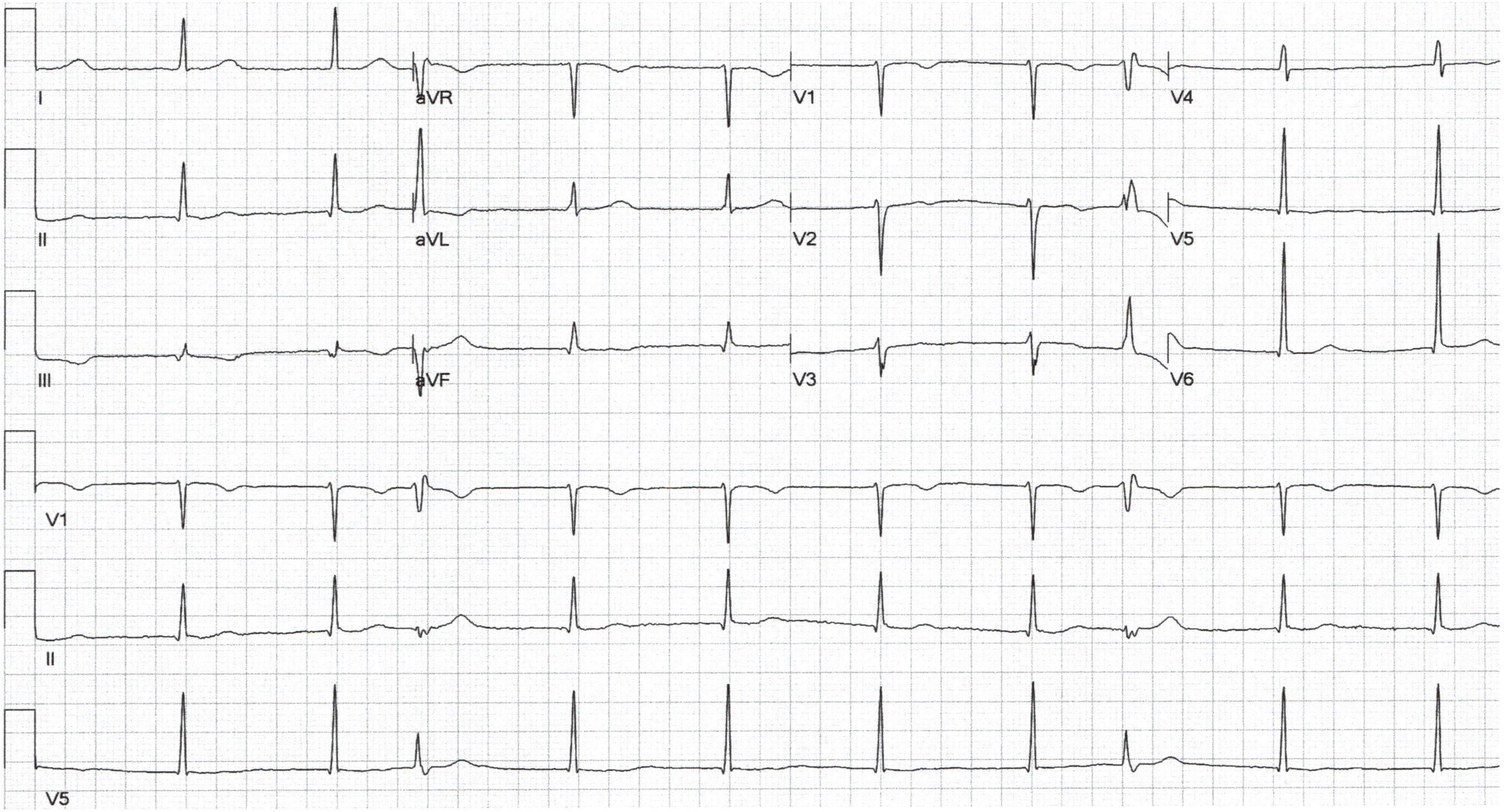

## Question 2-14

The “junctional” rhythm shown in **Figure 2-14A** is most likely to originate in:

1. Slow AV nodal pathway
2. RBB
3. Compact AV node
4. His bundle

## Answer

The rhythm is regular without a preceding P wave. The QRS is clearly normal so that an origin in the RBB is easily eliminated, as it would generally be expected to have a bundle branch block pattern. The only clue we have to answer the question is centered on the behavior of the rhythm to the 2 relatively narrow PVCs, and we focus on one of these in **Figure 2-14B**.

The PVC is relatively narrow with a very rapid initial deflection and this is most compatible with origin in the His-fascicular system. When measurements are made, it is noted that the PVC advances or "resets" the next destined junctional beat. We further notice that the interval after the PVC, analogous to the "post-pacing interval," virtually equals the junctional cycle length (1031 vs. 1011 ms). This can only happen if the PVC has intimate access to the origin of the junctional pacemaker (be it reentrant or automatic). This would make a His bundle site of pacing more likely than an AV nodal site, and therefore Option 4 would be the most logical of the options presented.

Figure 2-14B

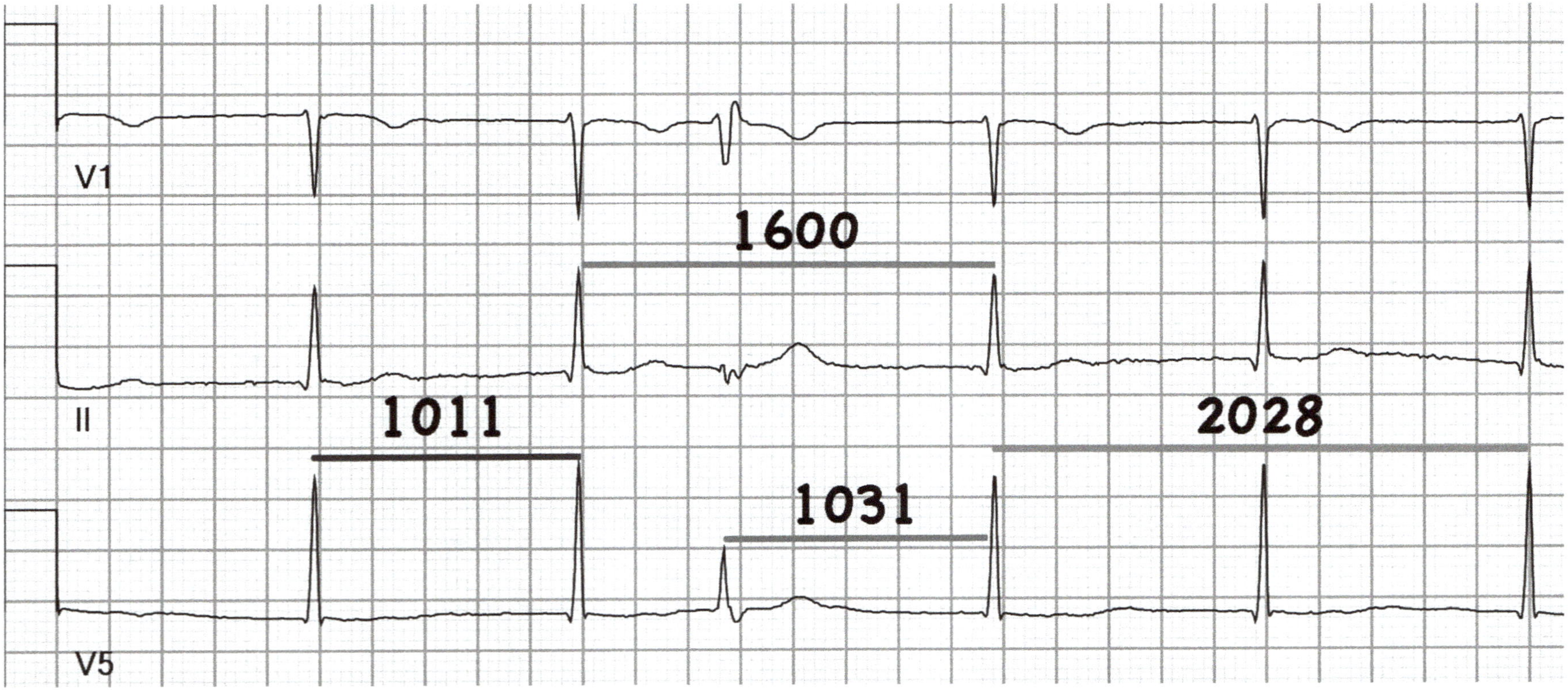

# Chapter 3

## The Narrow QRS Tachycardia

Figure 3-1A

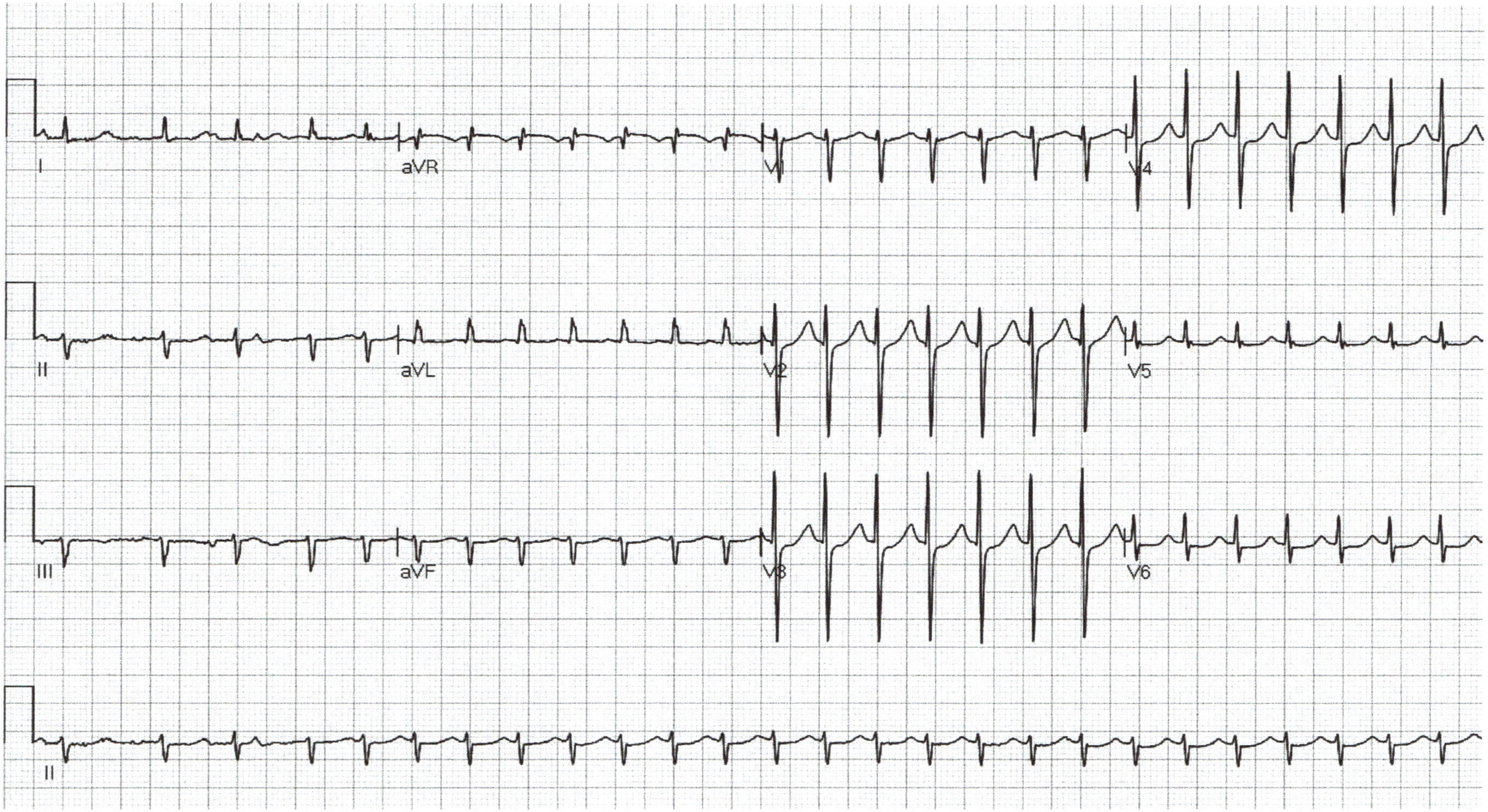

## Question 3-1

The tachycardia shown in **Figure 3.1A** is:

1. Atrial tachycardia (AT)
2. Atrioventricular nodal reentrant tachycardia (AVNRT)
3. Atrioventricular reentrant tachycardia (AVRT)
4. Atrial flutter (AFL)

## Answer

The key to this tachycardia is found at the onset, as is frequently the case. The tachycardia starts after 2 premature atrial contractions (PACs) and is regular with no obvious P waves. The initiating PAC, indicated by the **horizontal line** in **Figure 3.1B**, has a very long PR interval, undoubtedly a slow AV node pathway. With no P waves seen in the diastolic segment during tachycardia, it is reasonable to presume that it is obscured within the QRS—and this, realistically, can only be AVNRT.

Although onset with PR prolongation is typical of AVNRT since AV node delay is necessary for the onset, orthodromic AVRT also generally requires AV conduction delay. Even AT can start with a prolonged PR interval, since that is the usual physiological response to closely coupled PACs, and yet have nothing to do with the tachycardia mechanism.

Figure 3-1B

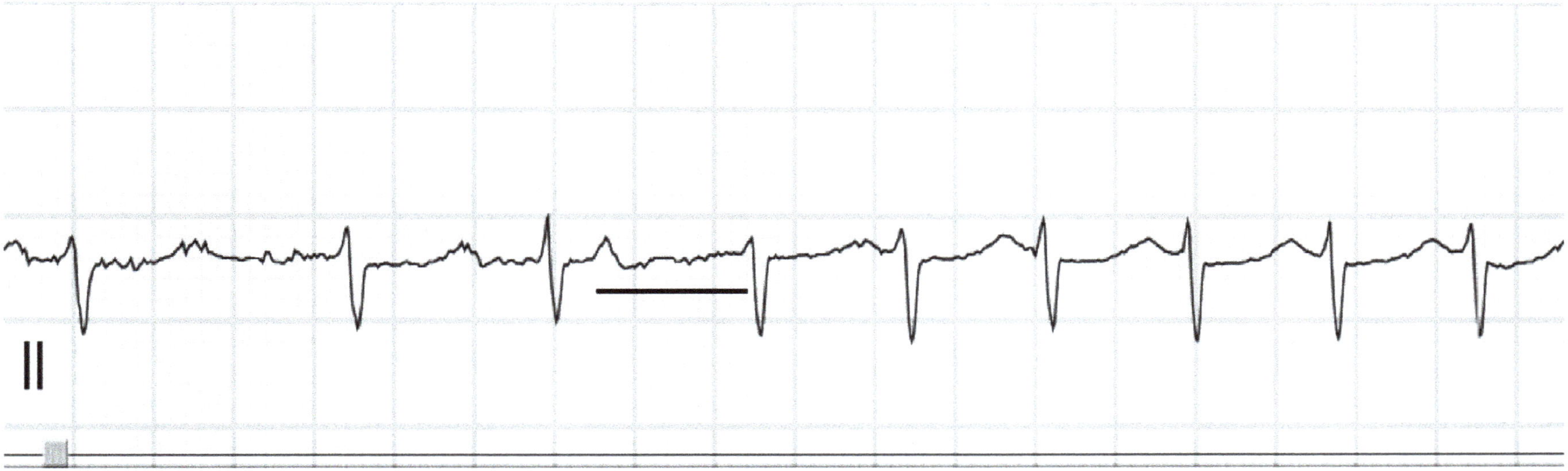

Figure 3-2A

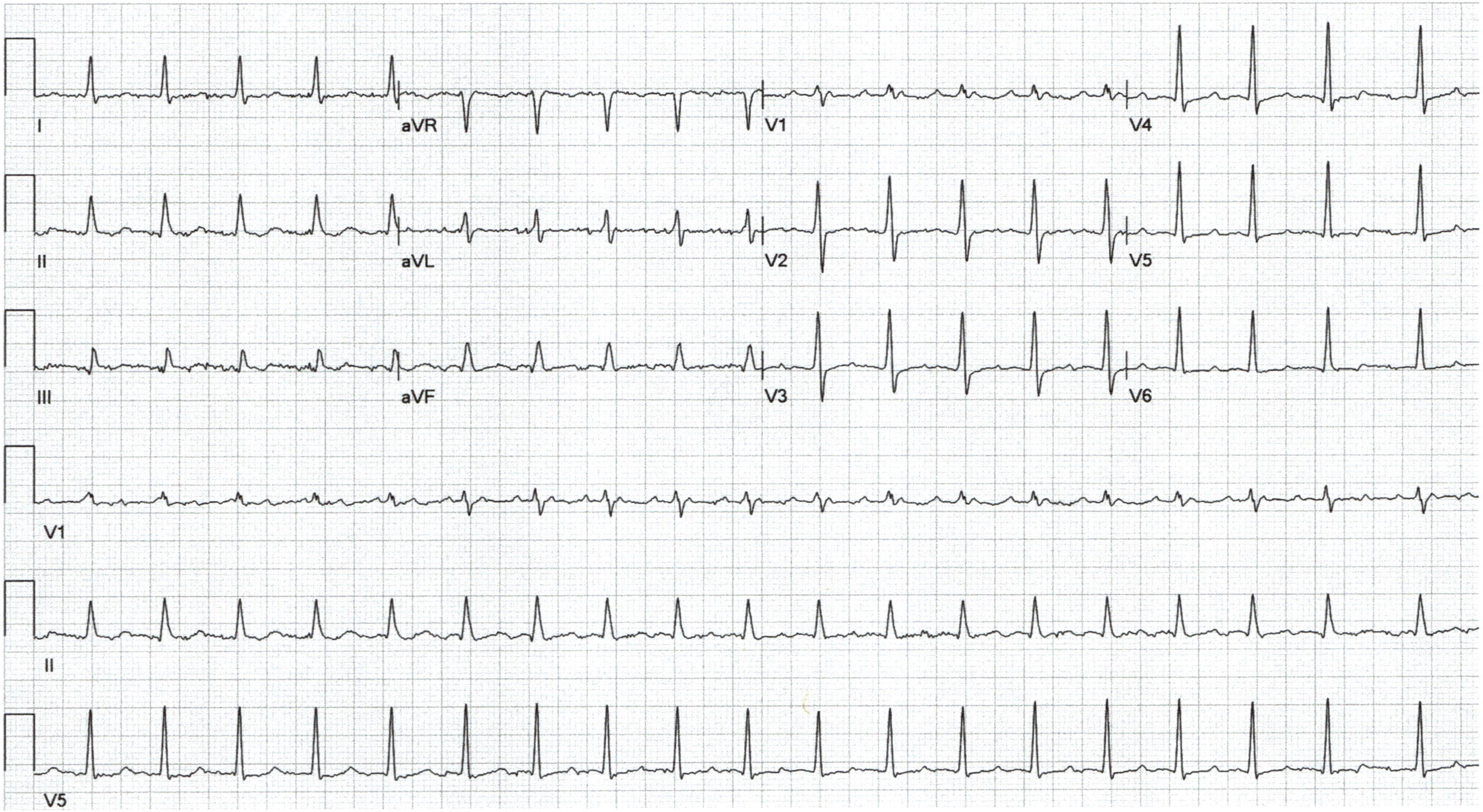

## Question 3-2

The tachycardia shown in **Figure 3-2A** is:

1. Sinus tachycardia
2. AVNRT
3. AVRT
4. Atrial flutter

## Answer

Figure 3-2A is not a pristine tracing, a circumstance we frequently must deal with. It was initially read as sinus tachycardia. This diagnosis is problematic, since atrial activity is usually more evident, and specifically, a positive P wave is usually seen in the frontal leads 1, 2, and 3. In this example, P waves are difficult to identify, but a P wave is arguably most evident in $V_1$.

The value of actually enlarging and honing in the area of interest again becomes evident in **Figure 3-2B**. I routinely will place calipers, electronic or otherwise, on 2 consecutive P waves and "seek the center"—in this case indicated by the dashed line. This is usually helpful in exposing a second P wave, which becomes more obvious when highlighted by the centerline. It is easy to miss a second P wave hidden in the QRS, but systematically "seeking the center" will decrease the odds of this happening. If the "center" falls within the QRS, a hidden P wave cannot be ruled out.

This ECG shows atrial flutter with 2:1 AV conduction.

Figure 3-2B

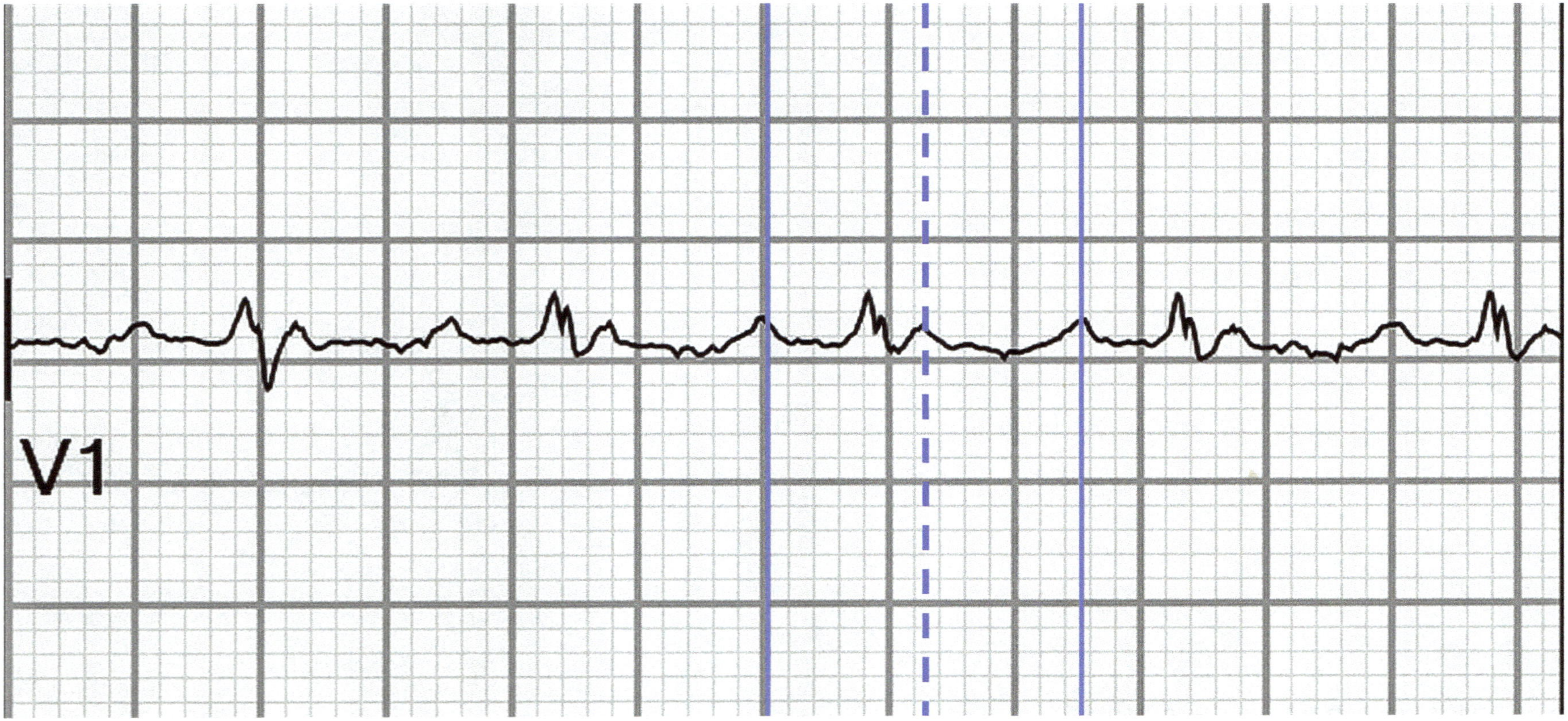

Figure 3-3A

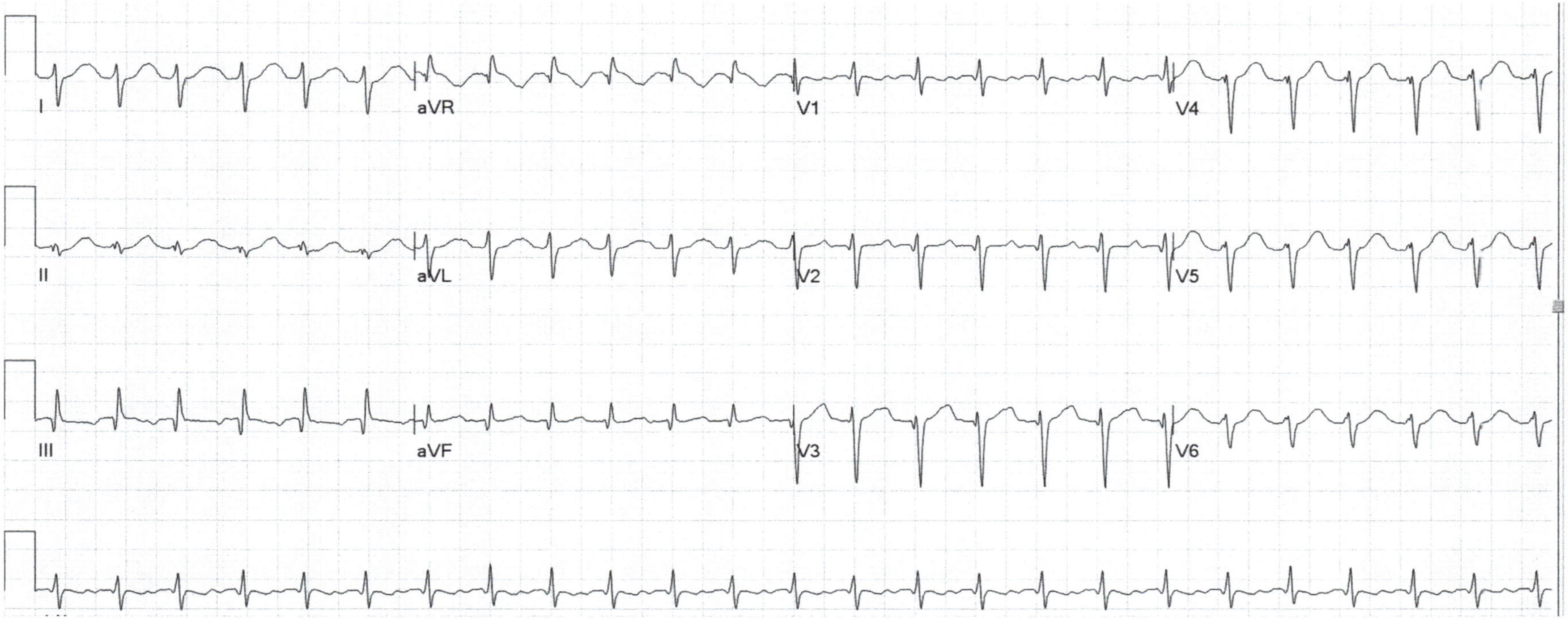




## Question 3-3

The tachycardia shown in **Figure 3-3A** is:

1. Sinus tachycardia
2. AVNRT
3. AVRT
4. AFL

## Answer

The tracing in Figure 3-3A falls into the category of "SVT with no obvious atrial activity."

It may be that the P wave is missing, low in amplitude, or obscured. If the latter, it is usually obscured in the vicinity of the QRS or T wave. P waves are often of higher frequency ("sharper") than T waves, but not invariably, and findings may be subtle.

In this example, one observes a subtle but clear variability in width of the T wave that is best appreciated in lead 1 (**Figure 3-3B**). Lead 2 shows a subtle, small, "sharp" glitch varying in location slightly on the T wave. This will happen if there is slight cycle length (CL) variation during a rhythm and the P and T are slightly and variably "fused" (electrocardiographically fused, obviously not mechanistically). The P is "hiding" on the downslope of the T wave, and this is evident during such CL variation, in this instance during sinus tachycardia.

Here, as elsewhere, the value of actually magnifying the area of interest is highlighted.

Figure 3-3B

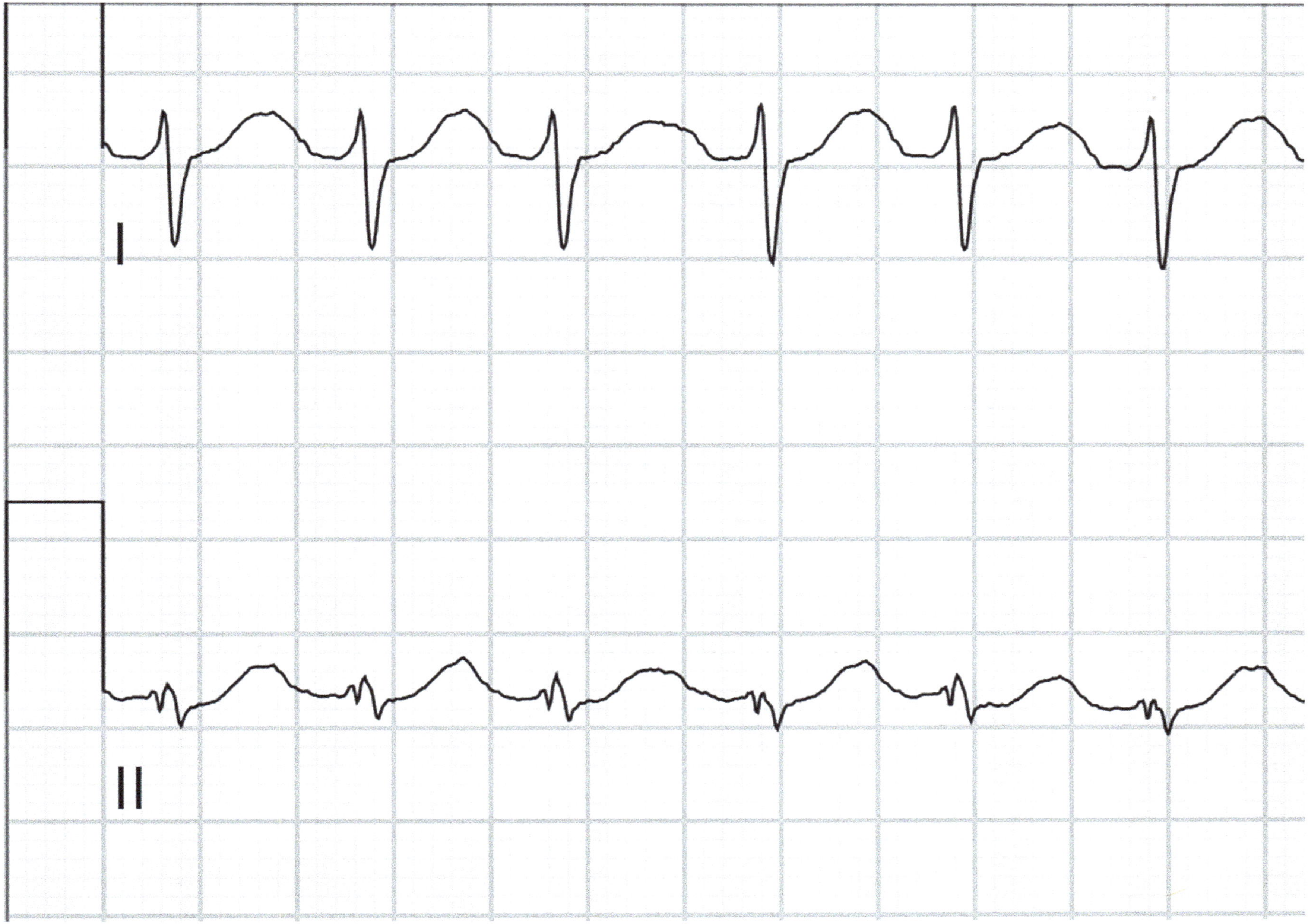

Figure 3-4A

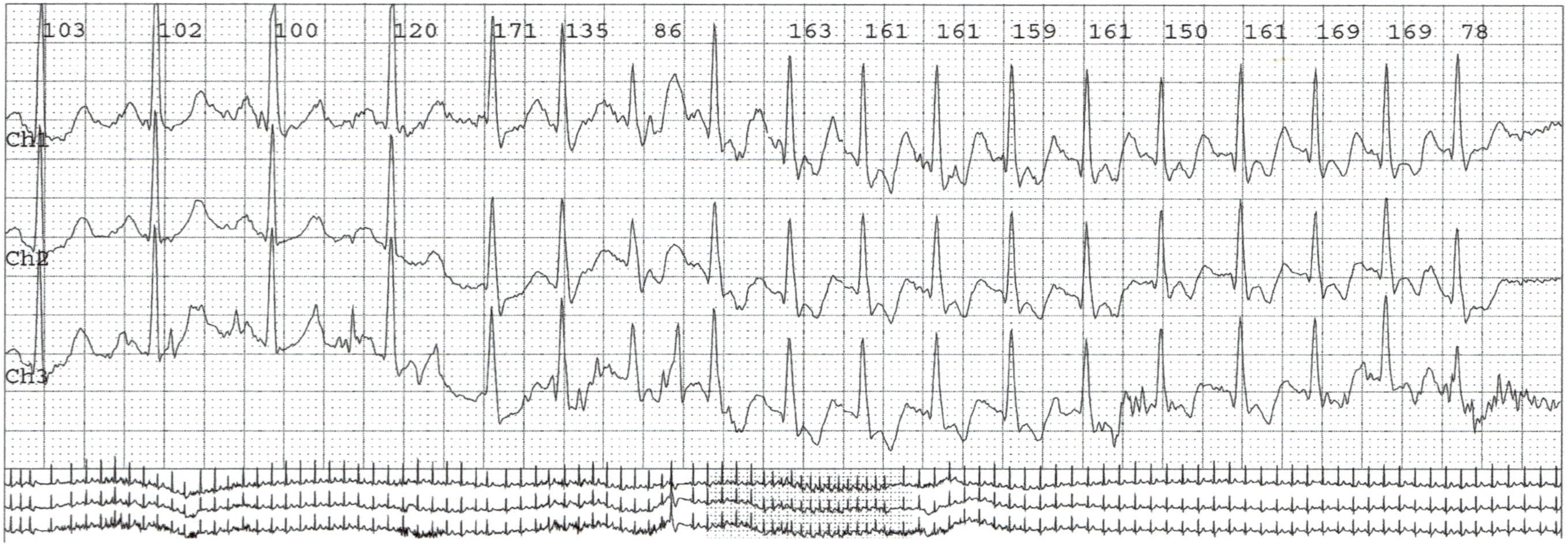


Question 3-4

## Question 3-4

The tachycardia mechanism in **Figure 3-4A** is:

1. AT
2. AVNRT
3. AVRT
4. Need more data

## Answer

This rhythm strip is clearly not the "cleanest" possible, but artifact and poor reproductions are a fact of life. In this example, there is no serious impediment to interpretation.

We see both onset and a termination of tachycardia, usually the most helpful in discerning the mechanism. The onset is especially laden with artifact and not of much value.

A relatively high-frequency deflection early in the ST segment during tachycardia is not present during sinus rhythm and is a P wave without much doubt (red dot in **Figure 3-4B**). Although the frontal leads are not identified, the P wave is opposite in polarity to the sinus P waves. We notice that the tachycardia ends with a QRS with no P wave seen after it. This is not helpful, being compatible with all our mechanism options. The reverse situation—that is, a tachycardia ending with a P wave—is more helpful when it occurs and would not be expected with an AT, since one would have to postulate spontaneous termination with coincidental AV block on that cycle.

The "body" of the tachycardia seems monotonously repetitive with no intervening ectopic activity or obvious "wobble" or CL irregularity. Nonetheless, it is useful to look for more subtle CL variability by careful measurement—and for these we magnify the region of interest. I interject again to say that *magnification of a region of interest is very valuable (I do it routinely!) and often exposes subtleties not apparent at the regular scale.*

In Figure 3-4B, it is apparent that the CL changes and the V changes precede the A changes. This of course cannot be an AT. Note that the statement was stated in the negative since it does not prove a mechanism. It only "disproves" one mechanism because the trailing chamber cannot be the instigator of the change. In our example, we have ruled out AT but it could still be AVRT or AVNRT. For that matter, it could theoretically also be junctional tachycardia (JT) or ventricular tachycardia (VT), but not AT.

*We can thus safely rule out AT but not AVNRT or AVRT. The correct answer to our question is therefore Option 4—we need more data.*

One can look at this a slightly different way. Figure 3-4B also shows that the RP interval during tachycardia stays relatively constant (red line, VA "linking"), while the CL varies slightly with the variability being in the PR interval. This suggests that the AV node is part of the circuit. This would not be expected in AT.

A careful look for CL variation or "wobble" can be most rewarding!

Figure 3-4B

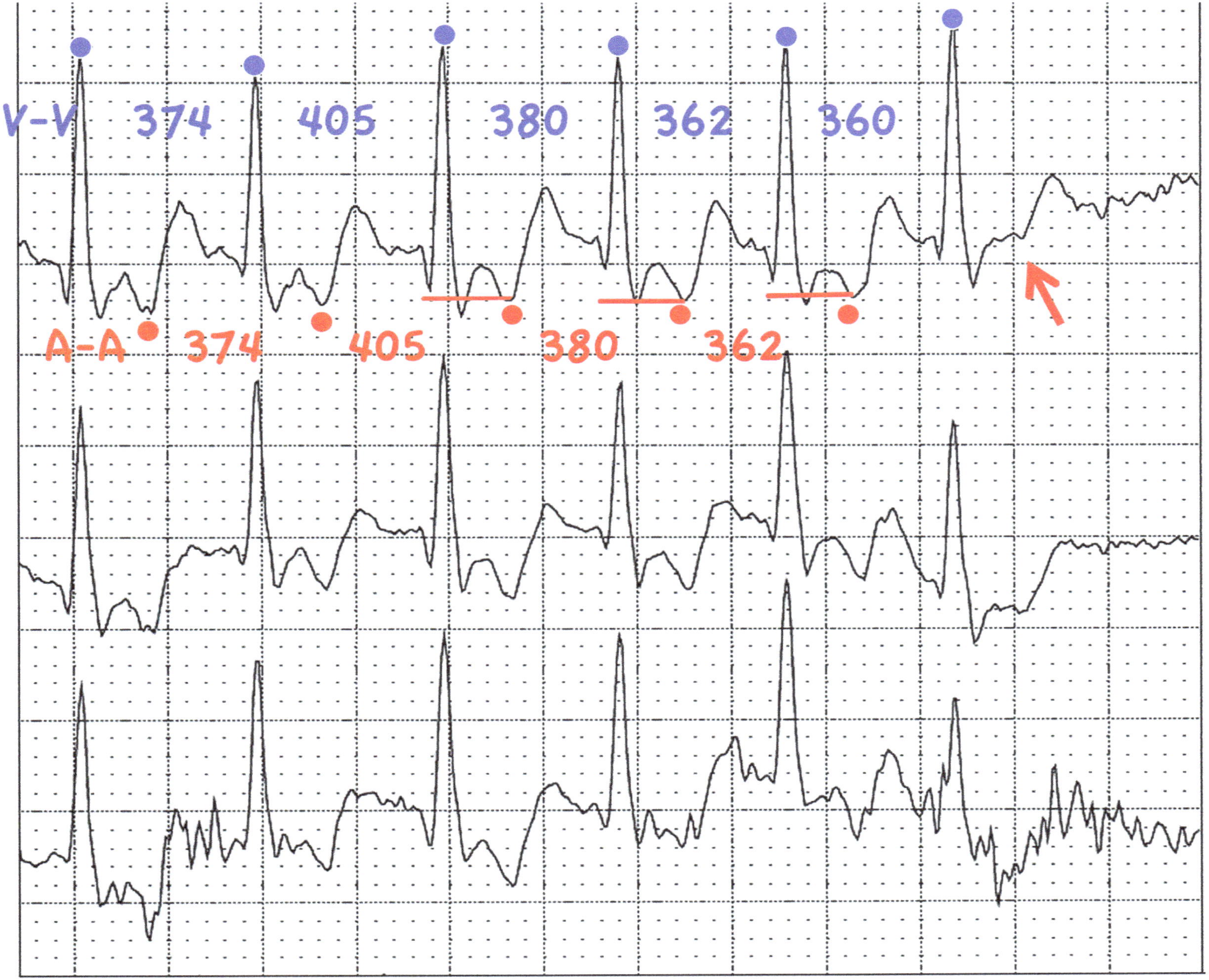
V-V
374
405
380
362
360
A-A
374
405
380
362

Figure 3-5A

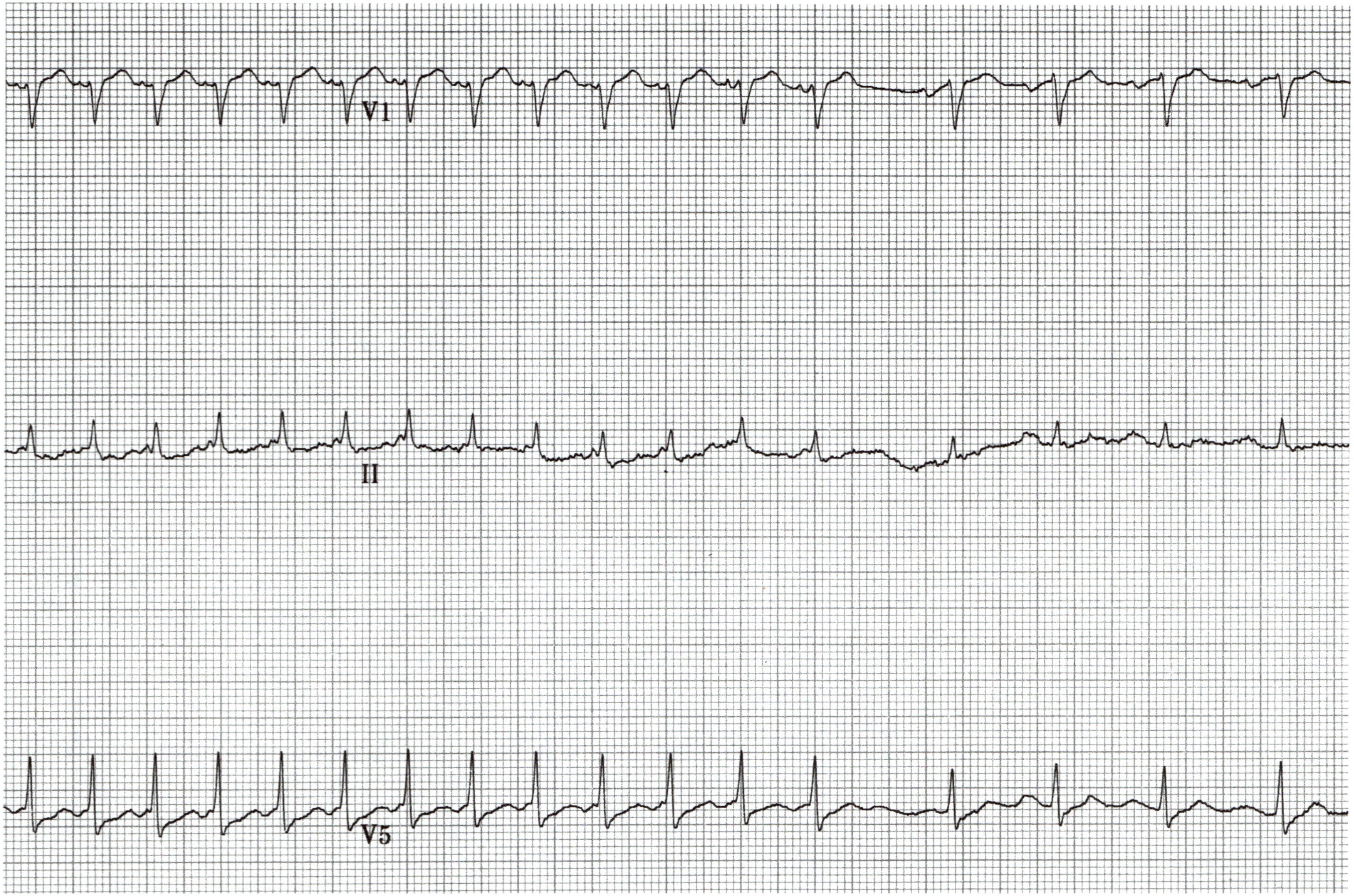


Question 3-5

## Question 3-5

The ECG shown in Figure 3-5A is recorded during adenosine administration in a 59-year-old woman with recurrent paroxysmal supraventricular tachycardia (PSVT).
The tachycardia mechanism is most probably:

1. AT
2. AVNRT
3. AVRT
4. Indeterminate

## Answer

The area of interest (the termination) is magnified as **Figure 3-5B** for clarity. The P wave is identified as preceding the QRS; hence the problem can be framed as "SVT with 1-to-1 AV relationship." It is difficult to characterize P-wave morphology from the available leads, so this will not be too helpful. We can call it a "long-RP tachycardia" a descriptor frequently used but not terribly helpful determining the mechanism.

The response to adenosine is usually very helpful and often diagnostic. Here we see a subtle lengthening of the CL prior to the break with a relatively constant PR interval. A QRS complex is the last event.

The tracing could be interpreted as compatible with AT with some CL prolongation prior to the break. The only difficulty with this interpretation is the very short PR interval in the range of 50 ms. Recall that the PR interval consists of both atrial conduction time to the AV node and traversing the normal AV conduction system to get to the ventricles. Even an atrial tachycardia "close" to the AV node must traverse the AV conduction system, and 50 ms simply seems too short an interval to allow this to take place (without postulating the existence of an accessory pathway (AP), such as an atrio-Hisian pathway).

"Typical" (slow-fast) AV node reentry would fit the observations the best. Recall that the VA interval in AVNRT is really a "pseudo interval," since conduction does not proceed from the ventricles to the atria. Rather, the reentrant circuit in the AV node region conducts both to the A and to the V but doesn't need either mechanistically. Thus, the "retrograde" P in AVNRT, although usually within or slightly after the QRS, can also slightly precede the QRS, especially if there is some conduction delay to the V. If we look at it this way, our P preceding the QRS is our usual "retrograde" P and the adenosine is terminating tachycardia with block to the next QRS!

The tachycardia would technically also be "compatible with" AVRT if we are dealing with a decremental AP with a long conduction time conducting retrogradely (a so-called "long RP tachycardia"). If such is the case, we still have the problem of explaining an exceedingly short conduction time from the exit of the AP at the atrium through the normal AV conduction system to the ventricle—which is the same problem as for the AT explanation.

Thus, the best answer would be Option 2, AVNRT.

It is noted that a "triggered" JT, potentially responsive to adenosine, must remain a theoretical possibility, although likely very rare indeed in a middle-aged woman with PSVT and not one of the options presented to the reader in the multiple choice question.

To the disappointment of her curious physicians, this patient chose medical therapy as opposed to ablation and the final diagnosis must remain unknown for the time being.

Figure 3-5B

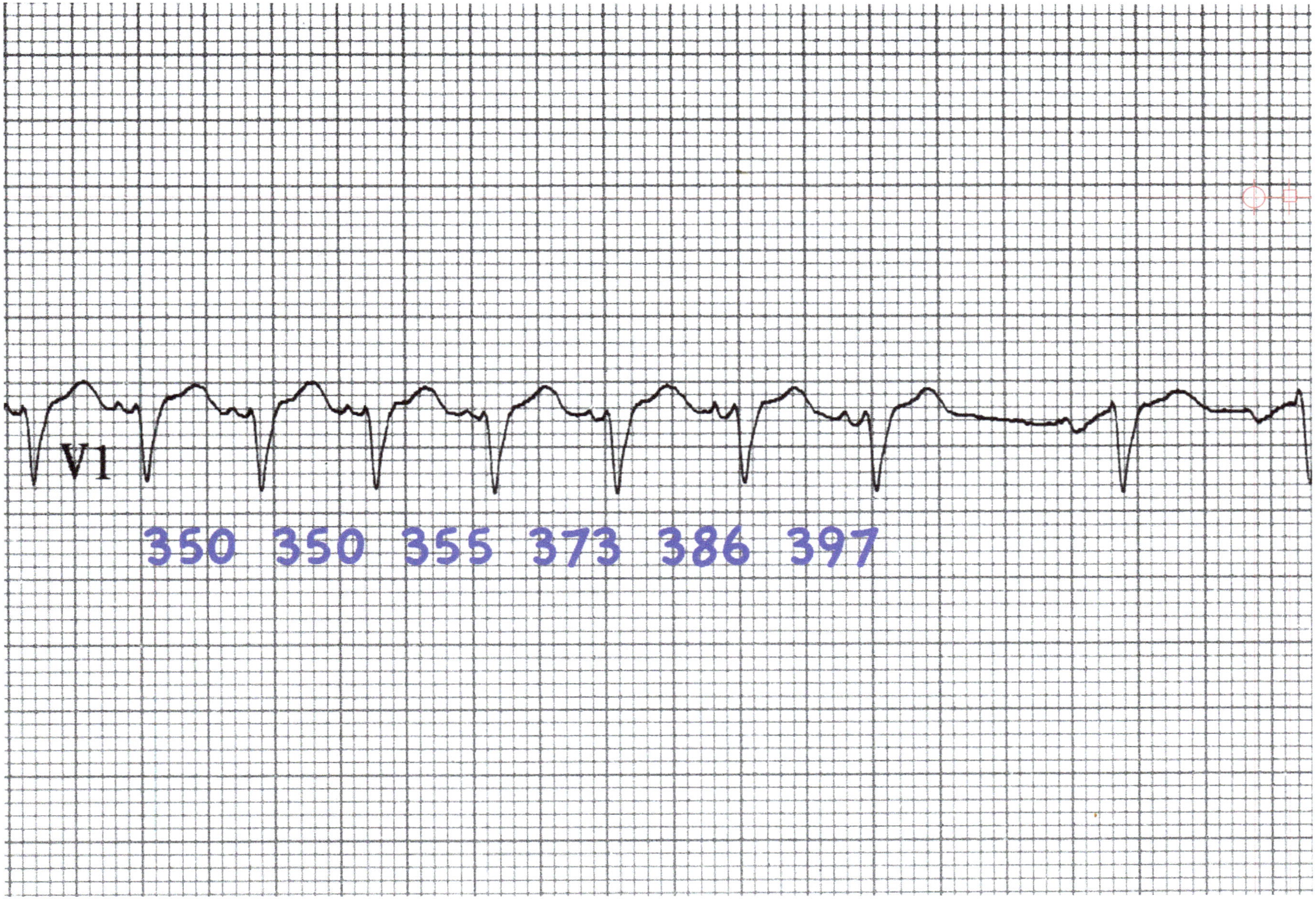

Question 3-6

Figure 3-6A

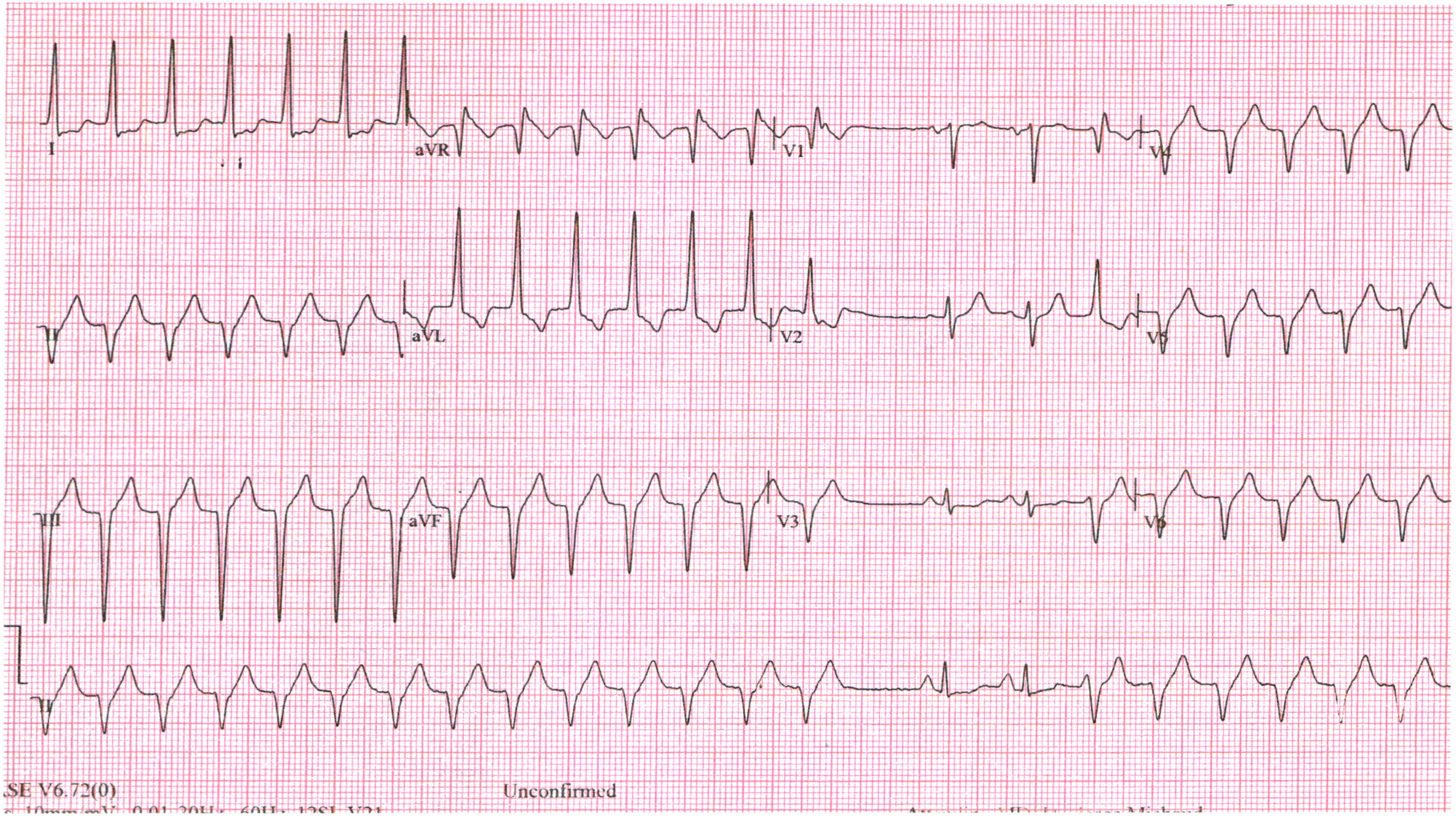

Question 3-6

## Question 3-6

The tachycardia mechanism in **Figure 3-6A** is:

1. VT
2. SVT with aberrancy
3. Preexcited tachycardia
4. Need more data

## Answer

This tachycardia is technically a "narrow" QRS tachycardia but is certainly not a "normal" QRS tachycardia. There are QS complexes in the inferior leads and QS complexes across the precordium except for a "jog" in $V_2$, which is positive. We see no evidence of anterior infarction in the few sinus beats available to us that have normal QRS morphology. *This is not consistent with a normal bundle branch block pattern.*

The negative QRS complexes across the precordium (essentially "concordant") are most consistent with a relatively apical origin of QRS depolarization. This would be unusual for any known preexcitation pattern. Thus, a "reflex" diagnosis of SVT (as was the admitting diagnosis in this case!) with a relatively narrow QRS is very inappropriate.

The "smoking gun" or absolute proof is apparent from the onset of tachycardia (**Figure 3-6B**). The P waves are indicated by **blue dots**, and it is seen that the first tachycardia QRS interrupts the P wave. The first cycle can therefore be only ventricular, and thus the tachycardia is VT.

It is noted that VT can be relatively "narrow" if there is aseptal origin with relative cancellation of forces or if the VT is closely related to the conduction system and depolarizes the heart faster than would be seen with only myocardial conduction.

Figure 3-6B

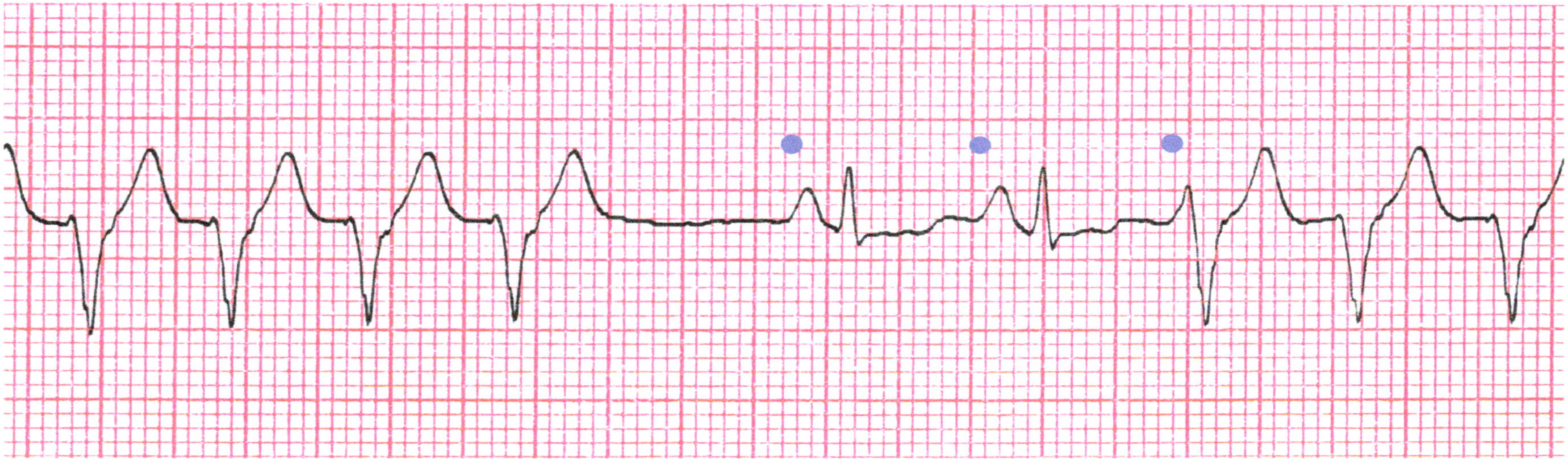

Figure 3-7A

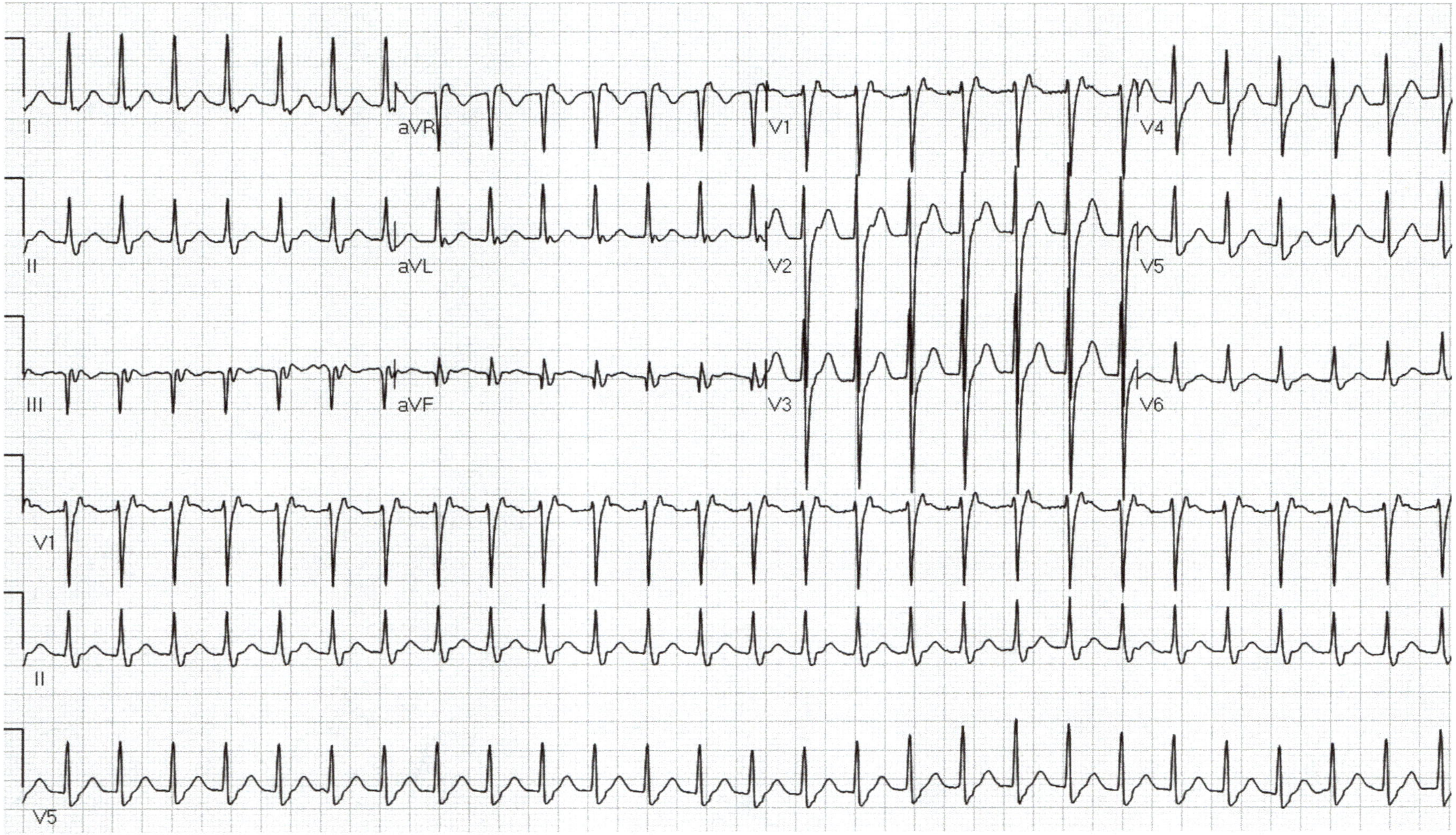

## Question 3-7

Question 3-7

The tachycardia shown in **Figure 3-7A** is most probably:

1. Sinus tachycardia
2. AVNRT
3. AVRT
4. AFL

## Answer

The tracing falls into the category of "SVT with no obvious atrial activity." In this example, there is a terminal deflection in the QRS that may be part of the QRS or could be a P wave hiding in the terminal part of the QRS.

A simple comparison of the ECG in sinus rhythm in **Figure 3-7B** rapidly clarifies this. The terminal part "disappears" in sinus rhythm in virtually every lead, confirming that it was not part of the QRS but a P wave. This is almost universally observed with typical AVNRT, although it's not always as obvious as our example. Of course, atrial tachycardia conducting over a slow AVN pathway with a long PR interval can't be ruled out absolutely but would be distinctly less common.

*It is important to compare the 2 tracings (tachycardia and sinus rhythm) side-by-side when the changes are more subtle.*

Figure 3-7B

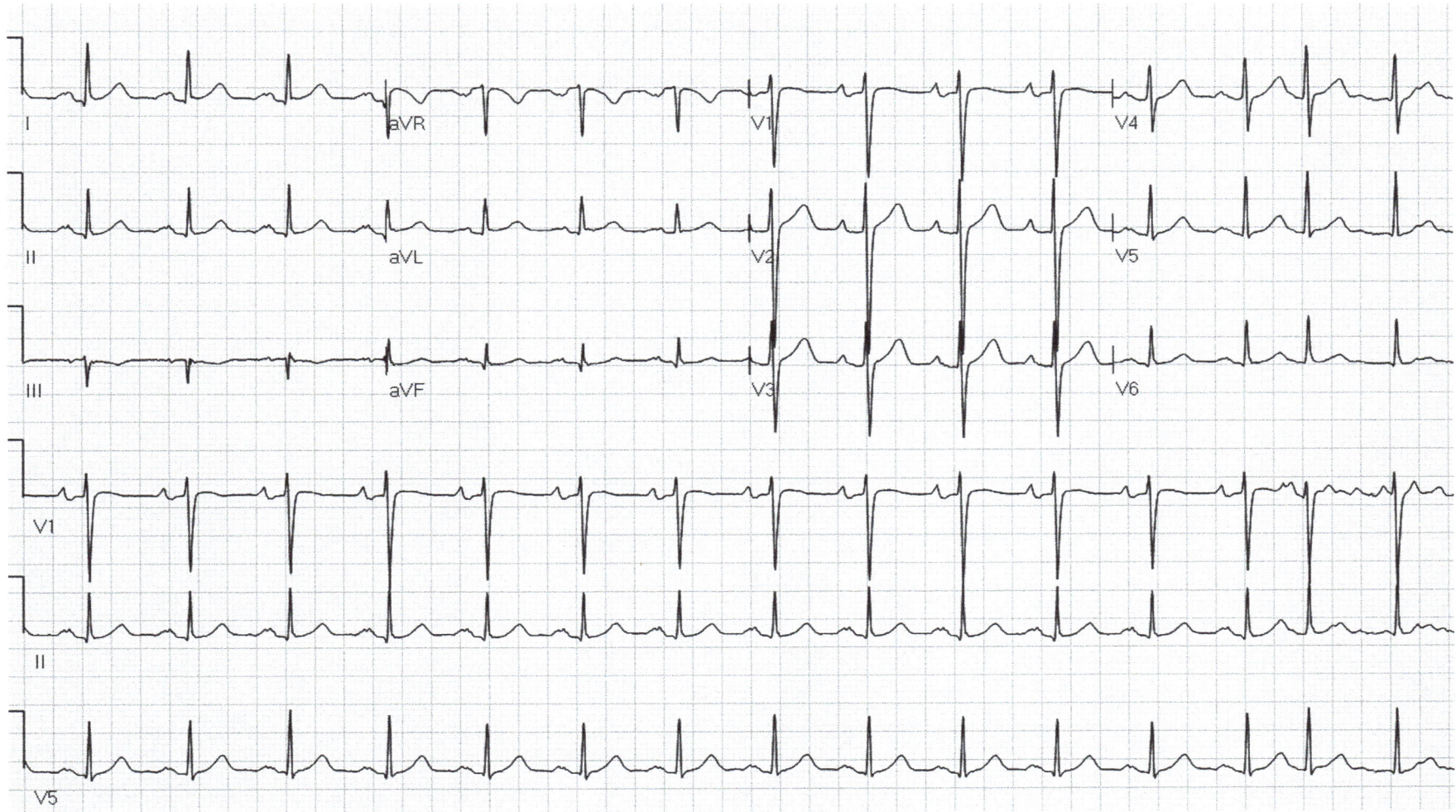

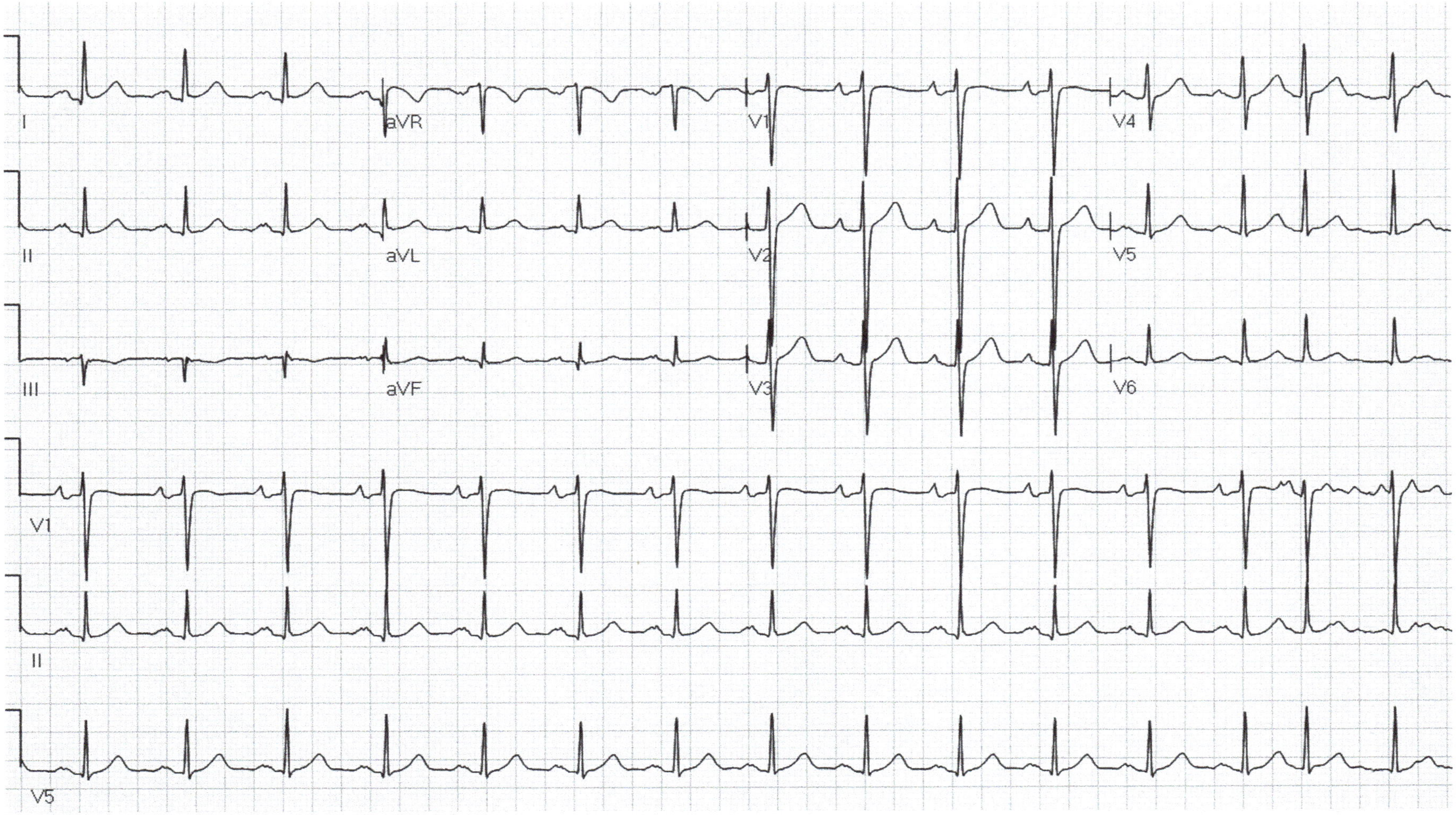


Question 3-7

Figure 3-8A

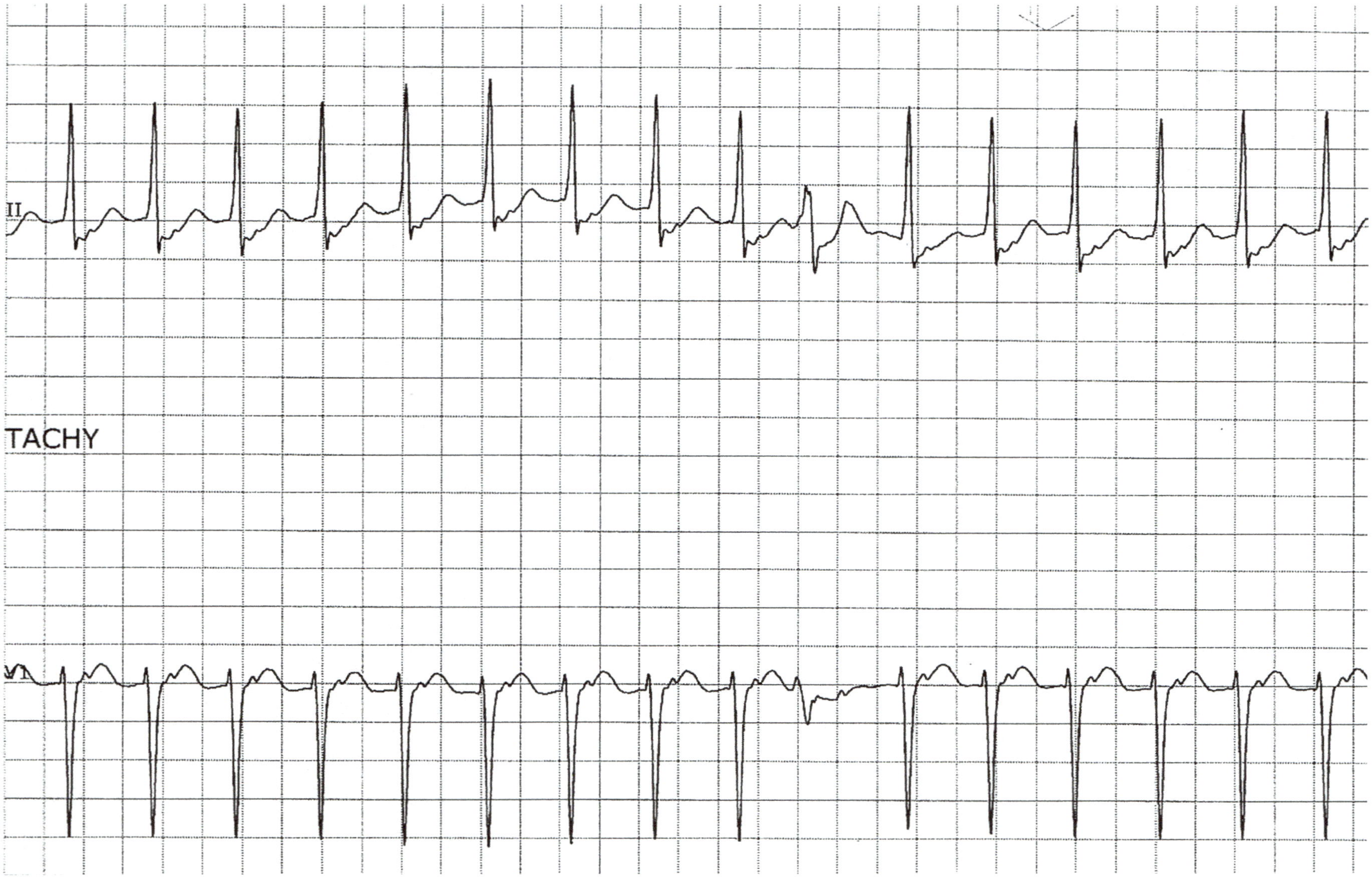


Question 3-8

## Question 3-8

The tachycardia mechanism shown in **Figure 3-8A** is most probably:

1. AT
2. AVNRT
3. AVRT
4. Need more data

## Answer

Figure 3-8A shows a regular, narrow QRS tachycardia at CL approximately 400 ms. There is a high-frequency deflection shortly after the QRS that is a candidate P wave but potentially also part of the QRS. We are fortunate to see a premature ventricular contraction (PVC). *This displaces the QRS and verifies that the deflection is not part of the QRS, but is instead a P wave.*

The VA interval during tachycardia is approximately 110 ms, a little short in general for AVRT. We note also that the PVC is largely negative in $V_1$ (left bundle branch block [LBBB] morphology), suggesting origin of the PVC in the right ventricle (RV).

**Figure 3-8B** is annotated and shows that the PVC is relatively early-coupled (hence the His would not be expected to be refractory), but even so, it does not move or "reset" the P wave or the tachycardia. Such would certainly be expected with an RV PVC with relatively close access to the tachycardia circuit, as might be the case if the tachycardia were AVRT using a right or posteroseptal AP. Failure of a closely coupled PVC makes the latter unlikely and is more suggestive of AVNRT, AT, or possibly AVRT over a left lateral AP, where the PVC is relatively far from the tachycardia circuit.

AT is less likely, since the PVC might be expected to invade the AV node retrogradely (concealed retrograde conduction into the AV node), prolonging the next PR interval—but here, the first QRS after the pause was not affected (i.e., no change in the PR interval after the PVC). Furthermore, the PR interval is very long so that one would have to postulate that the AT would be occurring coincidentally over a slow pathway—certainly possible, but less probable, since AT over a slow pathway is seen relatively rarely compared to AVNRT.

The correct answer to our question is thus Option 2, AVNRT. Note that the question includes the word "probably" since there is no absolute proof in this example but rather several bits of physiological circumstantial evidence. If the word "probably" were removed from the question, the correct answer would be "need more data," but in this case, the patient did have AVNRT.

The example serves to highlight a physiological approach to interpretation depending on the phenomena expected with differing mechanisms of tachycardia.

*Ectopic activity during tachycardia is a gift and will frequently be helpful, if not frankly diagnostic.*

Figure 3-8B

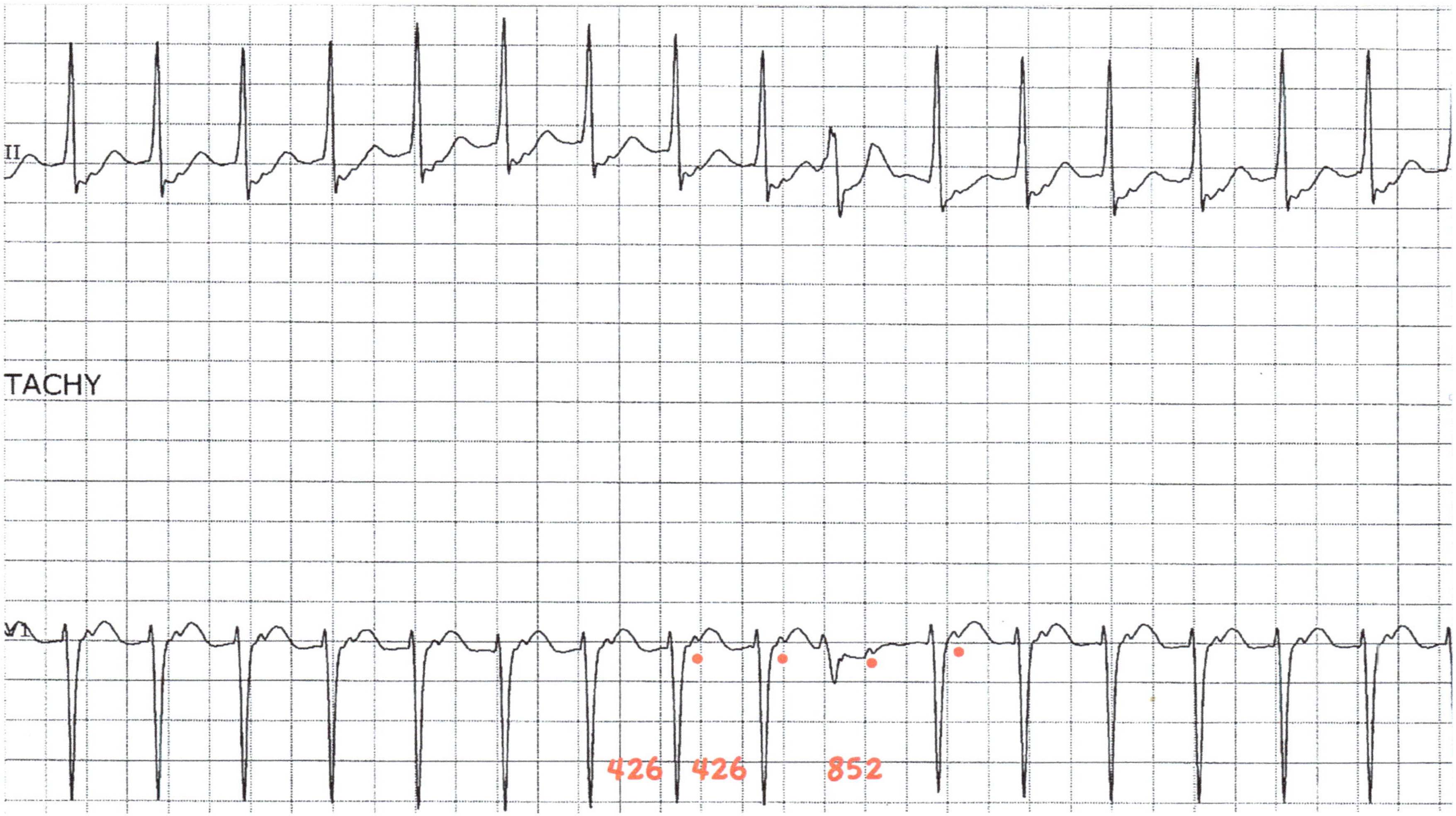

Figure 3-9

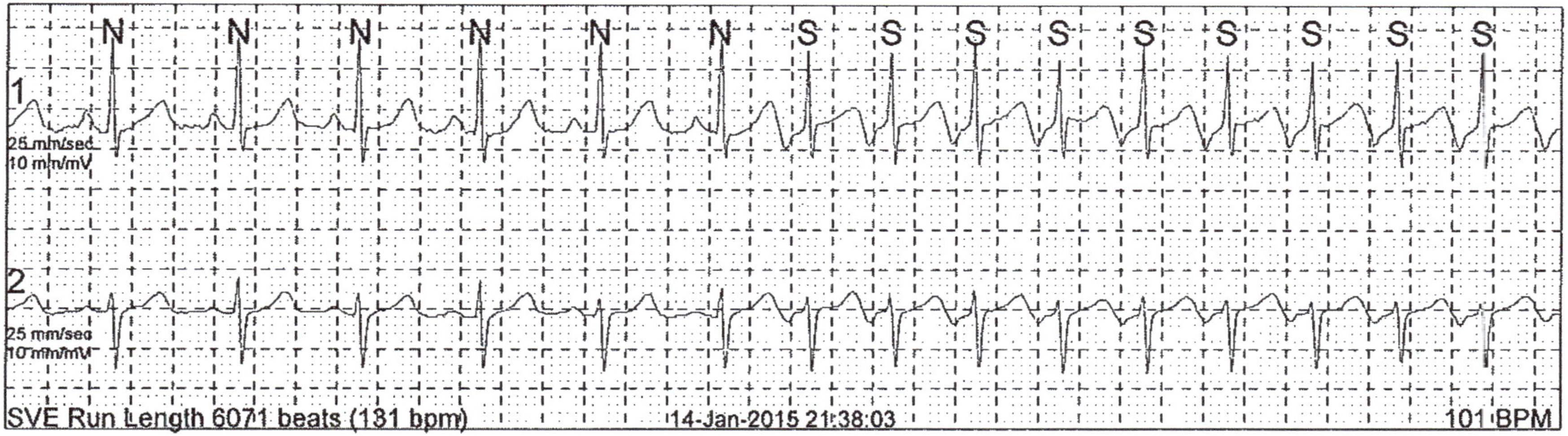


## Question 3-9

This patient had very frequent SVT. A typical onset is seen in **Figure 3-9**.
The mechanism of tachycardia is:

1. AT
2. AVNRT
3. AVRT
4. Need more data

## Answer

Atrial activity during tachycardia is readily recognized by the distortion of the T wave during tachycardia (compare the T wave relative to that in sinus rhythm). The tachycardia apparently starts with a relatively late-coupled PAC with no significant PR prolongation of the initial cycle. This would generally make AT more likely, since the junctional reentrant tachycardias (AVNRT and AVRT) usually require some PR prolongation at the onset of the tachycardia induced by atrial ectopy.

This type of tachycardia is commonly referred to as a "long RP" tachycardia for obvious reasons. As stated previously, I don't find this designation very useful, since the differential diagnosis remains essentially the same, namely our first 3 options above (AVNRT is obviously "atypical" by definition). For that matter, it might just as reasonably be called a "short PR" tachycardia, right?

The semantic issues aside, there is really no hard diagnostic evidence to venture a strong opinion from this tracing, and the correct answer to the question is Option 4—we need more data.

The next 2 examples (Questions 3-10 and 3-11) are drawn from the same patient and clarify the diagnosis.

Figure 3-10A

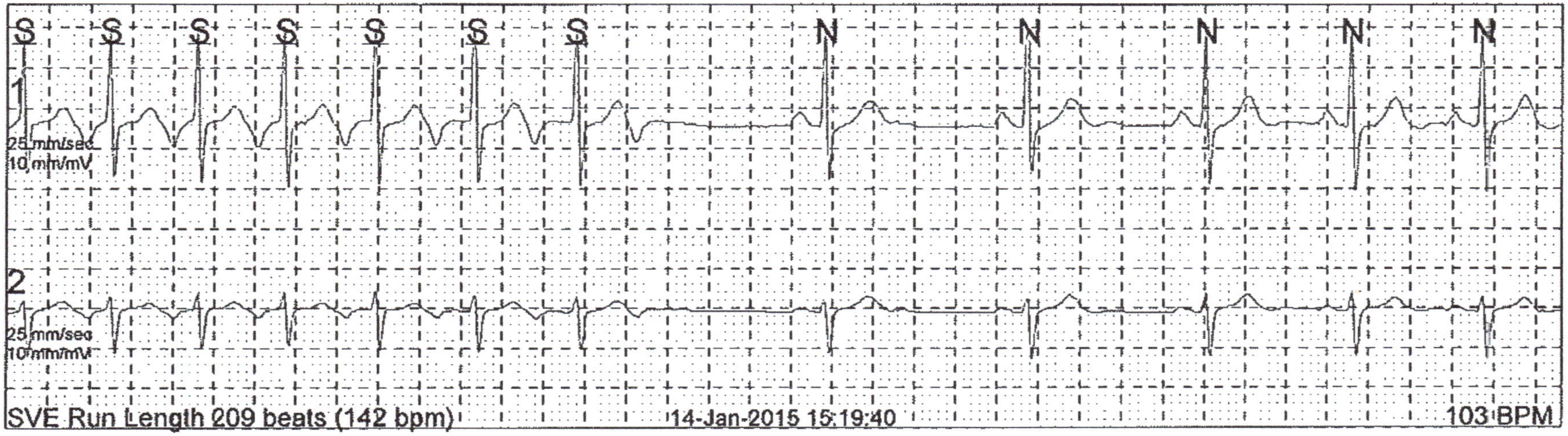




## Question 3-10

The mechanism of tachycardia in **Figure 3-10A** is:

1. AT
2. AVNRT
3. AVRT
4. Need more data

## Answer

The tracing in Figure 3-10A is from the same individual presented in Question 3-9. This pattern of spontaneous termination of tachycardia was observed repeatedly.

The initially apparent observation is that the tachycardia terminates with a P wave. This would make AT statistically unlikely, since one would have to postulate spontaneous termination of atrial tachycardia with concurrent coincidental block in the AV node.

However, there is indisputable evidence ruling out AT as illustrated in the magnification of the relevant area of interest in **Figure 3-10B**. Here we see that there is slight slowing of tachycardia prior to the break, and the *prolongation of the AA interval follows prolongation of the VV interval* (see also discussion of Question 3-4). This does not *prove* any mechanism, since several mechanisms may be involved if the VV change precedes the AA change, but it ***absolutely*** *rules out* AT.

Another way of looking at this observation is that PR prolongation slows the tachycardia; hence the AV node (anterogradely) must be part of the circuit.

We still can't distinguish between AVNRT (obviously atypical by definition) and AVRT, however; hence the correct answer here remains Option 4—that is, we need more data.

Figure 3-10B

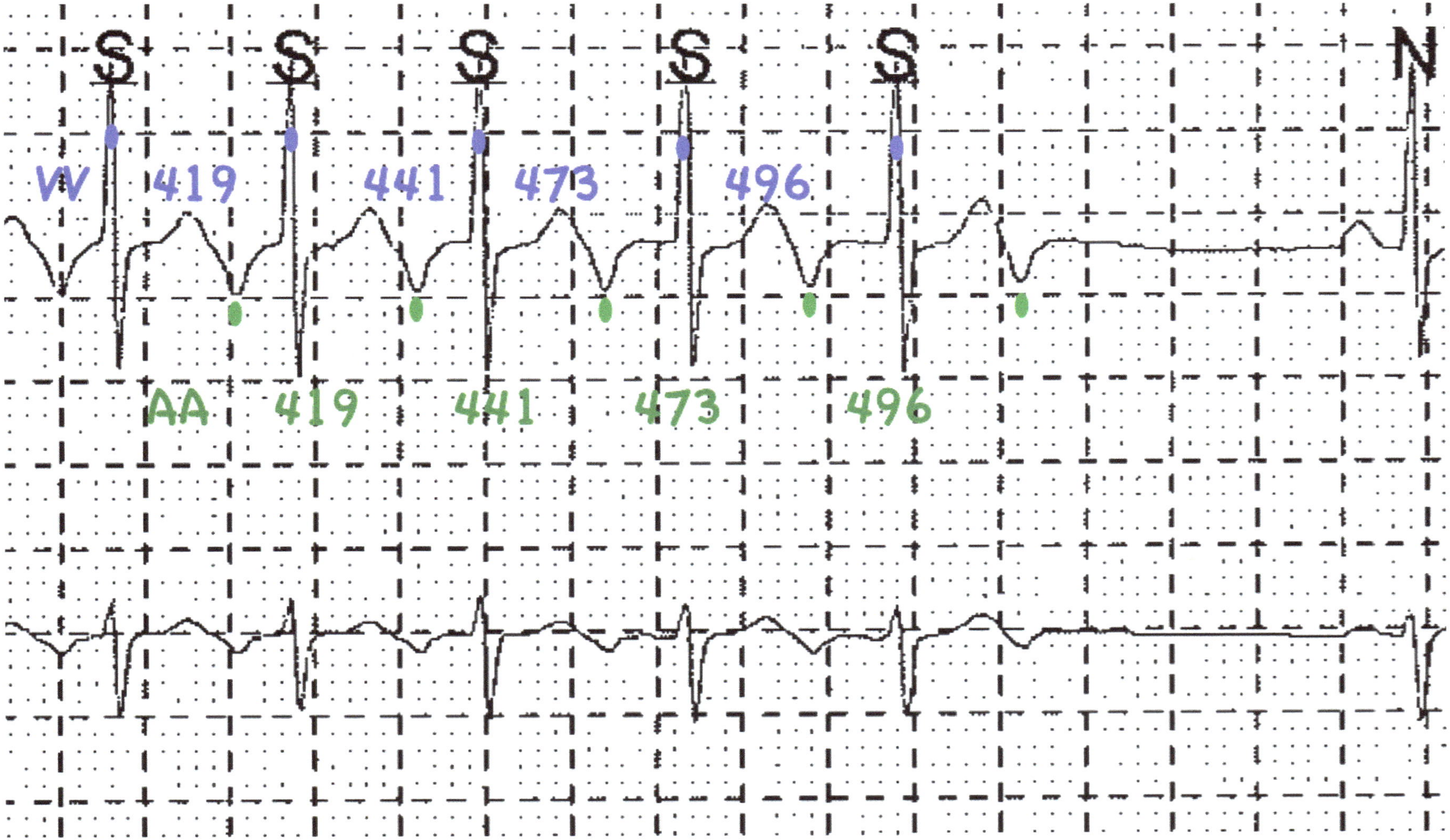

Figure 3-11A

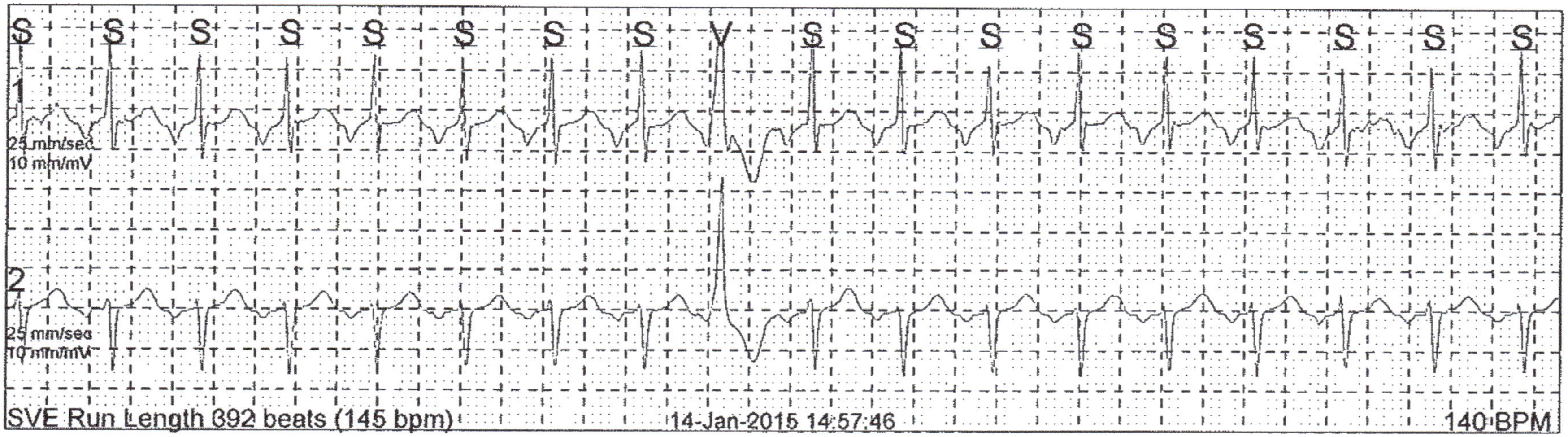


## Question 3-11

The tracing in **Figure 3-11A** is taken from the same patient presented in Questions 3-9 and 3-10.

Are we further informed?

The tachycardia mechanism is:

1. AT
2. AVNRT
3. AVRT
4. Need more data

## Answer

We are now very fortunate to see a PVC during the tachycardia, which allows us to see how it perturbs the mechanism, just as a PVC inserted into the tachycardia cycle during tachycardia during an electrophysiology study would. All our focus now shifts to magnifying the area of interest (**Figure 3-11B**) and careful measurement.

The CL is very stable, such that small changes after the PVC are meaningful and can be appreciated. The first observation is that the PVC is relatively late-coupled and interrupts the inscription of the preceding P wave. This results in advancement of the *subsequent* P wave (**red lettering**) and QRS; that is, it *resets* the tachycardia. One also appreciates that the CL surrounding the PVC (**black lettering**) is less than 2 cycles.

*Resetting the tachycardia mechanism with a relatively late-coupled PVC virtually rules out AT and AVNRT, which is the "big picture" conclusion of this tracing.*

The PVC has excellent access to the excitable gap of the circuit. Hence, we are left with AVRT, a tachycardia mechanism with a relatively large circuit and excitable gap.

To be a little more academic, and for the more advanced reader, we can consider whether or not the His bundle was refractory at the time the PVC arrived. Of course, we can't know that without the His bundle recording, but it doesn't matter since we can measure the VA interval (or "RP" interval) during tachycardia and compare it to the VA interval after the PVC. We note that the VA interval after the PVC is only 33 ms longer than that during tachycardia, and thus the ventricle is undoubtedly "in" the circuit.

Advancement of the circuit with the single PVC essentially "entrains" the circuit for a single cycle, and we should remember that the usually accepted interval difference (VA of PVC minus VA of tachycardia) for considering the PVC being "in" the circuit during entrainment in the electrophysiology laboratory is less than 85 ms.

A PVC that resets AVNRT would have a much longer VA interval, since the distance and time to get to the A from a PVC would be much longer than from the AVNRT circuit (unless one postulated the concomitant existence of rare nodoventricular or nodofascicular pathways).

Figure 3-11B

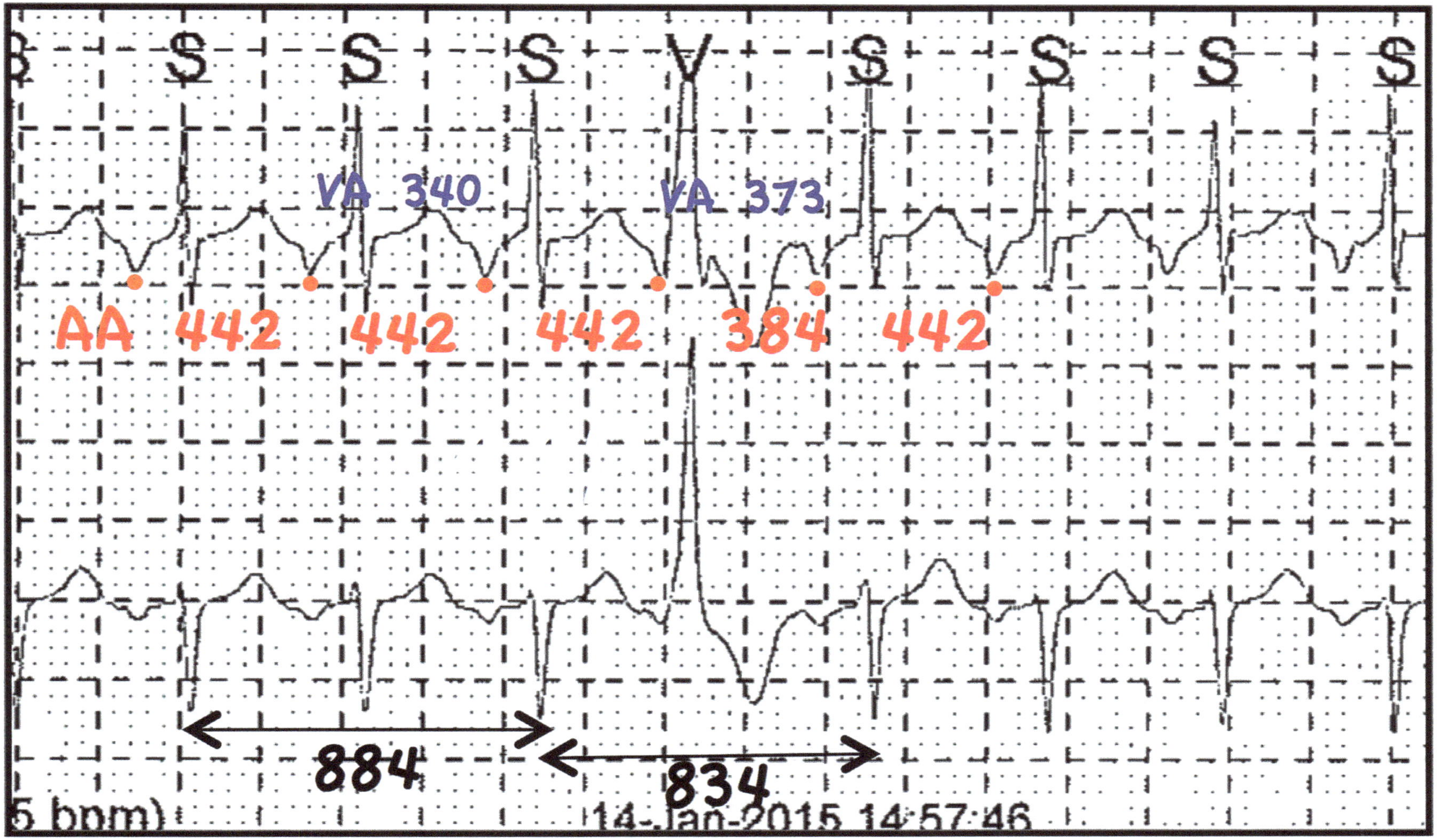
S
S
S
V
S
S
S
S
VA 340
VA 373
AA 442
442
442
384
442
884
834
5 bpm)
14-Jan-2015 14:57:46

Question 3-12

Figure 3-12A

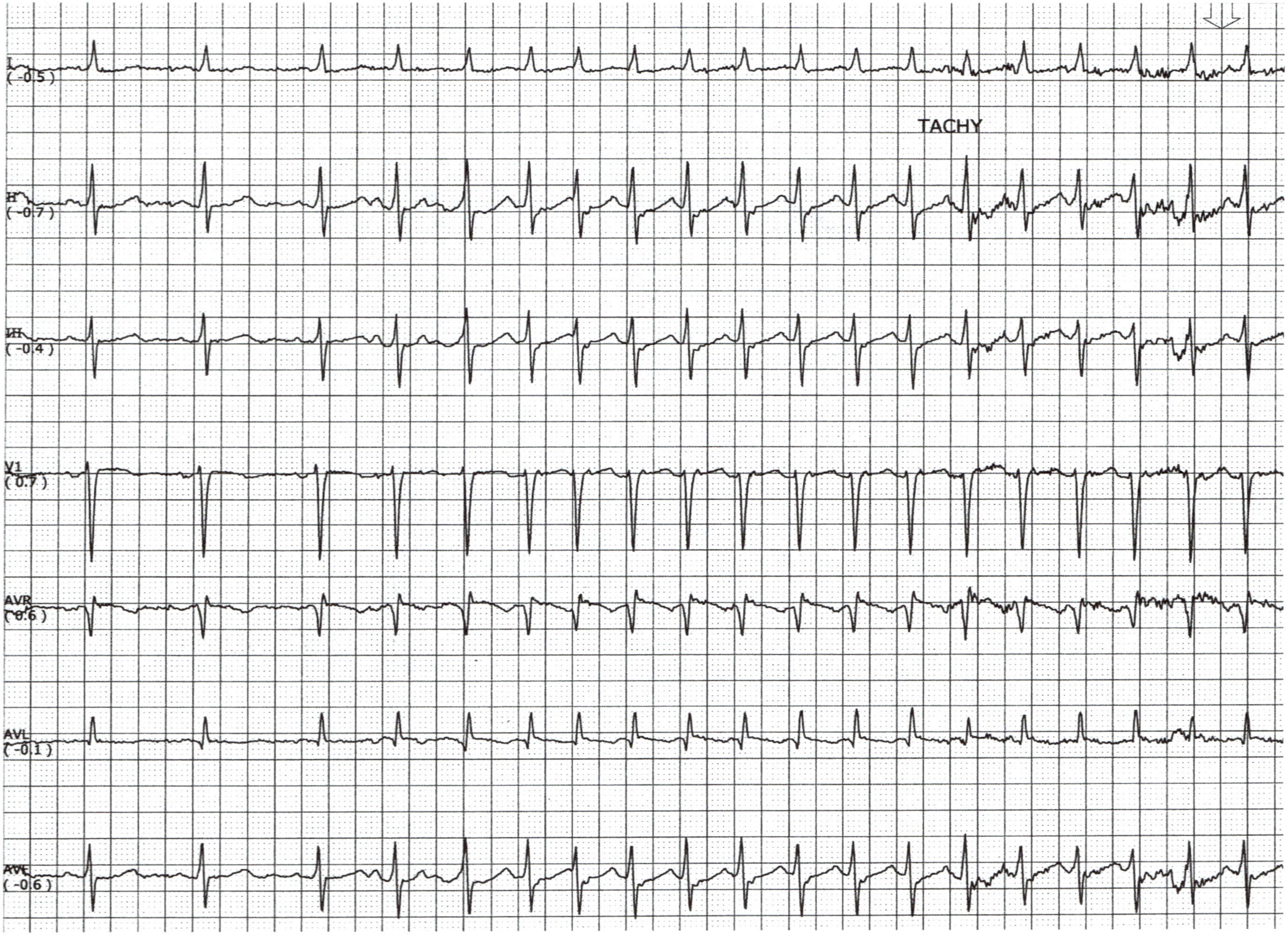

## Question 3-12

The tachycardia mechanism shown in **Figure 3-12A** is:

1. AT
2. AVNRT
3. AVRT
4. Need more data

## Answer

The onset of this relatively regular SVT is a little complicated, and we will begin by searching for P waves during the tachycardia. None are obvious in the diastolic interval, so we will search for P activity that might be obscured by the QRS complex.

To facilitate this, we must carefully compare the QRS during sinus rhythm to the QRS during stable tachycardia (**Figure 3-12B**). It then becomes obvious that there is a sharp terminal deflection in the QRS during SVT that is not there during sinus rhythm (**red circles**), and this is undoubtedly a P wave. This is very useful as it narrows the diagnosis essentially to AVNRT or AT with a long PR interval (i.e., over a slow AV nodal pathway not related directly to the tachycardia mechanism).

We then carefully look for some irregularity in the CL ("wobble") and observe some at the onset of SVT (**blue** and **black annotation** on the third channel). A small prolongation of CL is observed and the change in the QRS (i.e., VV) precedes the change in the PP interval (AA). *This is very helpful since it rules out AT.*

An alternate way of looking at the same event is to observe that the PR prolongs and the next A is proportionally prolonged; that is, the AV interval prolongs but the VA interval stays the same (the VA is "linked"). See also discussion in **Question 3-4**.

The onset of the tachycardia is a little more difficult to sort out, but tachycardia begins with at least 2 PACs (downward **red arrows**) and the PR interval after the second PAC is 320 ms, indicating the presence of a slow AV nodal pathway. This of itself doesn't prove the mechanism of the SVT (AVNRT), which only becomes evident later in the record.

Figure 3-12B

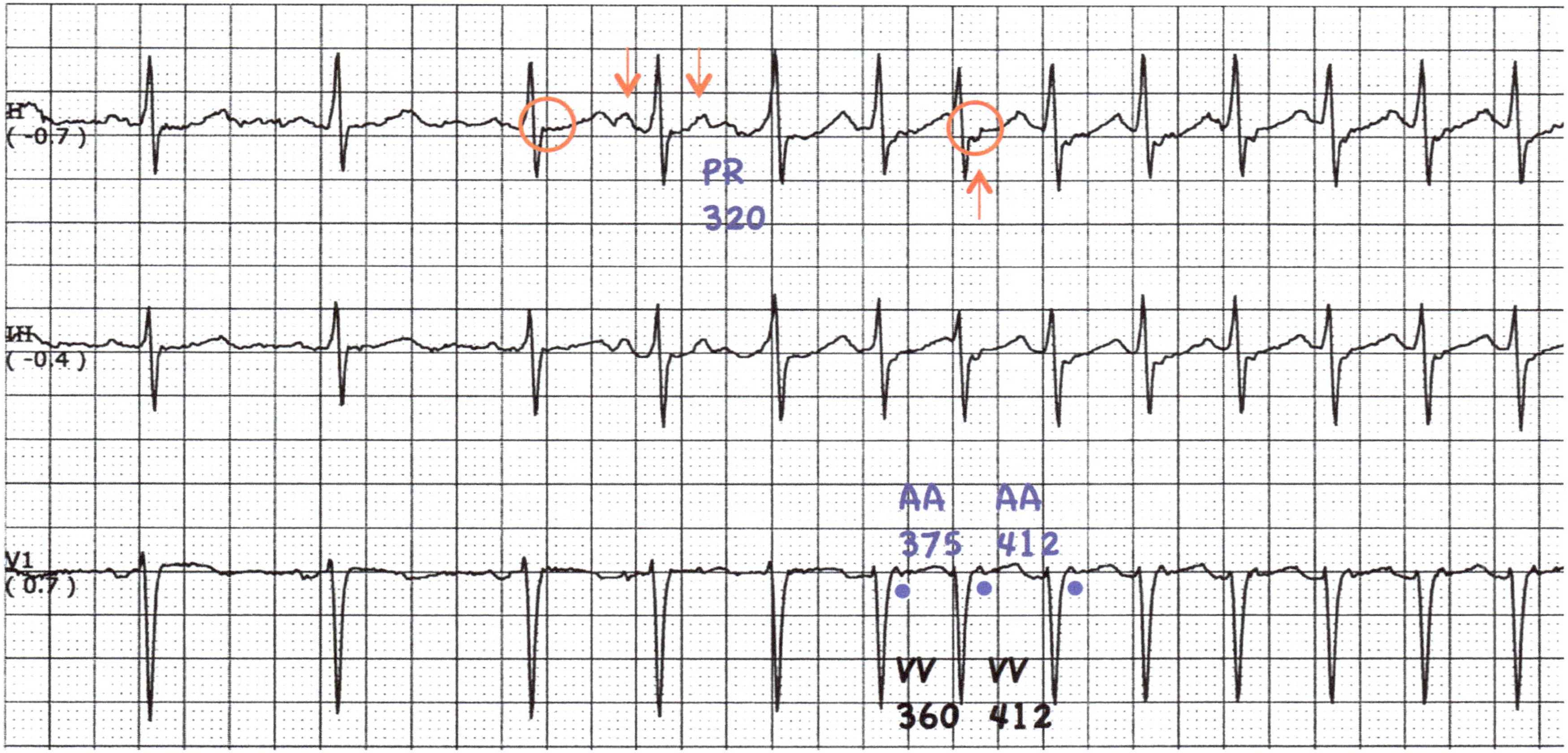

Figure 3-13A

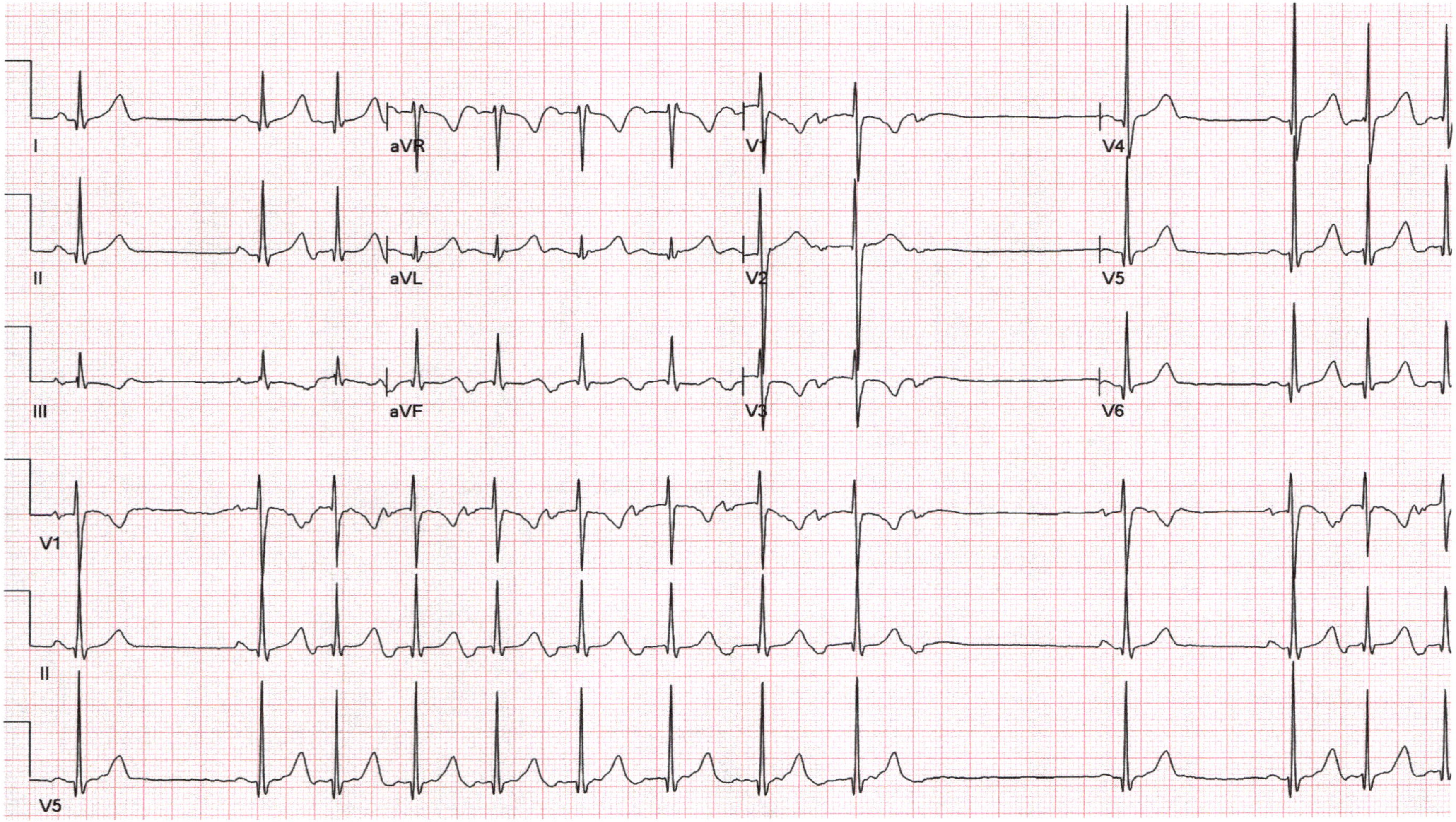

## Question 3-13

Similar runs of tachycardia were observed on many occasions during the monitoring period in this asymptomatic individual.

The tachycardia mechanism shown in **Figure 3-13A** is:

1. AT
2. AVNRT
3. AVRT
4. Need more data

## Answer

This is again a so-called "long-RP tachycardia," but as I pointed out elsewhere, this designation doesn't help us in determining the mechanism, which includes all the "usual suspects" as per Options 1–3. We are nonetheless fortunate in observing both tachycardia onset and offset, which, we are told, is reproducibly observed. In addition, we see slight irregularity in the CL.

The termination is useful in that it ends with a P wave, and there is no reason for an AT to block in the AV node on the exact cycle that it terminates; AT is thus very unlikely. Second, we see 2 onsets, and both begin with a preceding sinus cycle after a relative pause. This is again less likely with AT, which will often be the first cycle after a pause. The apparent "need" for a preceding sinus cycle or ectopic "inducer" is more in favor of AV or AVNRT.

Finally, we have definitive evidence for ruling out AT by focusing on the areas where the cycle length is a little variable and magnify a termination (**Figure 3.13B**). We note that the VV interval (**red**) prolongs near the end and the next AA interval (**blue**) prolongs proportionally and tachycardia stops. *This absolutely rules out AT.*

Another way of looking at this as emphasized elsewhere is that the PR interval (**black**) prolongs just before the break and resets the following P wave (prolongs the AA interval) so that *the AV node must be a part of the circuit.* Alternately, one may think of it as the RP interval being maintained (linked) in spite of prolongation of the PR interval.

The correct answer to our question nonetheless remains Option 4—namely, need more information, since the mechanism can be either AVRT over a retrogradely conducting AP with a long conduction time or, less commonly, AVNRT also utilizing a retrograde AV nodal pathway with a long conduction time.

Figure 3-13B

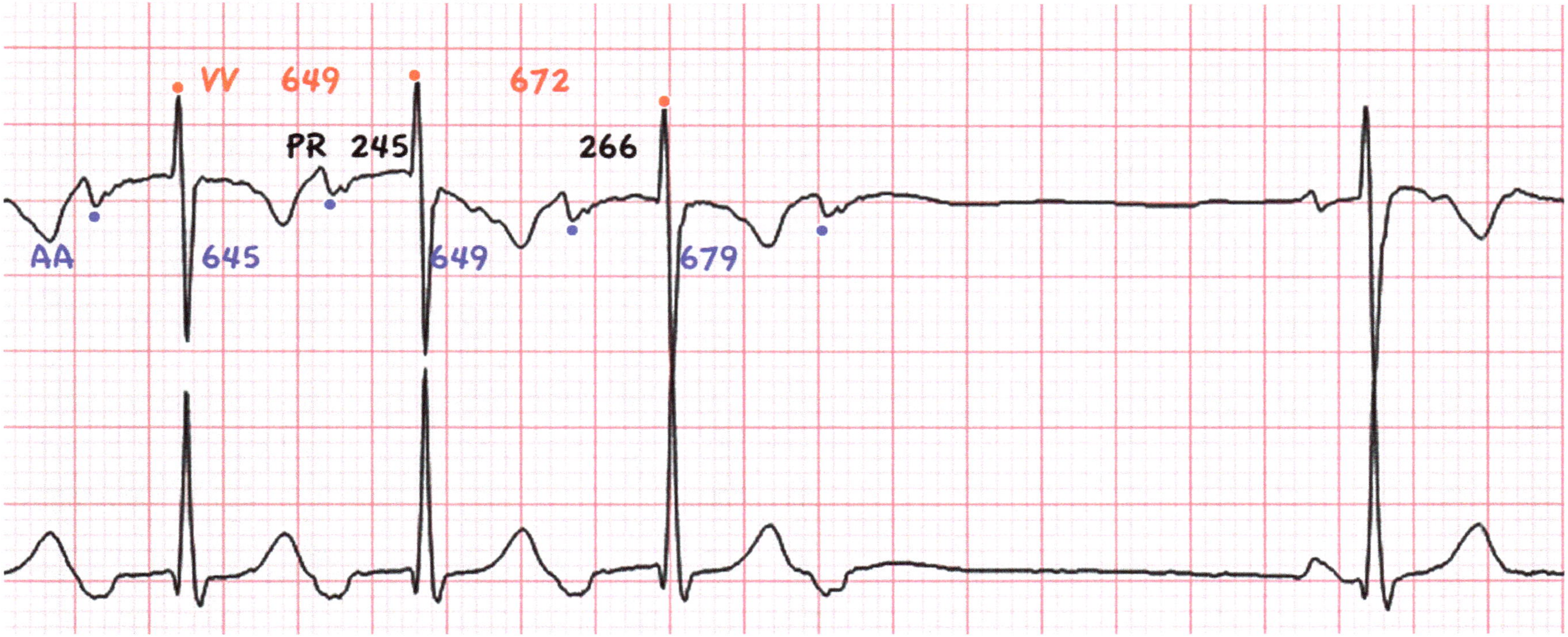

Figure 3-14A

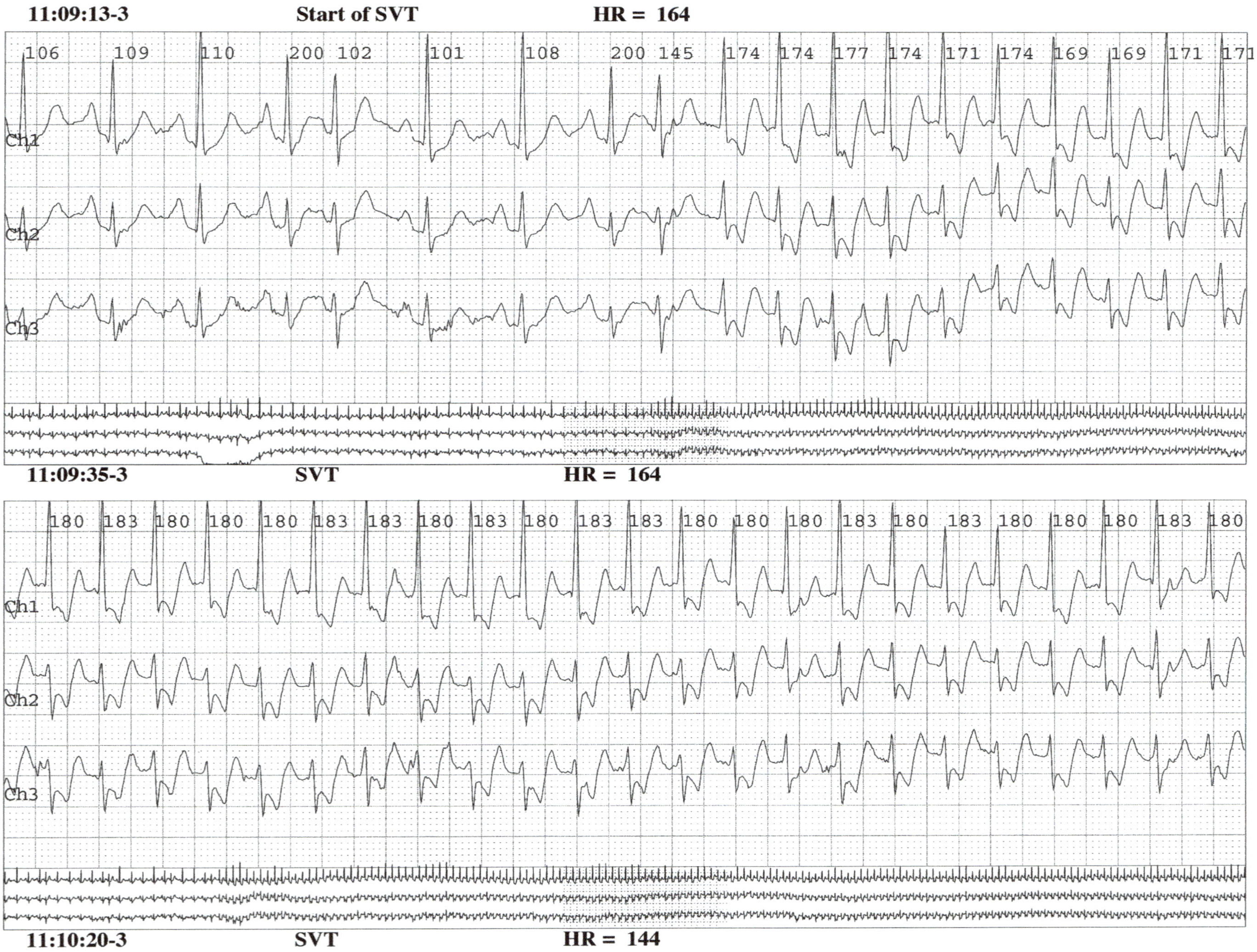
11:09:13-3
Start of SVT
HR = 164
106 109 110 200 102 101 108 200 145 174 174 177 174 171 174 169 169 171 171
Ch1
Ch2
Ch3
11:09:35-3
SVT
HR = 164
180 183 180 180 180 183 183 180 183 180 183 183 180 180 180 183 180 183 180 180 180 183 180
Ch1
Ch2
Ch3
11:10:20-3
SVT
HR = 144

## Question 3-14

This patient had very frequent SVT. A typical onset is seen in **Figure 3-14A**. The mechanism of tachycardia is:

1. AT
2. AVNRT
3. AVRT
4. Need more data

## Answer

The most useful information on this tracing comes from the mode of onset and we will magnify this part for clarity (**Figure 3-14B**). The tachycardia is initiated after 2 PACs (**red arrows**), after which we see a regular SVT with an inverted P in the ST segment (**circle**). The second PAC conducts with a very long PR interval, that is, over a slow AV nodal pathway. This suggests that AV node conduction delay was needed for the tachycardia and favors AV node reentry as the diagnosis. Of course, AV reentry also generally needs AV node conduction delay to start the tachycardia with a PAC.

AT is most unlikely with this onset, since we see that the VA interval is constant from the very first QRS ("linked"). It would be a significant coincidence if the first P wave of AT has the same VA relationship to the *preceding* QRS (to which it is not mechanistically related) as to the subsequent SVT and that it should occur coincidentally after a very long PR interval.

The correct answer to our question is thus Option 4; that is, we need more data. The next example (**Question 3-15**) is drawn from the same patient and may clarify the diagnosis.

Figure 3-14B

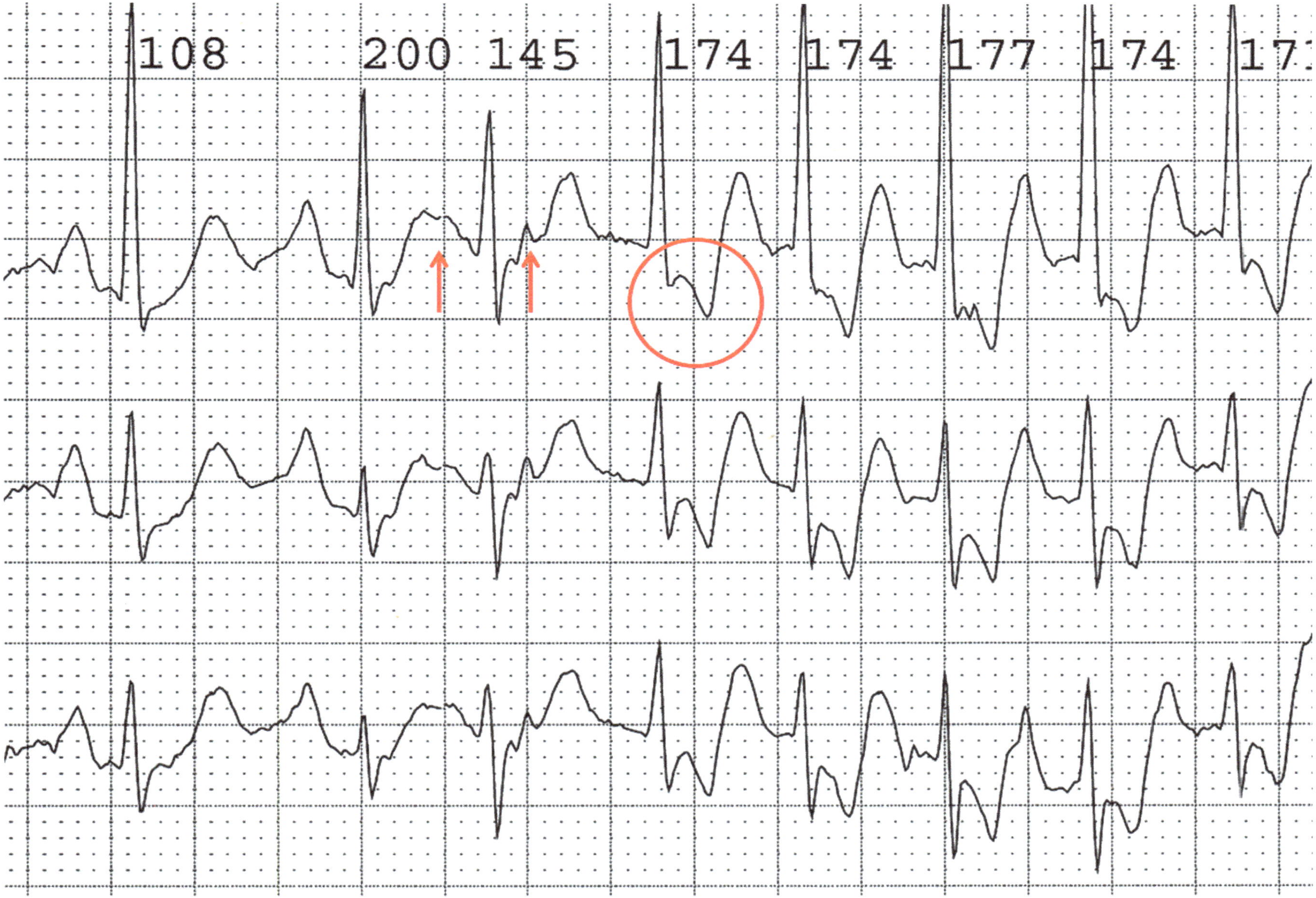

Figure 3-15A

**11:10:29-3** **End of scan** **HR = 144**

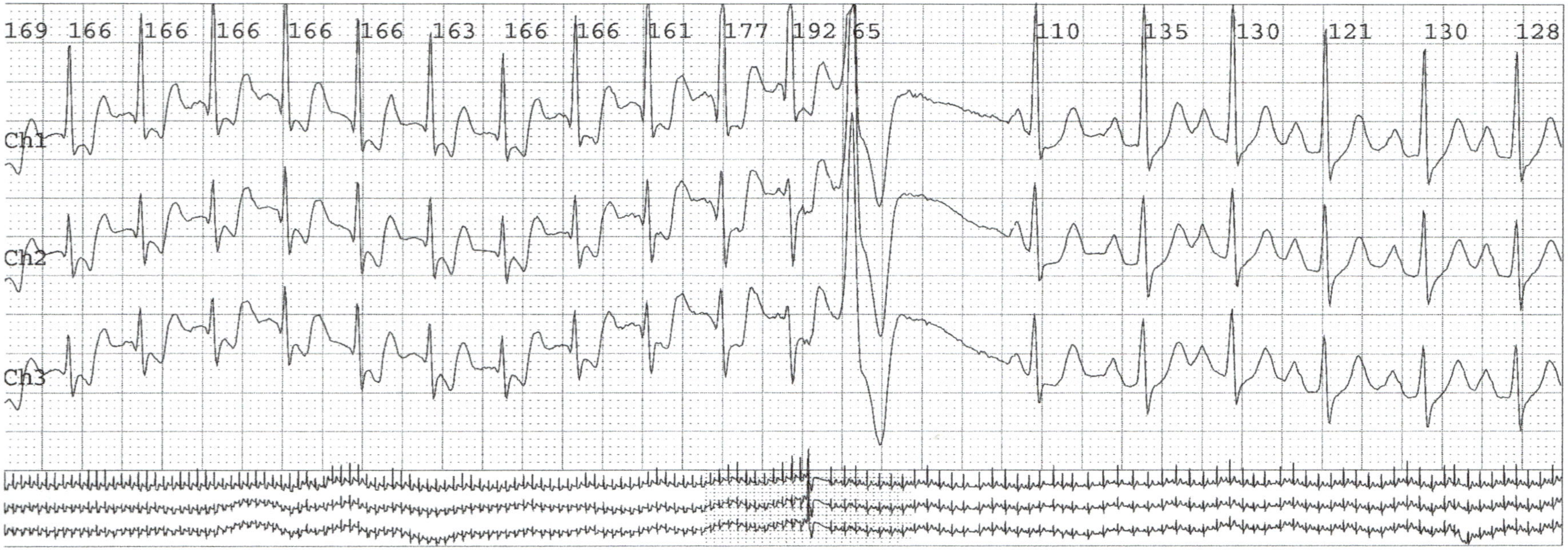


Question 3-15

Question 3-15

## Question 3-15

**Figure 3-15A** is a further recording from the patient discussed in Question 3-14.
The mechanism of tachycardia is:

1. AT
2. AVNRT
3. AVRT
4. Need more data

## Answer

We have now been given the "gift" of a PVC that terminates the tachycardia, which was observed on more than one occasion (assuring us that the termination was not just coincidental, i.e., a spontaneous termination). One hardly needs to make any measurements at this point, but we will do so to complete the exercise (**Figure 3-15B**).

There is no identifiable P wave after the QRS, but that is not critical here. What is striking is that the PVC is relatively "late-coupled." We can't see the His electrogram, of course, but the tachycardia is regular, and we can estimate how premature the PVC is relative to the next anticipated QRS during tachycardia (**blue vertical lines**). It is obvious that the PVC anticipates the next QRS by 60 ms or so.

The His bundle surely must be refractory at this point, yet the PVC resets (breaks) the SVT so that retrograde conduction must be proceeding over an AP! This makes AV reentry utilizing an accessory AV pathway as the retrograde limb most probable—although an atypical pathway such as a nodoventricular can't be ruled out when a His refractory PVC terminates tachycardia.

*A message here is that one can generally assume a His-V time of 50–60 ms in most individuals to approximate the His position and allow analysis as if it were the equivalent of a PVC programmed into SVT during a full electrophysiology study.*

Figure 3-15B

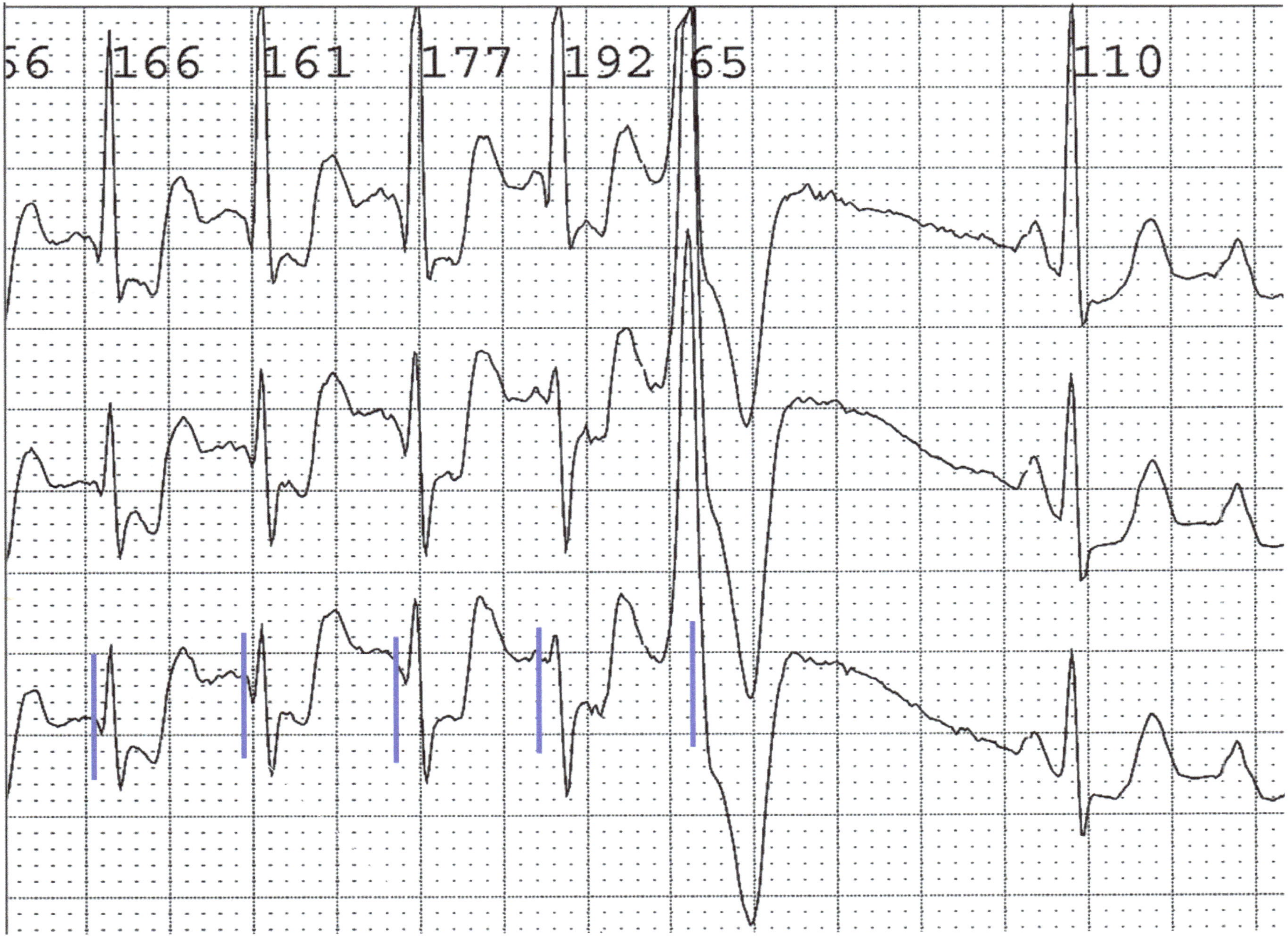

Question 3-16

Figure 3-16A

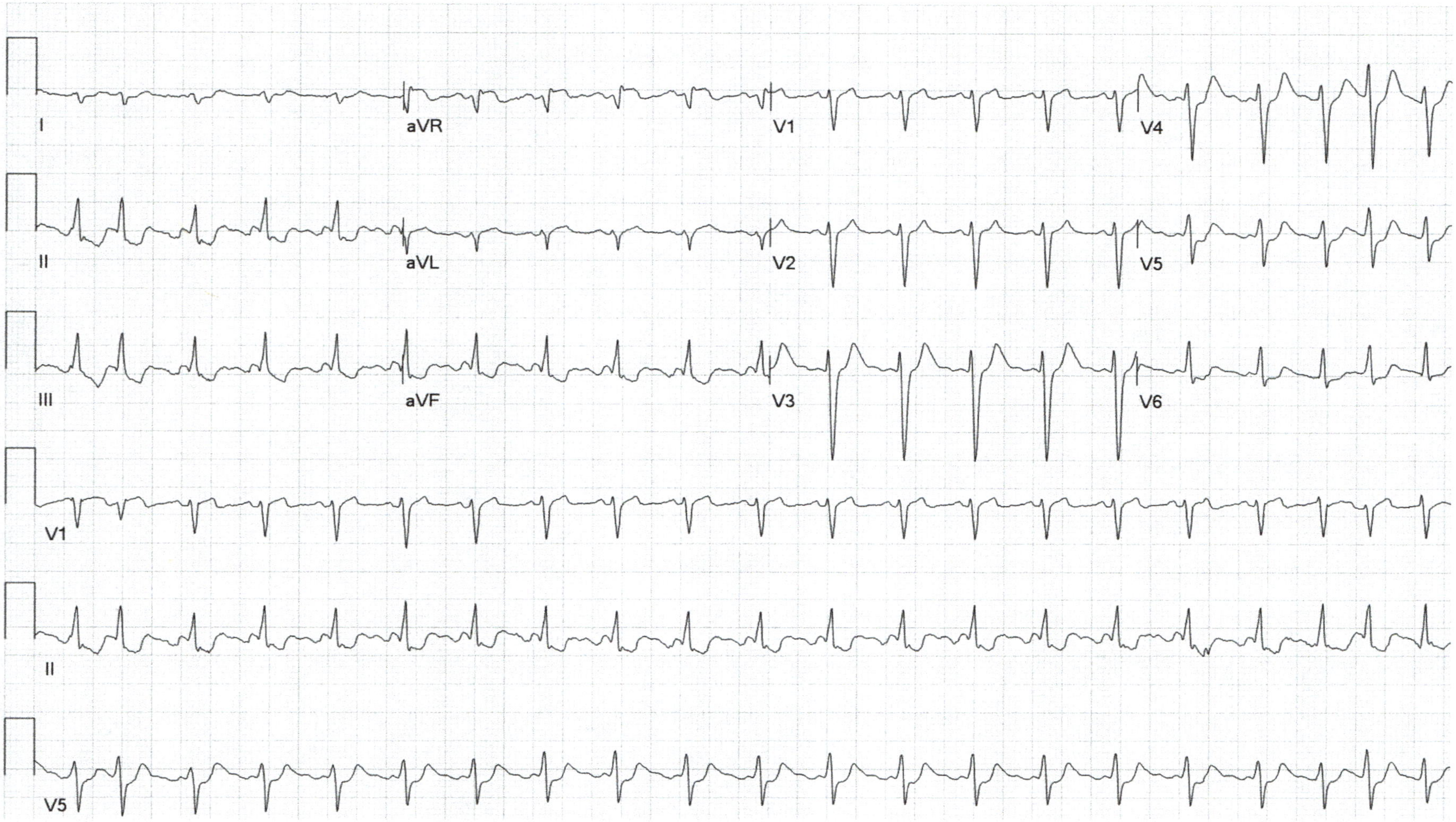

Question 3-16

## Question 3-16

The tachycardia mechanism in **Figure 3-16A** is probably:

1. AT
2. AFL
3. AVNRT
4. AVRT

## Answer

At first glance, this appears to be AT with a short PR interval. In fact, the PR is quite short, in the range of 100 ms (the PR during sinus rhythm in this patient was 190 ms at a heart rate of 60). The morphology of the P wave is not quite clear but appears to be "low to high" with negative initial forces in the inferior leads. A PR interval significantly shorter than that during sinus rhythm at much slower heart rates has a limited list of possibilities since, all things being equal, one would expect a *longer* PR during SVT.

The finding of a substantively shorter PR during tachycardia than sinus rhythm can occur if:

1. An atrial focus is closer to the AV node or the fast input into the AV node.
2. Flutter waves during typical atrial flutter enter the AV node by the AV node input near the coronary sinus (CS) os and will exhibit a relatively shorter PR because of this more direct input. Thus, in AFL with 2:1 AV conduction, the PR of conducted beats may actually be shorter than in sinus rhythm.
3. The P wave preceding the QRS may not be the one that conducts to it. For example, in AT with 2:1 AV block, the P wave actually conducting to the QRS may be the *prior* P wave to the one immediately preceding the QRS. Similarly, in AVNRT, the P wave in typical AVNRT may appear slightly in front of the QRS since the P wave in AVNRT does not conduct directly to the AV node.

In our example, this short PR with a low-to-high atrial sequence alerts us to the possibility of AFL and a careful search for a second P wave is warranted (as it should be, anyway). Magnifying the area of interest (**Figure 3-16B**), the **solid red lines** line up with visible P waves and the **dashed red lines** are at their halfway point, where P waves should be if it were AFL. A slight deformity of the T wave suggests that a second P wave may be concealed here, but it is difficult to be sure without seeing the T wave during normal rhythm for comparison. We now note a slight irregularity in the rhythm at the onset of the tracing. The first QRS has a different ST-T wave than the second and subsequent beats.

*The first QRS thus provides us with a "baseline" ST segment, which is smooth for over 200 ms, making it most probable that the earlier distortion of the ST segment in the subsequent beats is really a P wave "hiding" in the ST segment.*

The correct answer here is Option 2, AFL (with a cleverly concealed P wave distorting the ST-T wave).

Figure 3-16B

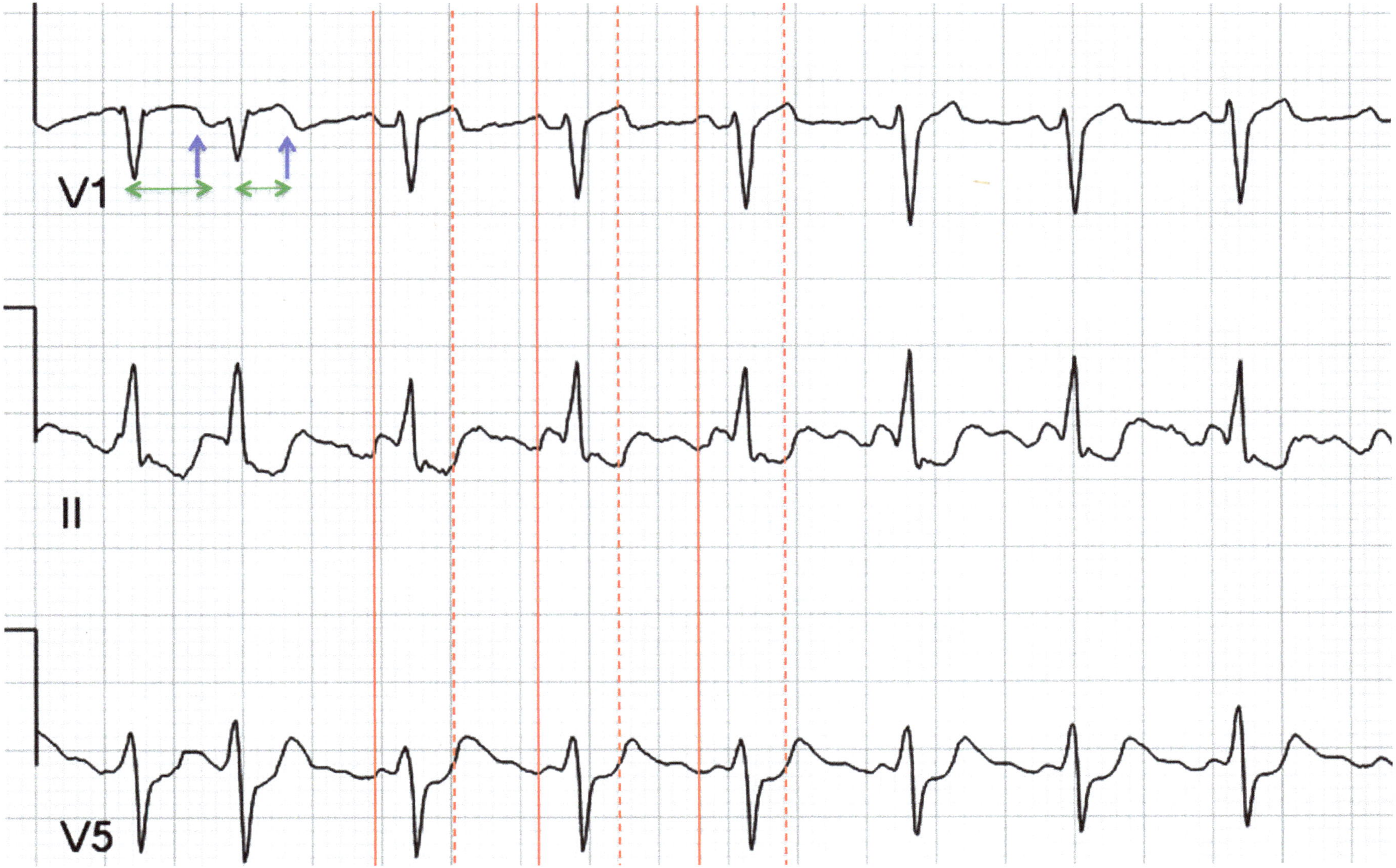

# Chapter 4

## The Wide QRS Tachycardia

Figure 4-1A

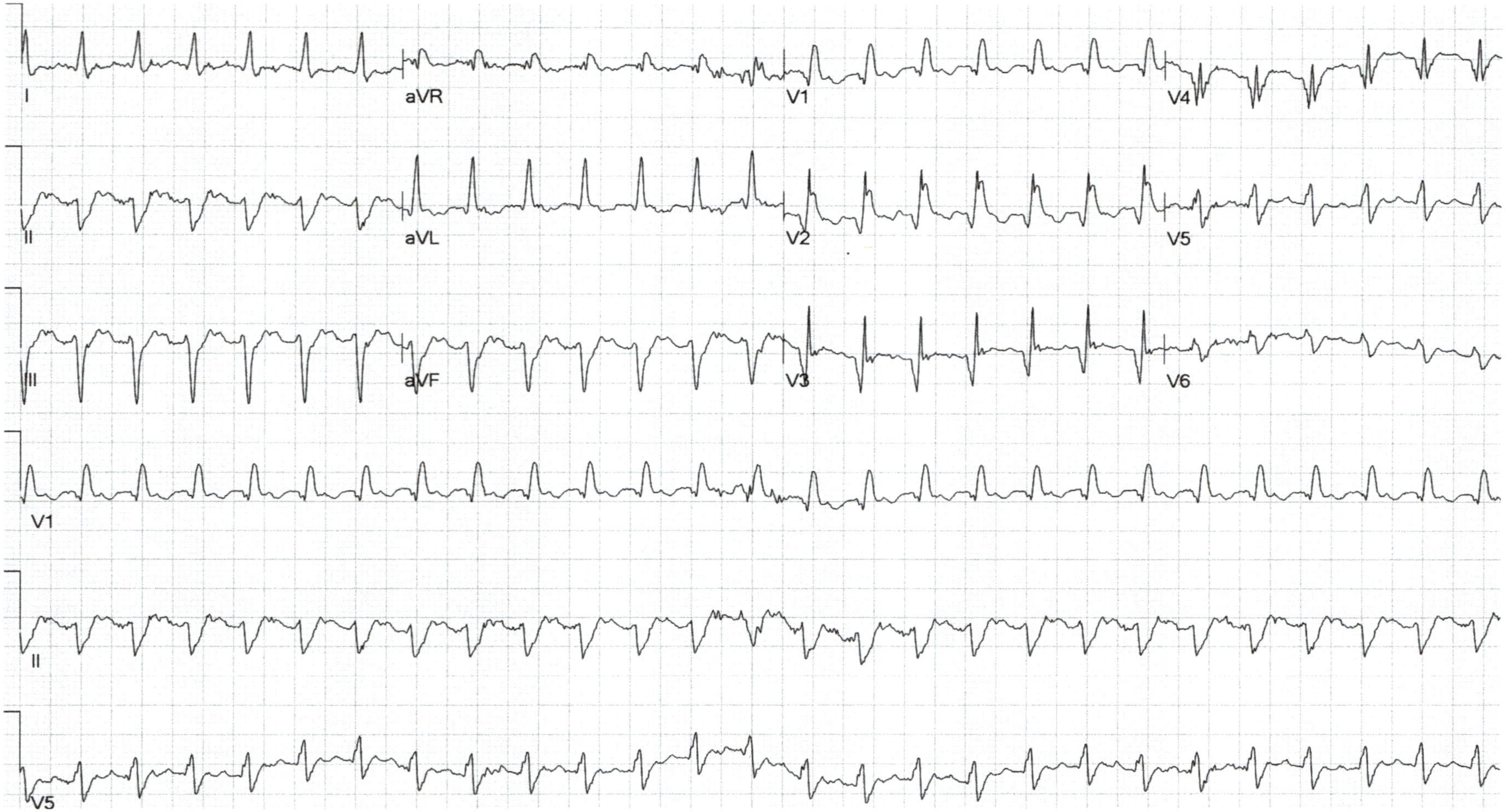

## Question 4-1

The ECG shown in **Figure 4-1A** is recorded from a 75-year-old man admitted for dyspnea in the context of a history of myocardial infarction.

The tracing is best interpreted as:

1. Ventricular tachycardia (VT)
2. Sinus tachycardia
3. Atrioventricular (AV) reentry
4. Need more data

## Answer

This wide complex tachycardia (WCT) has right bundle branch block (RBBB) morphology with left-axis deviation. In the experience of the author, bifascicular block is a rare aberrancy pattern and favors VT unless the patient had previous left anterior hemiblock or bifascicular block. A candidate P wave is seen in early repolarization (for example, in lead 2) and the tracing would thus be labeled as WCT with a 1:1 VA relationship and a "short-RP"(or "mid-RP," depending on where the P is judged to begin) tachycardia. This latter nomenclature, although widely used, is not terribly helpful, since we still need to determine whether the A is leading the V or vice versa.

The P-wave morphology would be helpful but the onset and offset of the P wave is not entirely clear. Cycle length (CL) irregularity would be helpful (i.e., is a CL change in the QRS followed by a similar change in the P wave, ruling out atrial tachycardia (AT), or vice versa ruling out VT?) but this tachycardia is quite regular. A truthful answer would really be Option 4, since most of us would want to see a little more data before committing firmly.

However, additional information is forthcoming in **Figure 4-1B**, which shows an ECG from a previous admission. It clearly shows sinus tachycardia with bifascicular block and a QRS similar to the one in Figure 4-1A (allowing for some variability in electrode positioning). In particular, the P wave can now be "seen" more clearly in our original tracing (compare leads 2 and 3 in each) with a high-to-low activation sequence and a long PR interval. The diagnosis is now more evident: sinus tachycardia.

Figure 4-1B

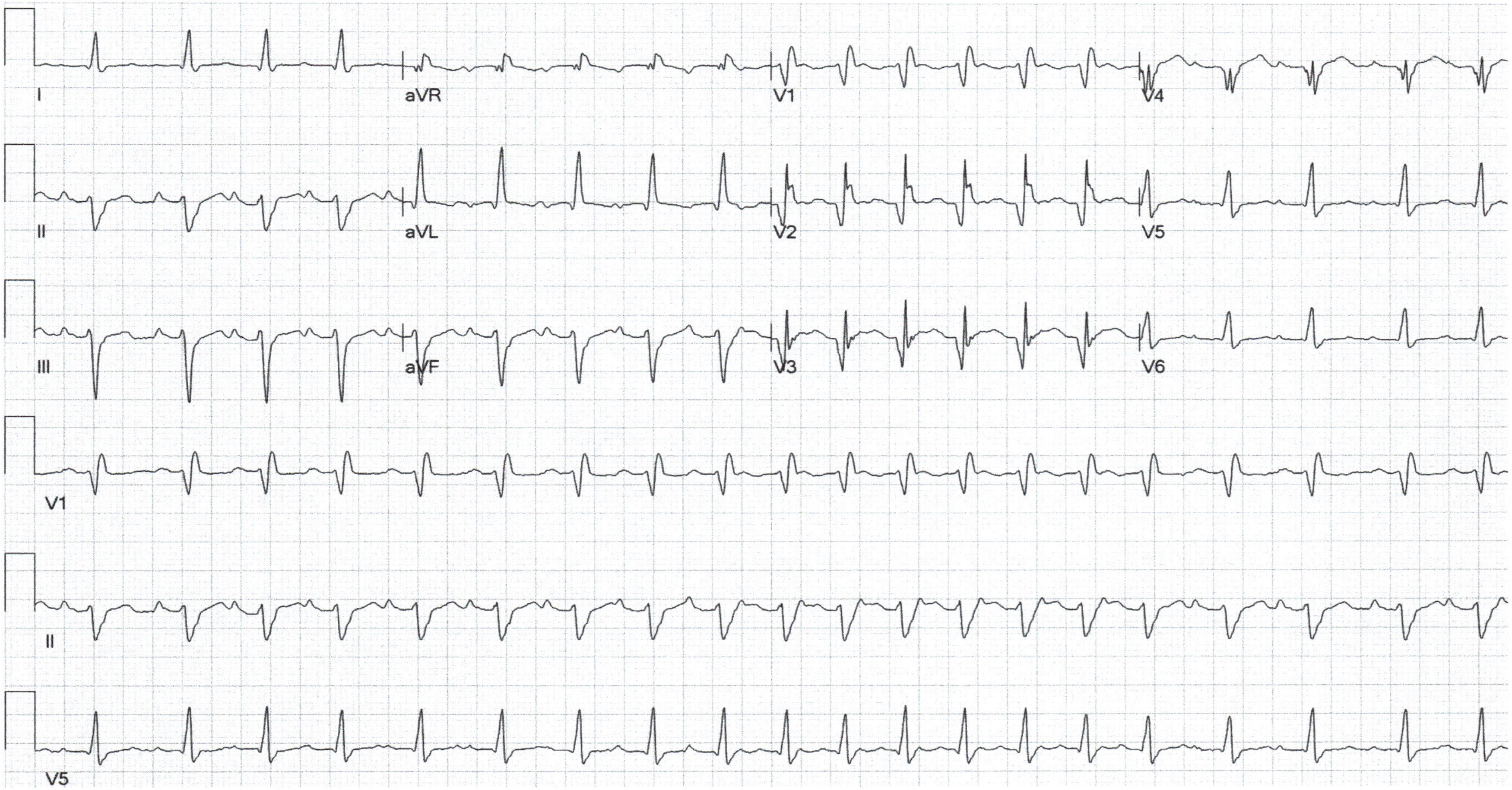

Question 4-2

Figure 4-2A

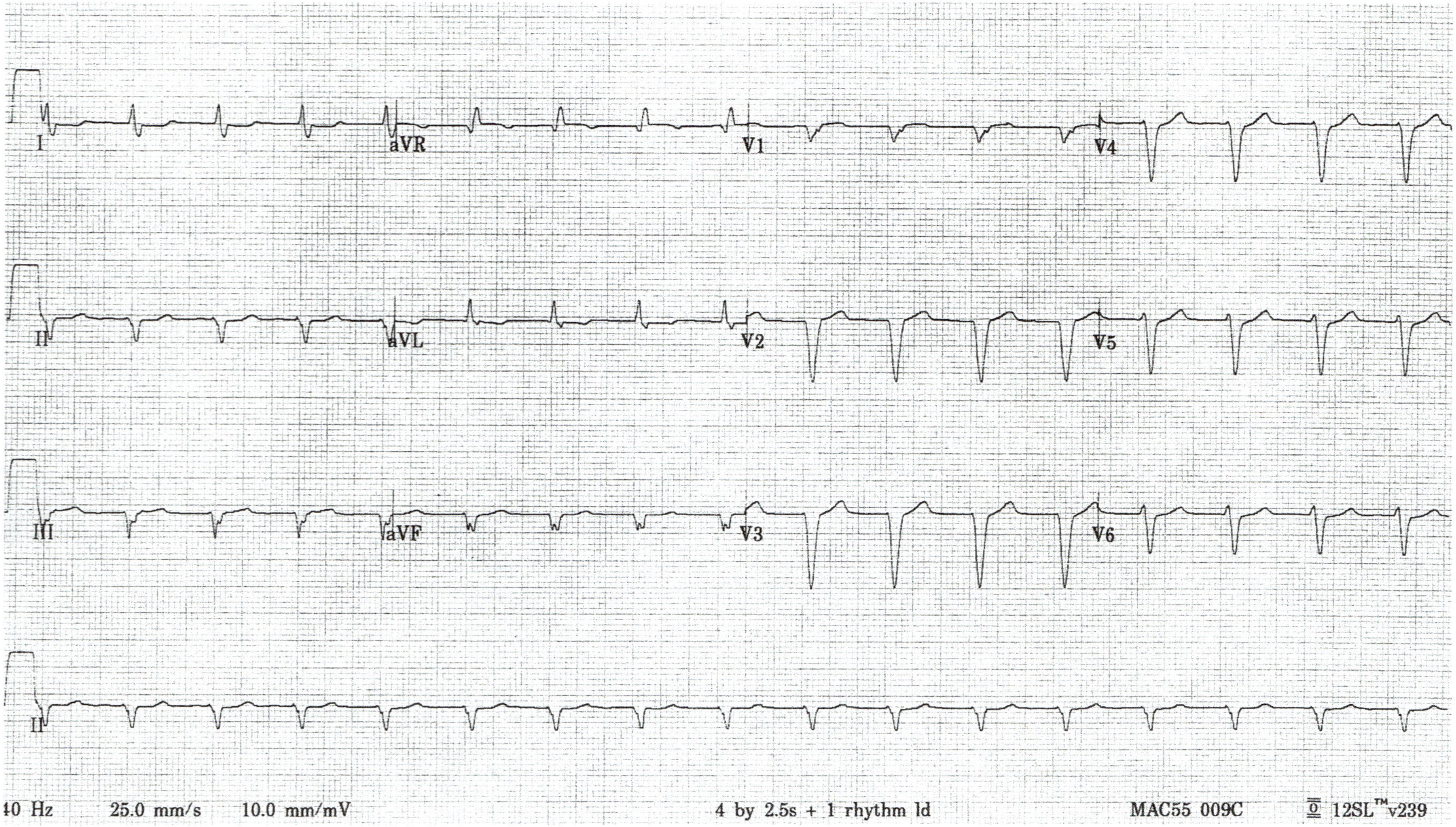

## Question 4-2

The rhythm shown in **Figure 4-2A**, at a rate of approximately 105 beats per minute (bpm), is most probably:

1. AV node reentry
2. Atrial flutter (AFL) with 2:1 AV block
3. VT
4. Need more data

## Answer

The rhythm in Figure 4-2A is technically a "tachycardia" by definition, but the QRS is neither narrow nor very wide (QRS duration approximately 110 ms). P waves are not evident. It is reasonably supraventricular tachycardia (SVT) with inferior and anterior infarction patterns and might well be AV node reentry. One might expect to see some atrial activity in the diastolic interval if it were AFL with 2:1 conduction, yet this is not seen. It is a little "narrow," but this certainly should never suffice to rule out VT. The correct answer must then be Option 4, as the diagnosis can't be reasonably made from the ECG without more information.

Useful additional information is found in the ECG taken just before the recording of the tachycardia, as seen in **Figure 4-2B**. *It is always worth the effort to hunt down previous ECGs as is evident in this example.* The Figure 4-2B ECG is strikingly normal, with no infarction or conduction defect. If such is the case, one would reasonably expect a relatively normal or conventional aberration pattern during tachycardia, i.e., generally resembling typical RBBB or left bundle branch block (LBBB). The pattern observed has a vertical, upward axis (extreme right or left) in the frontal plane. It has QS complexes over virtually all the precordial leads, which would also be most unusual for a bundle branch block pattern in a relatively normal heart. One might also call this precordial "concordance," which is an often-quoted "VT criterion" precisely because concordance would not be seen with usual bundle branch block patterns.

The ECG in Figure 4-2A can now reasonably be diagnosed as a ventricular rhythm, or more accurately, as "accelerated idioventricular rhythm," since it is not quite fast enough to be VT by definition.

Figure 4-2B

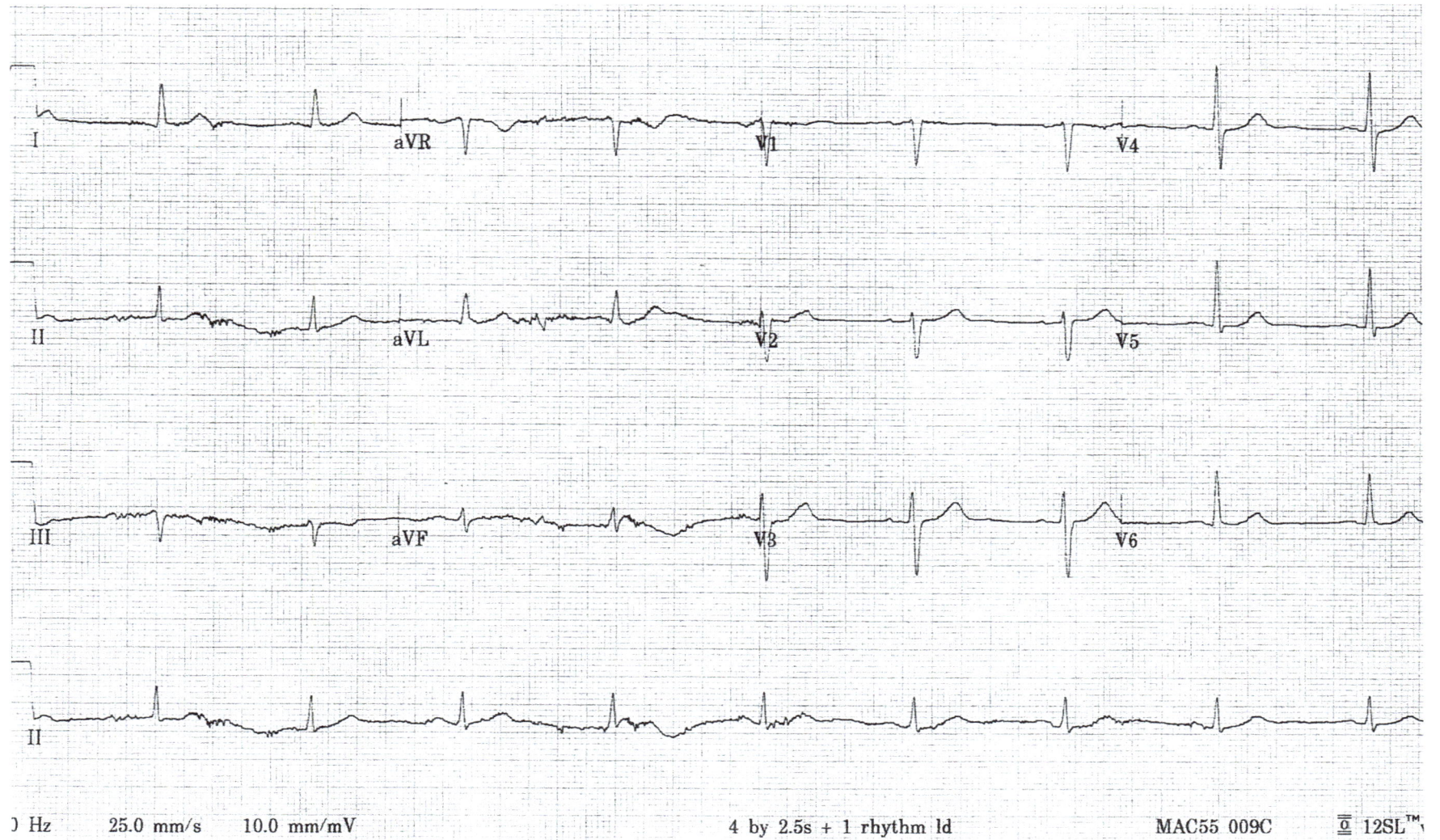

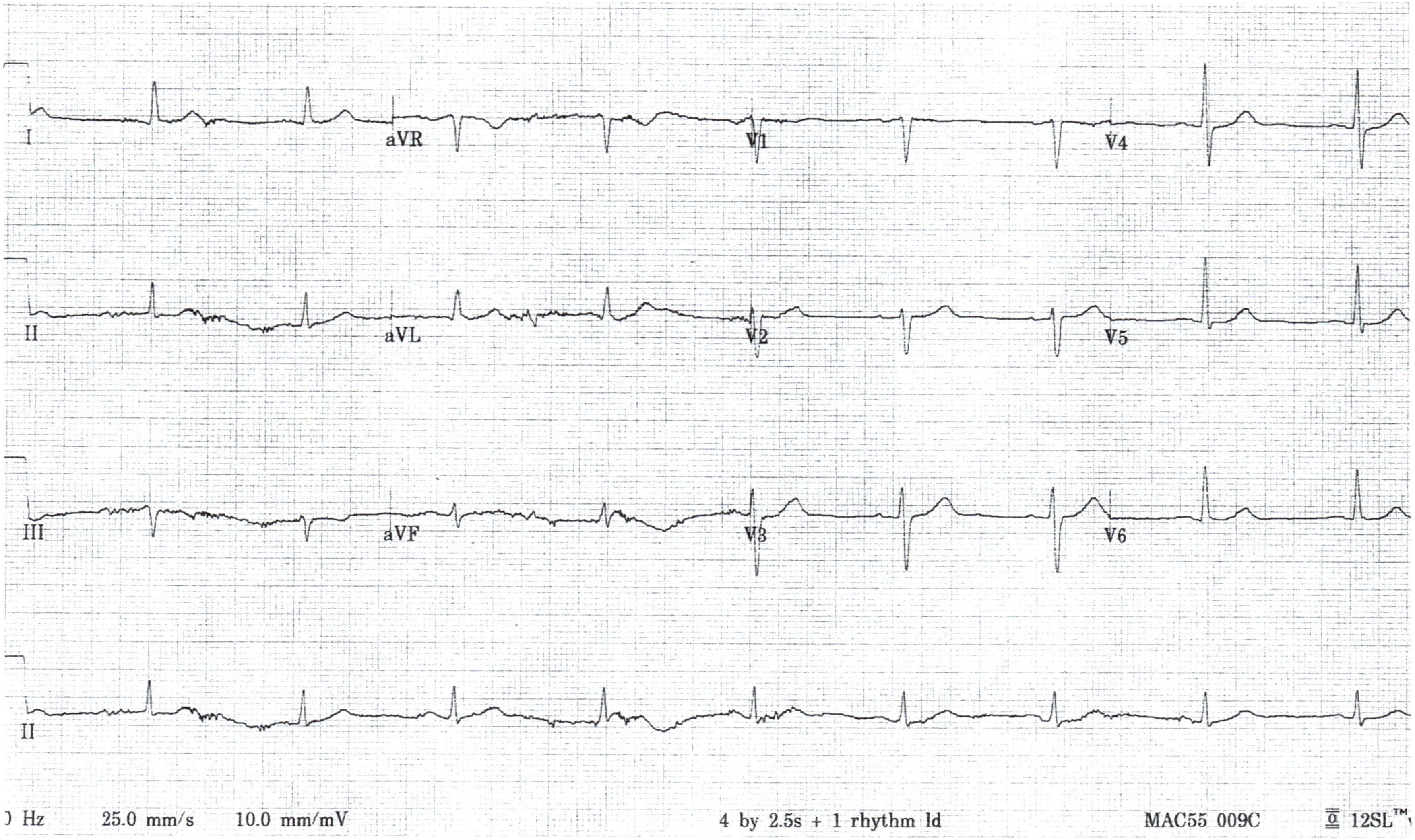
I
aVR
V1
V4
II
aVL
V2
V5
III
aVF
V3
V6
II
Hz
25.0 mm/s
10.0 mm/mV
4 by 2.5s + 1 rhythm ld
MAC55 009C
12SL™

Figure 4-3A

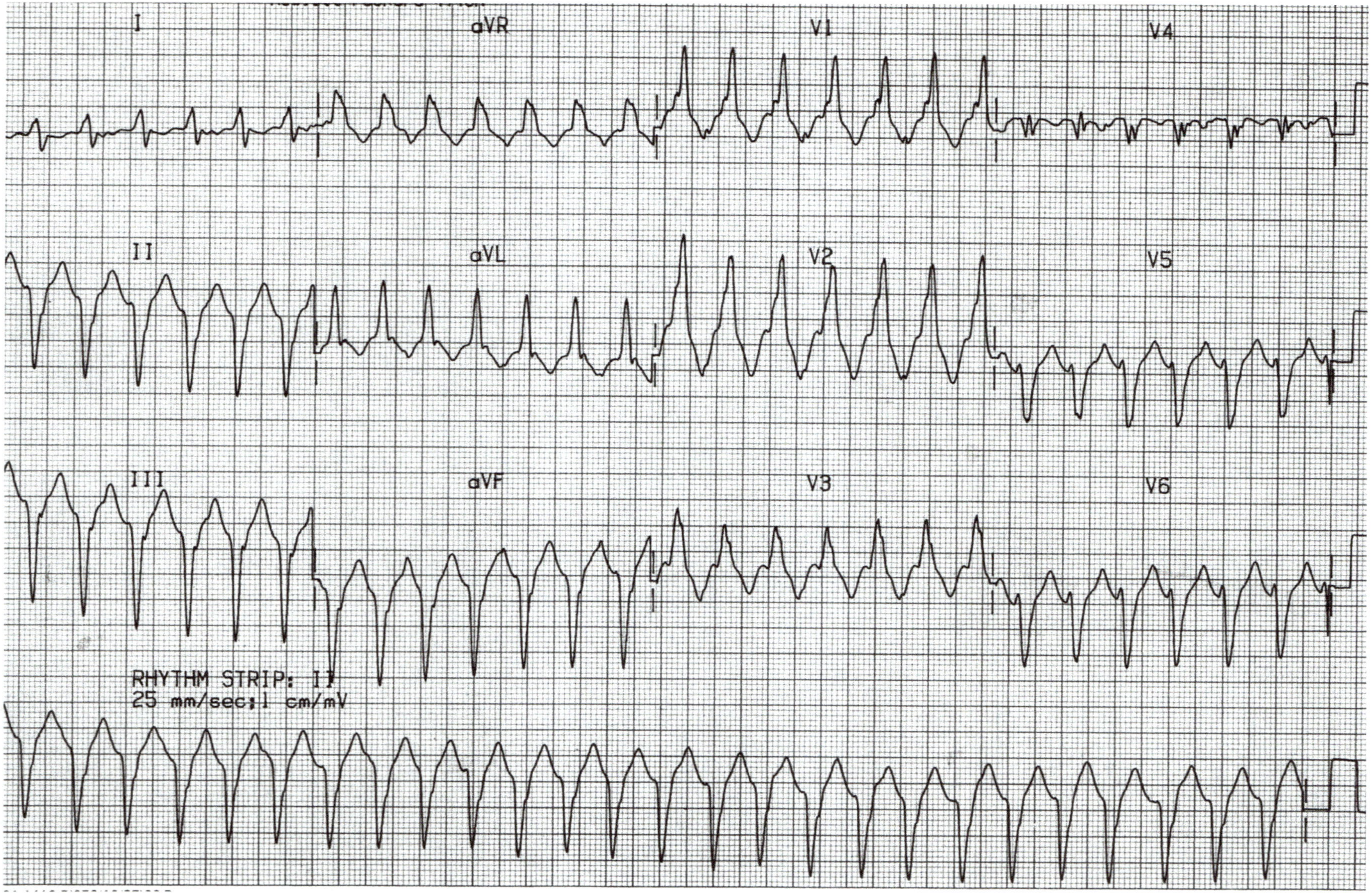
I
aVR
V1
V4
II
aVL
V2
V5
III
aVF
V3
V6
RHYTHM STRIP: II
25 mm/sec;1 cm/mV

## Question 4-3

The rhythm shown in **Figure 4-3A** is:

1. VT
2. Preexcited tachycardia
3. SVT with aberrancy
4. Need more information

## Answer

This rhythm has a RBBB-like pattern but is very atypical for RBBB. $V_1$ is monomorphic ("single-peaked") with slight slurring at the beginning of the upstroke. There is no terminal slurring in leads 1 or aVL, and R waves are greatly diminished in $V_4$–$V_6$. The axis is "northwest," which would be very unusual in a bundle branch block pattern. Thus, we are quite confident that it is not SVT with aberrancy.

We might then make a careful search for P waves. In general, *all* the leads available should be carefully examined but especially those leads where the QRS is relatively smaller and do not obscure the smaller P waves (**Figure 4-3B**). If we examine lead $V_4$, the P waves become more obvious, occurring after every second QRS (**red dots**), and are also seen in $V_1$, although a little more subtle. This, of course, essentially clinches the diagnosis as VT.

*Note that the atrial activity could not be confidently identified in all the other leads.*

Figure 4-3B

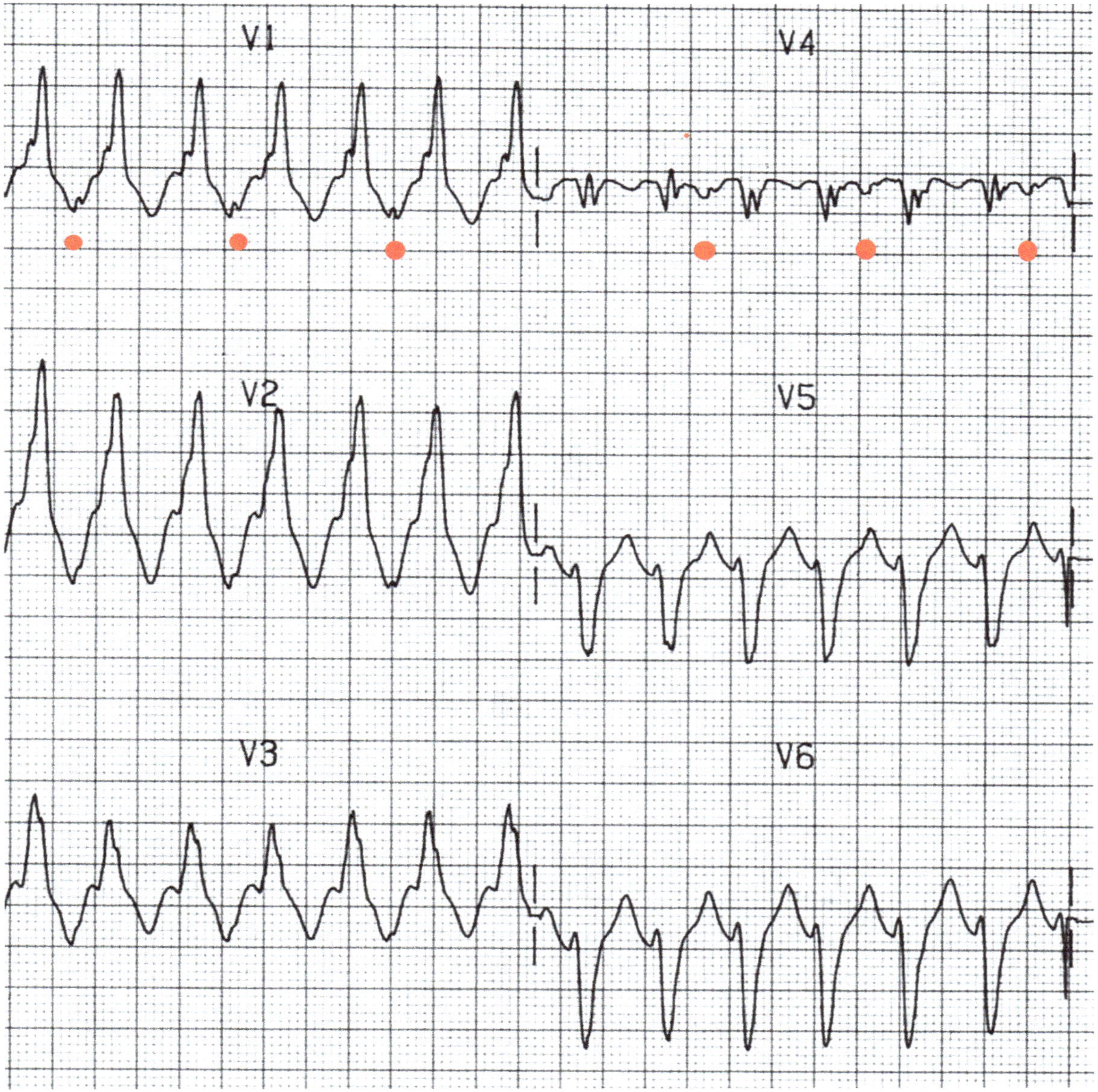

Figure 4-4A

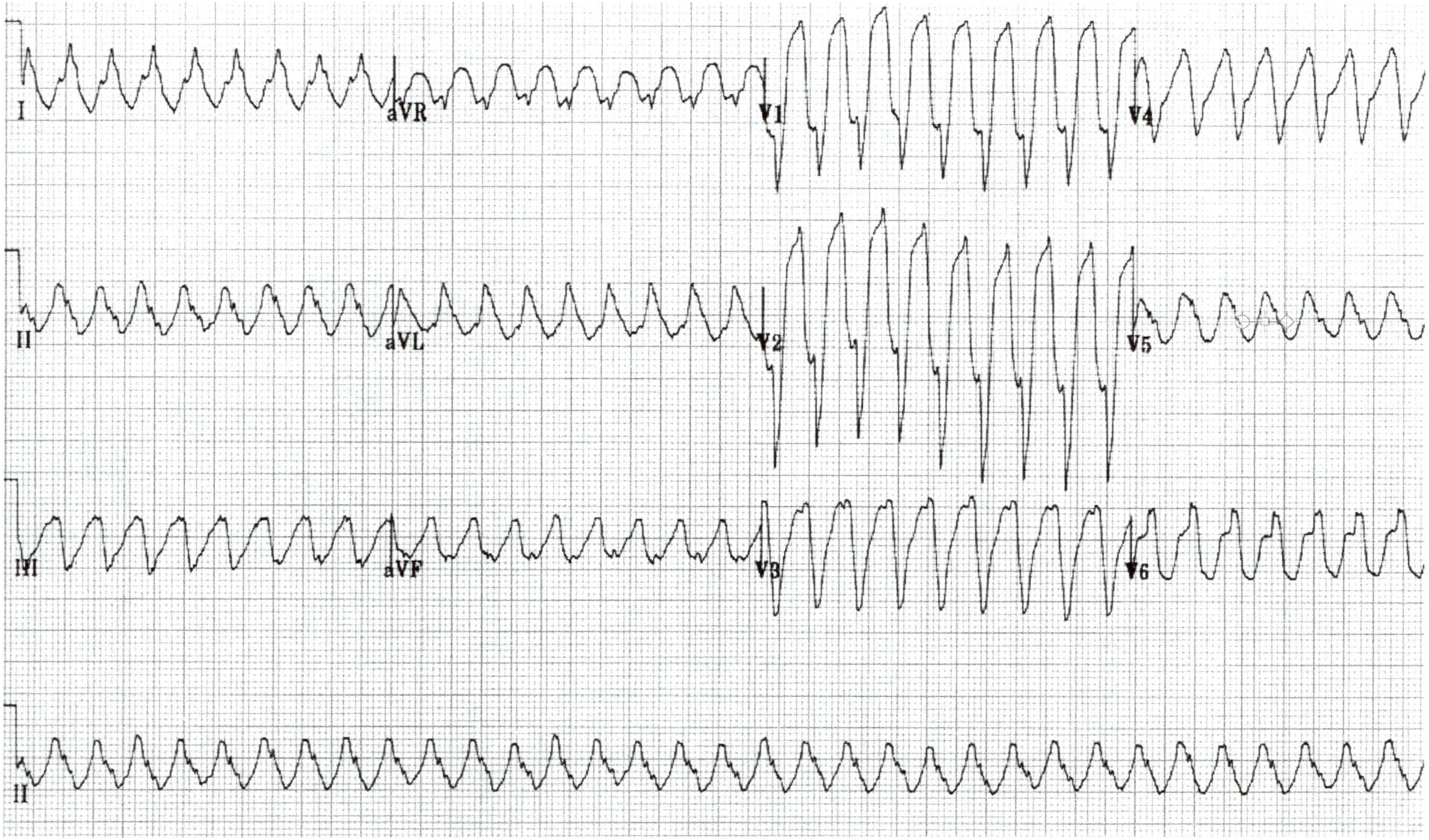

Question 4-4

## Question 4-4

The patient whose ECG is shown in **Figure 4-4A** presented to the emergency department with palpitations of 3 hours duration.
The tachycardia mechanism is:

1. VT
2. SVT with aberrant conduction
3. Preexcited tachycardia
4. Need more data

## Answer

The tachycardia was well tolerated, but this, of course, does not assist in our assessment of mechanism. It is rapid with LBBB morphology with marked repolarization abnormality, making it seem almost "sine wave"-like. Although there are multiple smaller rapid deflections (for example, lead 2), these are not clearly in the diastolic interval. Identification of P waves within the "borders" of the QRS complex—i.e., timing with the QRS—would be very problematic, since many notches in the QRS may be interpreted as P waves. The morphology of the QRS would be reasonably considered as a LBBB pattern so that VT could not be ruled in or out on this basis. In truth, the correct diagnosis would be Option 4, that is, more data required.

The next figure (**Figure 4-4B**) is recorded shortly after cardioversion. It shows sinus rhythm with a relatively typical RBBB morphology. In general, it would be very unusual (although not theoretically impossible) to have SVT with a LBBB pattern in this context with RBBB during sinus rhythm, and this observation makes it highly likely that the tachycardia in Figure 4-4A is VT.

In fact, *any* different QRS morphology during tachycardia (narrower, wider, or other) in the context of a resting bundle branch block makes VT highly probable. This is a very useful diagnostic aid, in our experience. This young man had repair of tetralogy of Fallot many years previously, and this tachycardia was indeed VT.

Figure 4-4B

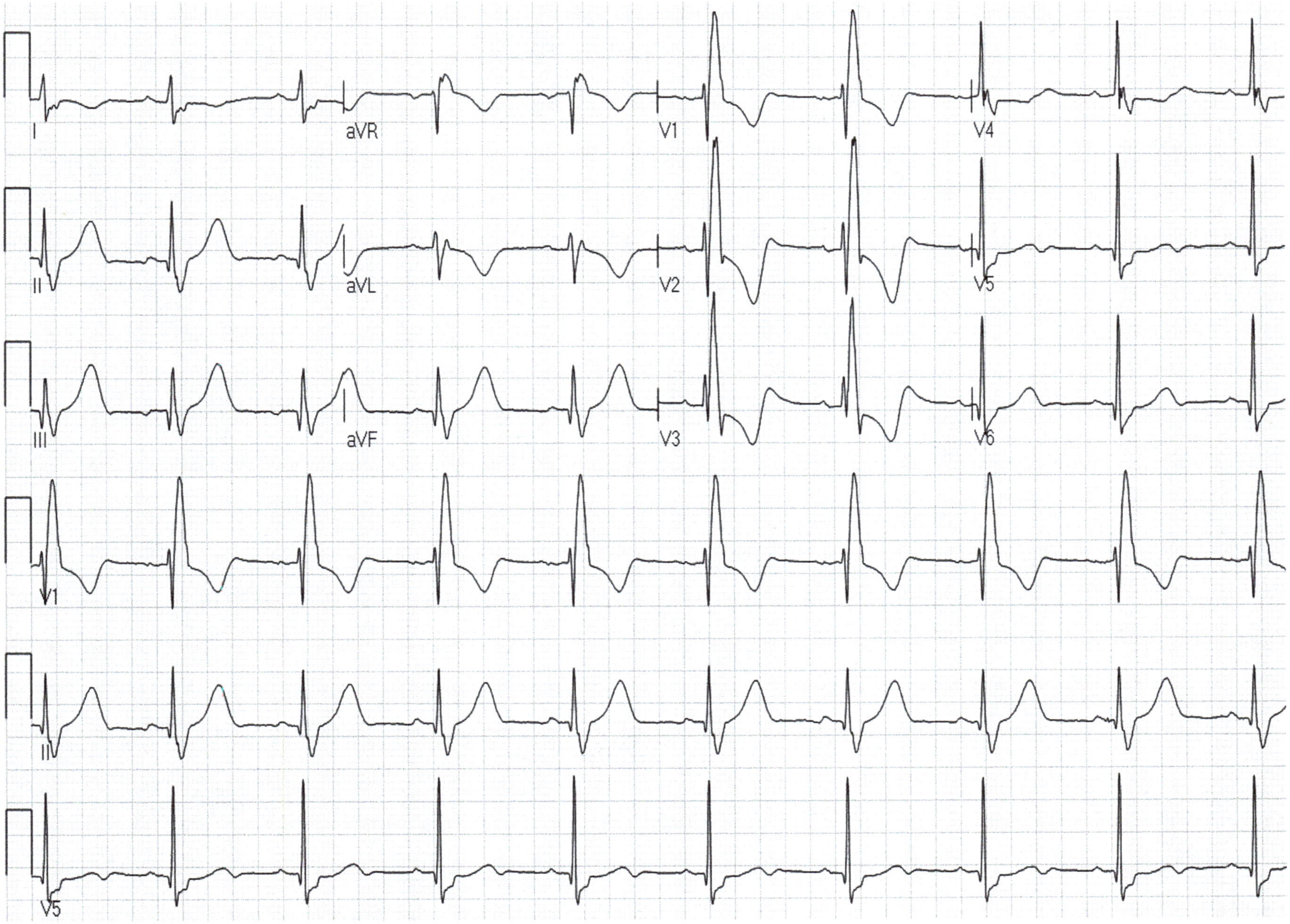

Question 4-5

Figure 4-5A

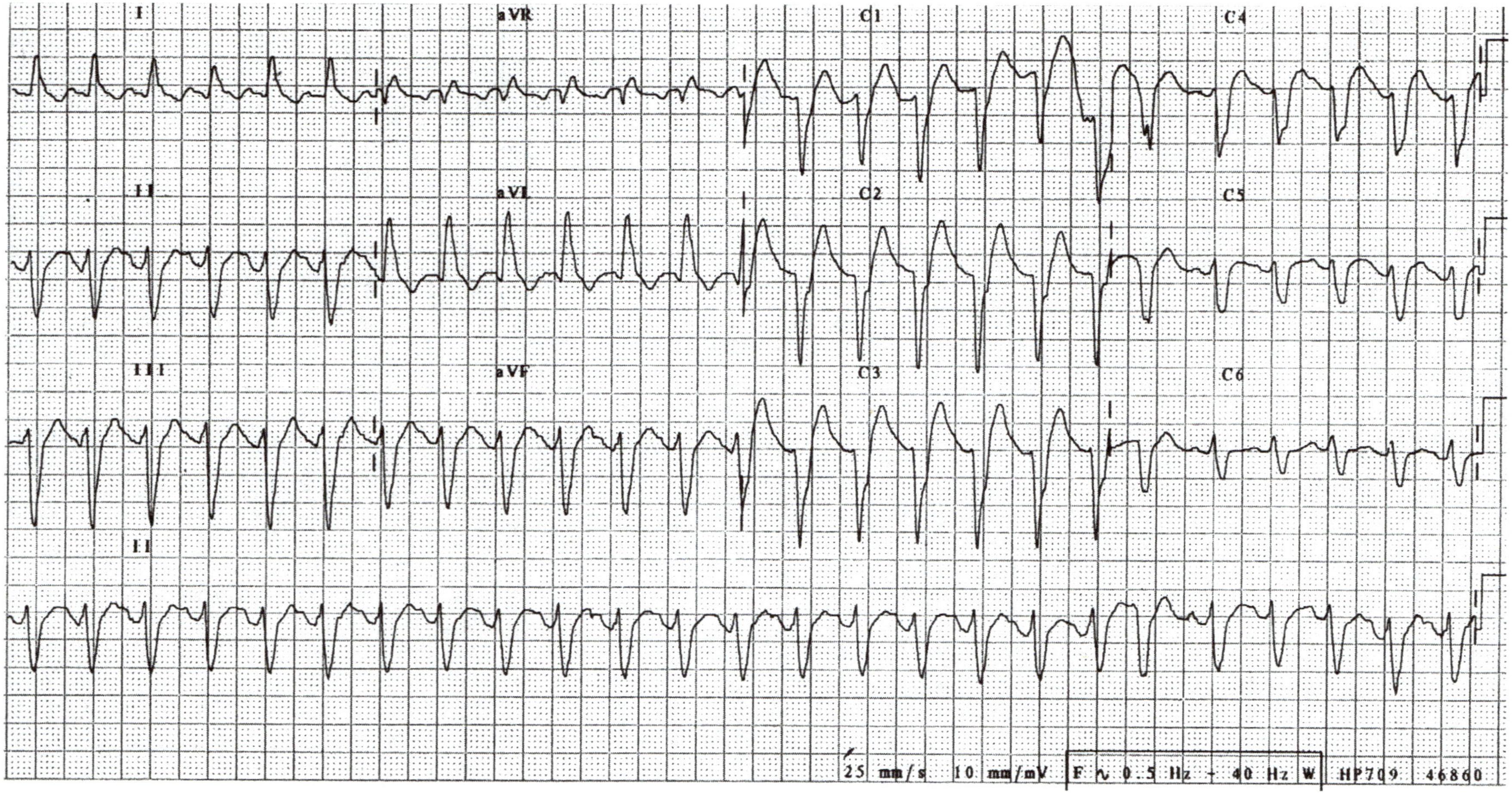

## Question 4-5

The mechanism of the tachycardia shown in **Figure 4-5A** is:

1. VT
2. SV rhythm with aberration
3. Preexcited AVRT
4. Need more data

## Answer

This WCT is relatively regular, with LBBB-type QRS morphology. The LBBB is reasonably "typical," with rS in $V_1$ and a very rapid downstroke in the S wave. This makes VT less likely, suggesting SV rhythm with LBBB aberration. We note that preexcited SVT over an atriofascicular accessory pathway (AP) may have a relatively "typical" LBBB-type QRS, but this would be a much more infrequent diagnosis than SVT with LBBB aberrancy if one is reduced purely to "playing the odds."

Atrial activity is not immediately apparent but is certainly suggested. **Figure 4-5B** enlarges the precordial leads and rhythm strip. The T wave appears to have a slightly variable "notching" diffusely, exemplified by the beats with vertical lines. This is suggestive of slightly variable fusion (electrical, not physiological) between the T and a subsequent P wave as might be seen as a result of slight irregularity in an atrial rhythm.

This impression is verified by the irregularity in the rhythm created by a premature ventricular contraction (PVC; **red dot**). The PVC advances the T wave and exposes the P wave, now clearly seen as a P wave consistent with sinus tachycardia. The PVC in essence opens the "window" slightly to allow visualization of the P wave. As evident in several other examples, a careful look for irregularity in the rhythm and ectopic activity in particular is well worth the effort.

Figure 4-5B

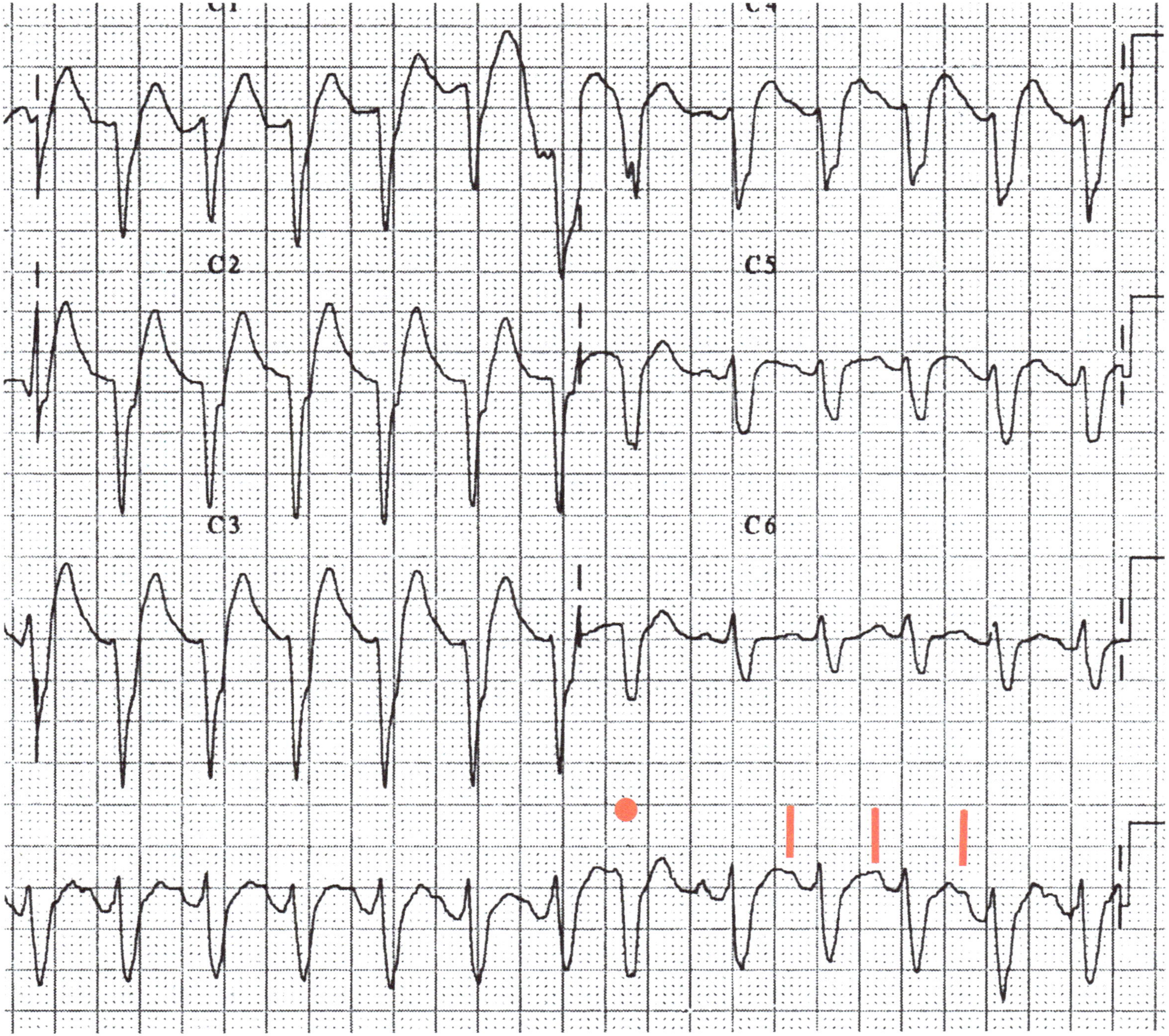

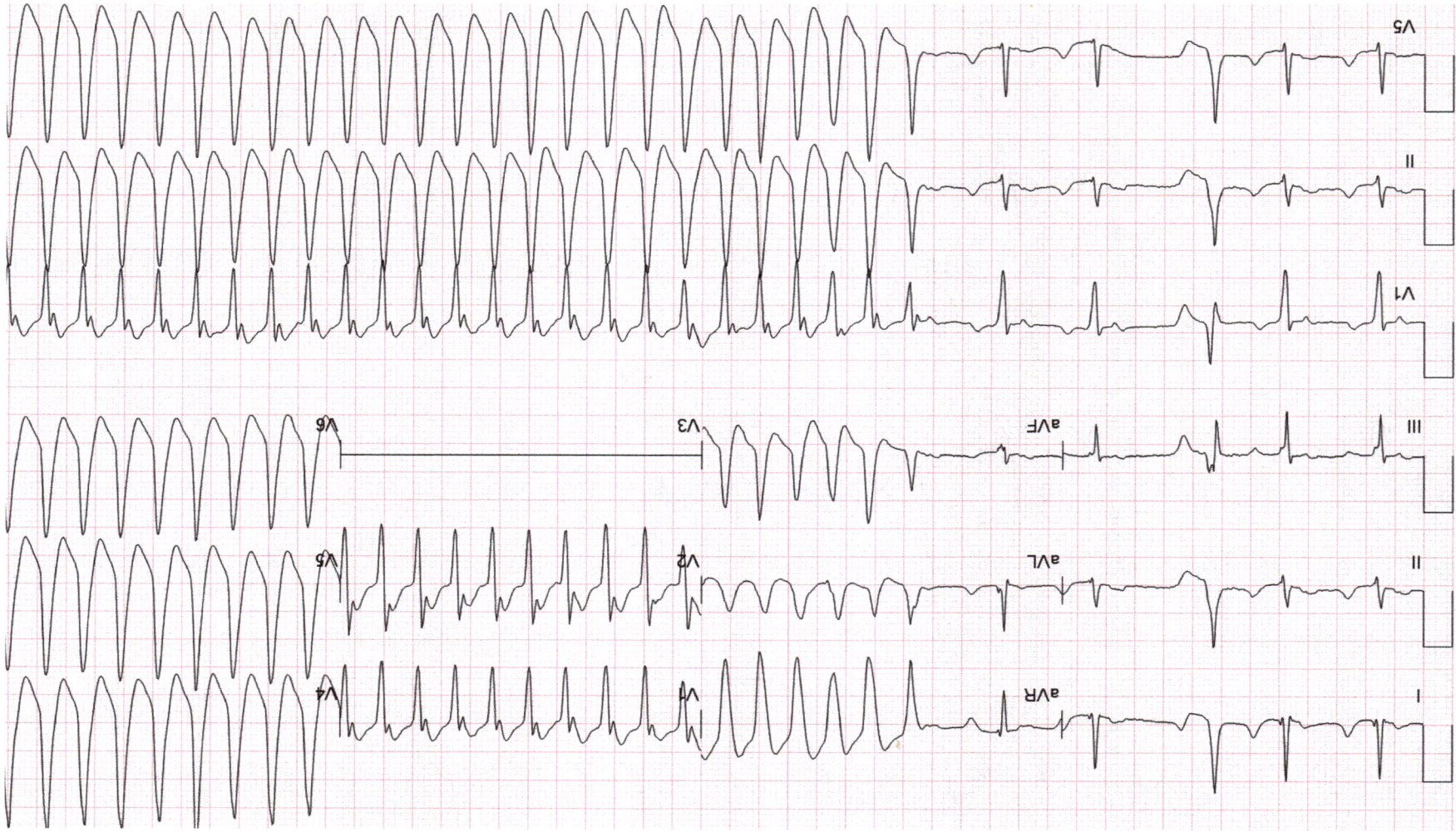

Figure 4-6A

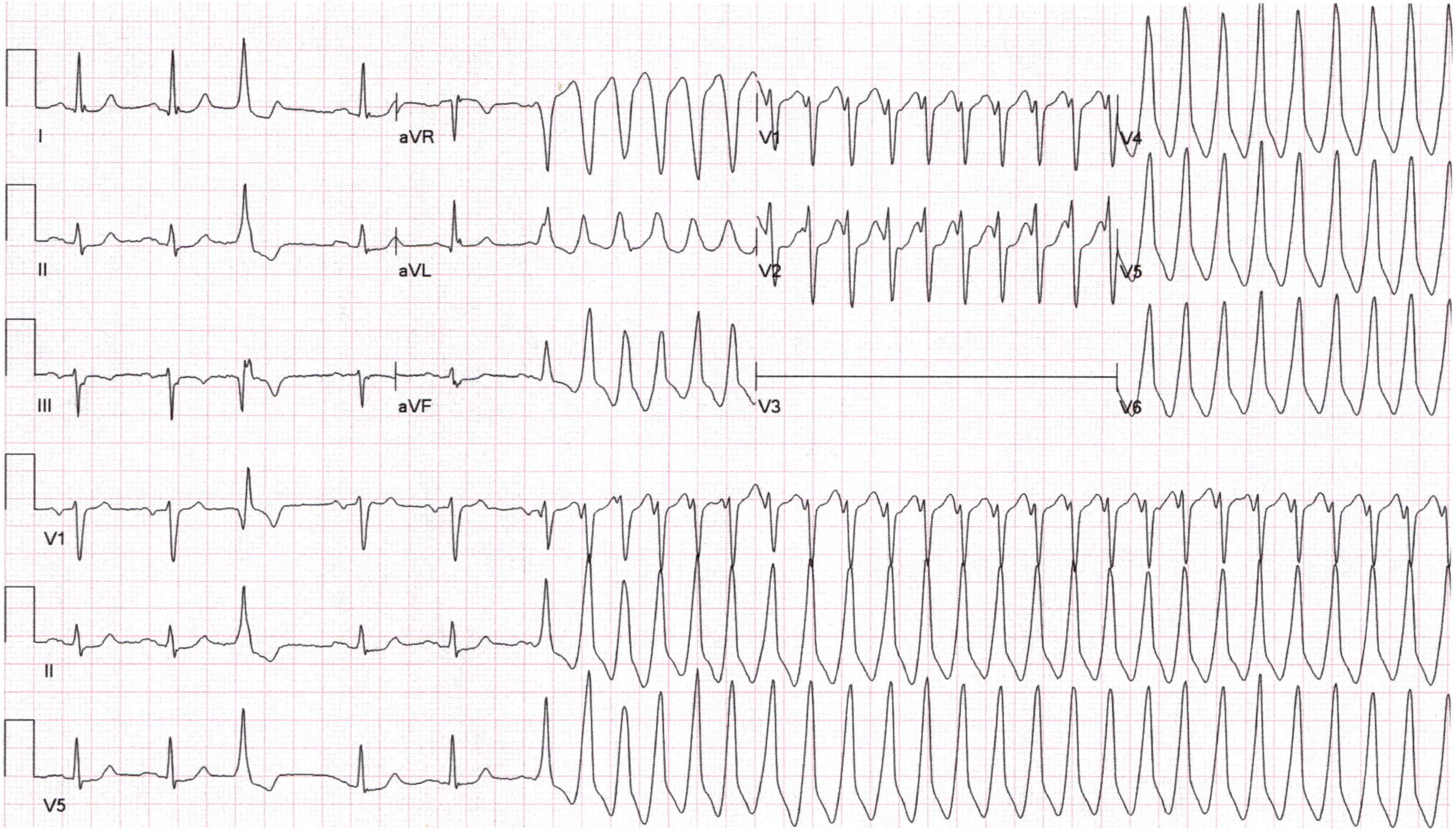

Question 4-6

## Question 4-6

The mechanism of tachycardia shown in **Figure 4-6A** is:

1. VT
2. Supraventricular rhythm with aberration
3. Preexcited AVRT
4. Need more data

## Answer

This WCT is regular, with CL approximately 300 ms. Atrial activity is not clearly evident. Tachycardia has LBBB morphology that is relatively typical. Any of our options are viable at this point.

There is an ectopic that is unequivocally a PVC (**Figure 4-6B, blue dot**), but the QRS morphology is different from our WCT, making this observation unhelpful. Clear identification of a PVC identical to the WCT would, of course, strongly favor VT as the mechanism of the WCT.

The answer comes from the onset of the WCT. The atrial rhythm is perfectly regular, but the PR interval (**horizontal line**) is interrupted by the QRS with a sudden apparent shortening of the PR interval. The first WCT cycle is also a little different (**narrower**) than the subsequent tachycardia, most compatible with a fusion beat. This can realistically only be VT.

Figure 4-6B

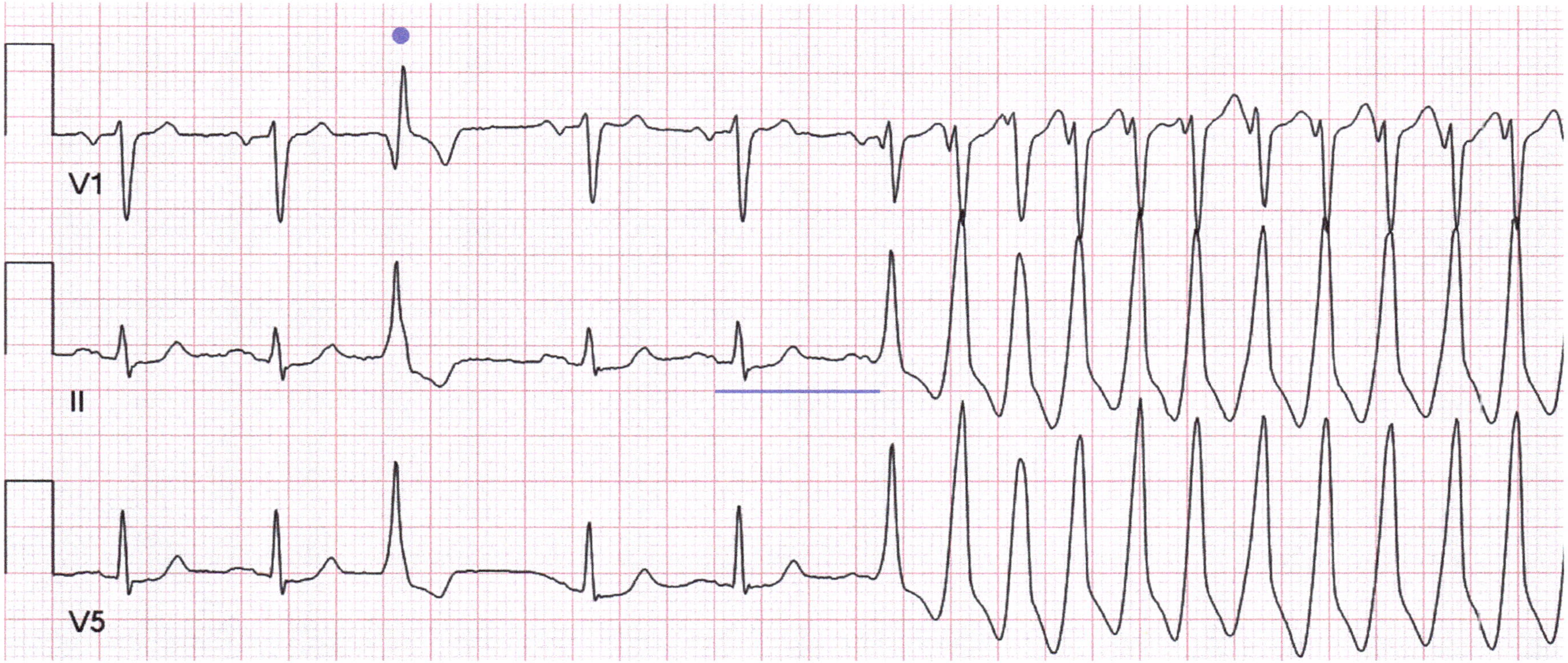

Figure 4-7A

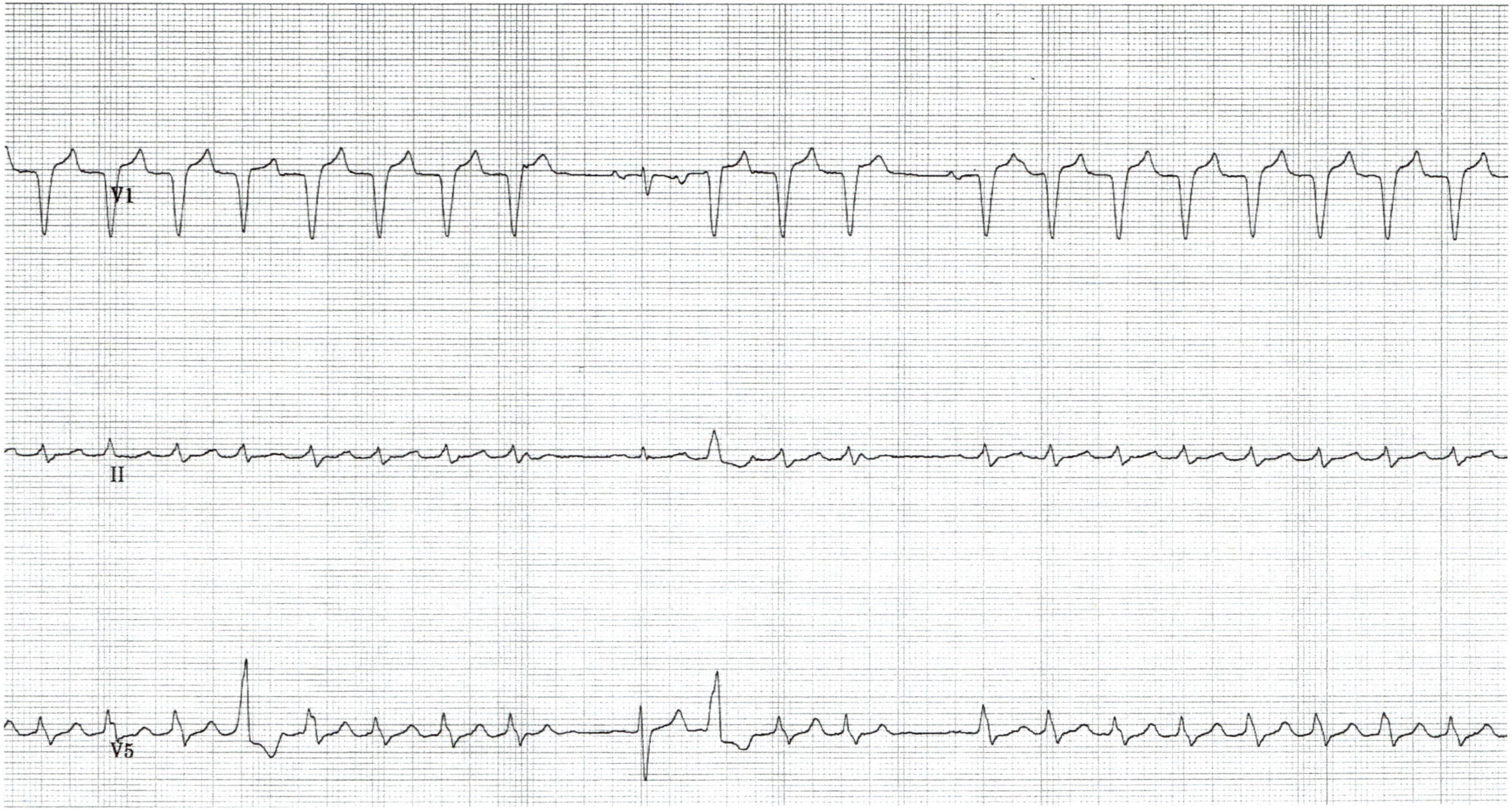


Question 4-7

## Question 4-7

The tachycardia mechanism shown in **Figure 4-7A** is:

1. VT
2. AV reentrant tachycardia (AVRT)
3. AV nodal reentrant tachycardia (AVNRT)
4. Sinus tachycardia

## Answer

Our tracing is very "clean" of artifact, and short runs of tachycardia are observed. We begin with the only clearly sinus beat (asterisk) and work from there. $V_1$ is very useful here, as a "sharp" deflection is seen in repolarization after the QRS, which has to be a second P wave. If one moves forward from this interval with calipers, one sees subtle "spikes" or peaks in the next 2 T waves in time with our initial interval (**dots**). The 3rd QRS has a little terminal notch (**downward arrow**) better seen in the lower lead 2 channel, most probably either an AV nodal echo or a premature atrial contraction (PAC). The pattern resumes after a slight pause. The horizontal arrow indicates that the next sinus beat after termination comes on time and the pause is fully compensatory (horizontal arrow), although that doesn't help us mechanistically here.

To summarize, we have sinus tachycardia (AT can't be ruled out from this tracing, but that was not provided as an option) with a long PR interval. LBBB, probably CL-dependent, is present. AV nodal echoes seem likely from the observations but not proven.

The main message of this tracing is to emphasize the importance of a careful search for P waves potentially lurking near the QRS or T wave. P waves totally simultaneous with the QRS would essentially be impossible to see, while those in the flatter part of diastole would generally be more obvious.

Figure 4-7B

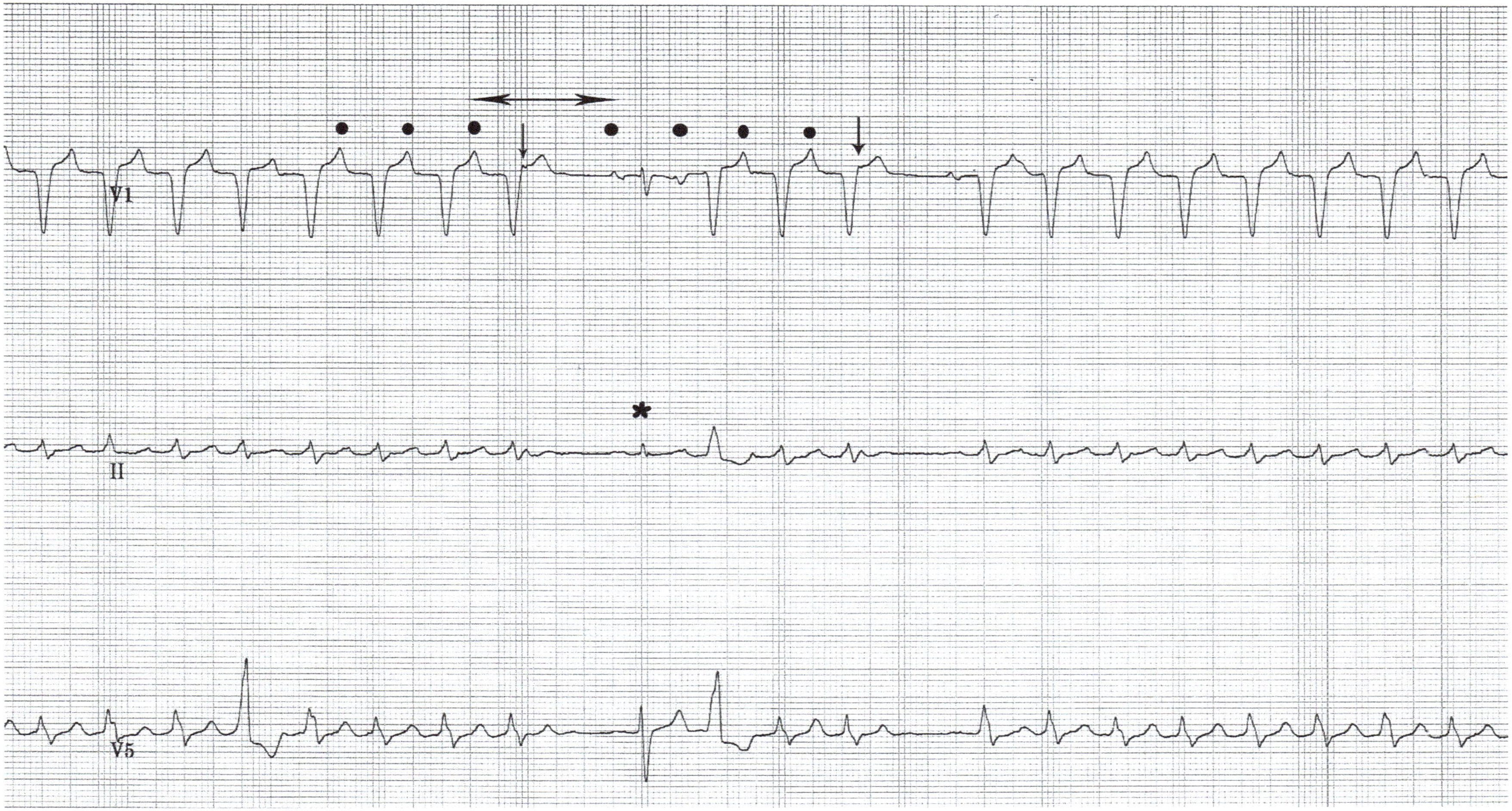

Figure 4-8A

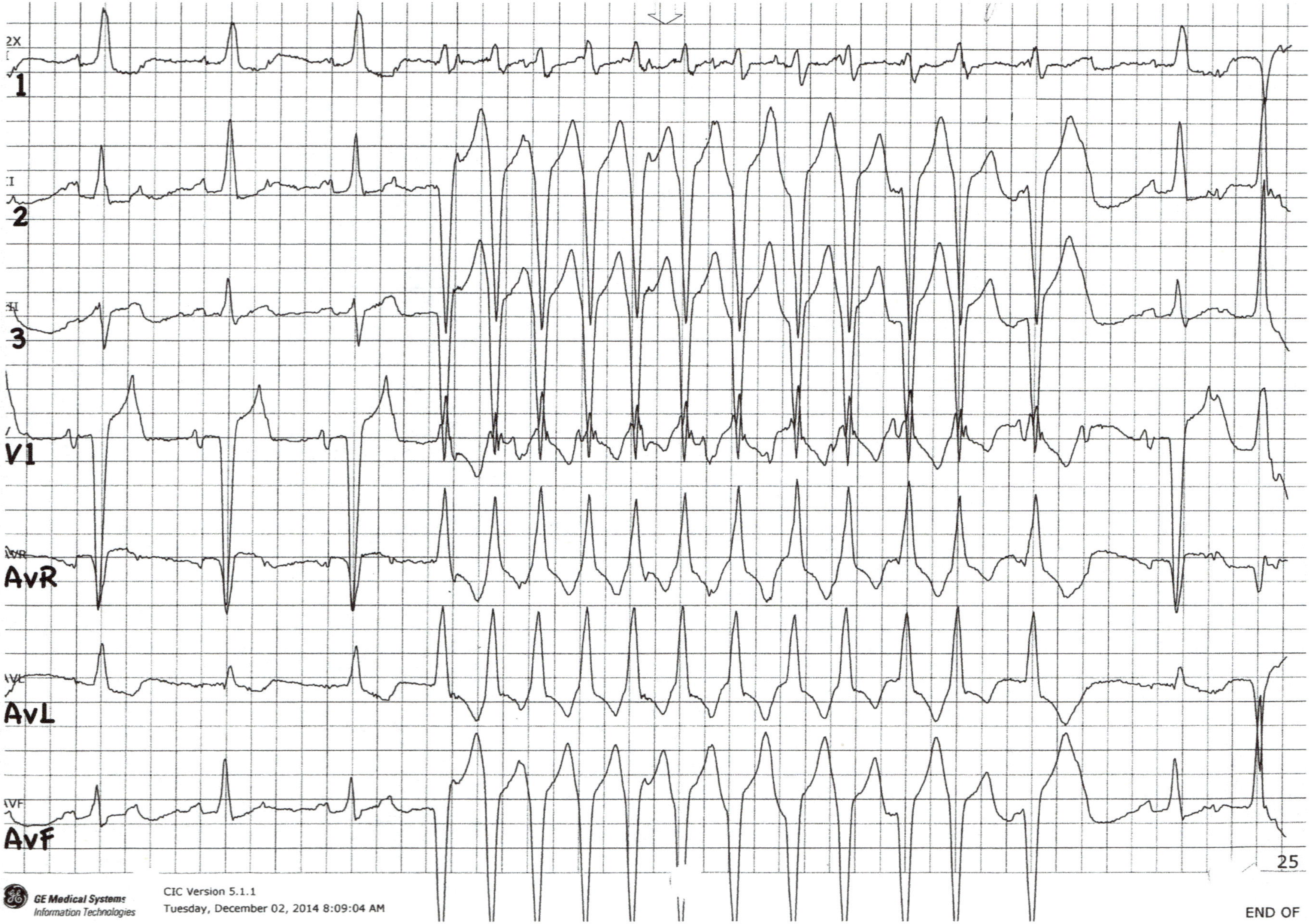
2X
1
2
3
V1
AvR
AvL
AvF
25
GE Medical Systems
Information Technologies
CIC Version 5.1.1
Tuesday, December 02, 2014 8:09:04 AM
END OF

## Question 4-8

The faster rhythm in **Figure 4-8A** is:

1. VT
2. SVT
3. Atrial fibrillation (AF)
4. Need more data

## Answer

Although not highly complicated, this tracing illustrates a compartmental or "zone" approach to a challenging tracing. We are very fortunate to have multiple leads available and both the onset and offset of the culprit rhythm. The latter provides 3 "zones" (left, right, and center) and 2 "transitions." It is not necessary to analyze from left to right, and in fact, *it is often easier to pick a zone that is relatively easy and understandable and build from that.*

Referring to the annotated version (**Figure 4-8B**), the *left* zone appears to show sinus rhythm with a suggestion of left ventricular hypertrophy (LVH). The tachycardia appears to start without an obvious P wave (*onset* transition zone).

Moving to the *right* zone after the offset of tachycardia, there is a pause after termination of tachycardia (the *offset* transition zone) that allows us to easily appreciate P waves (**arrows**) compatible with sinus origin (P-wave vector inferior and to the left), although "ectopic" atrial tachycardia is also possible. The P waves are now readily identified in all zones. It is now clear that atrial tachycardia is the baseline rhythm with 2:1 AV conduction, also now readily apparent in the *left* zone ("spiky" T waves due to "P on T") and in the *center* zone showing AV dissociation. This is, then, obviously VT in spite of the slight irregularity of CL.

One might note that the QRS during tachycardia also strongly supports VT. A total QS in the inferior leads with Rs at baseline would not be expected with RBBB. In fact, SVT at this rate would not be expected in the face of baseline 2:1 AV block during a relatively slow atrial or sinus tachycardia.

Dividing a complicated tracing into zones, starting in a zone that appears the least complicated, and focusing on the transitions provides a useful strategy for tackling the more complicated tracings. This strategy is equally useful for intracardiac tracings, which in principle can be thought of as just electrocardiograms with more leads.

Figure 4-8B

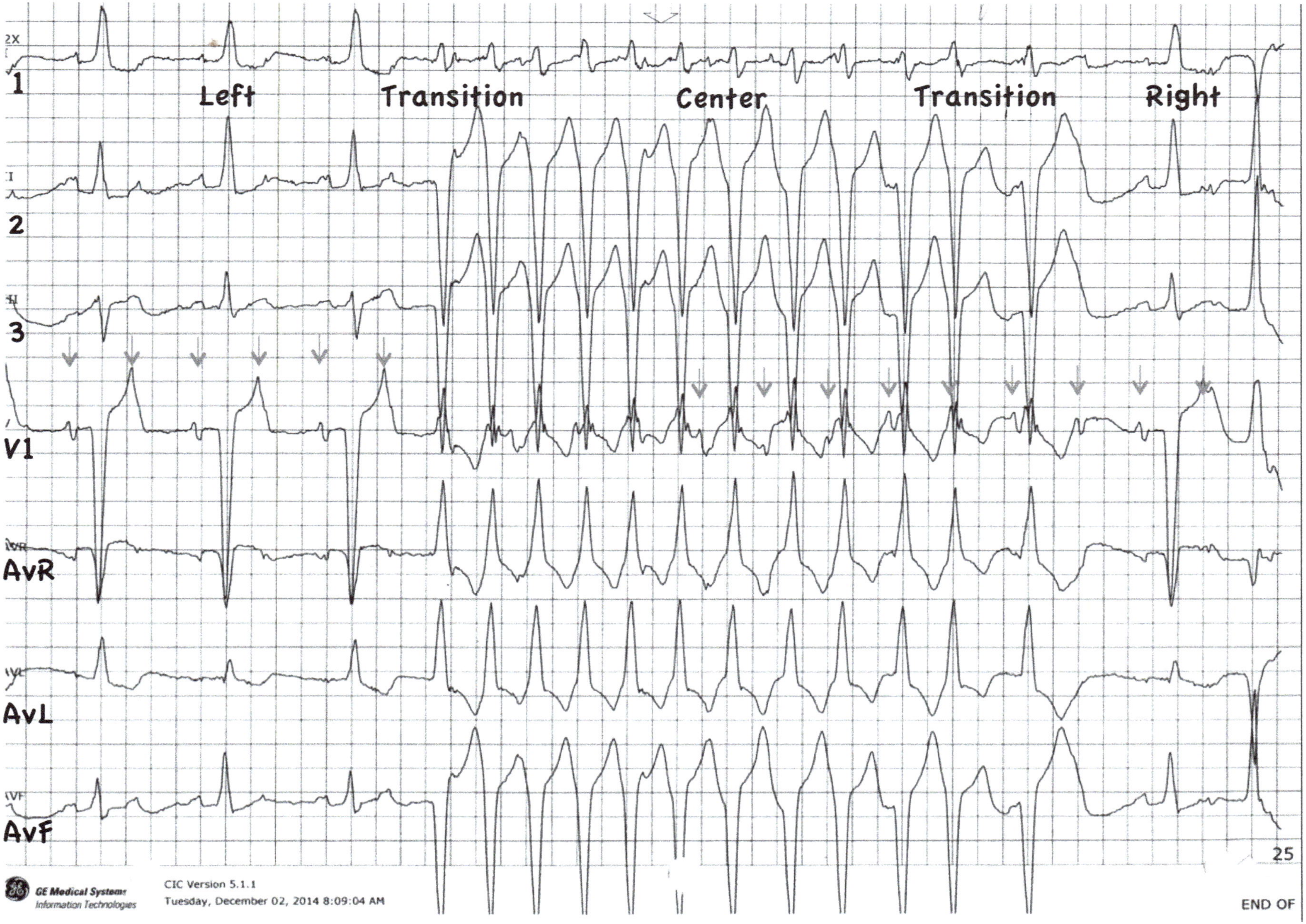
1
Left
Transition
Center
Transition
Right
2
3
V1
AvR
AvL
AvF
25
GE Medical Systems
Information Technologies
CIC Version 5.1.1
Tuesday, December 02, 2014 8:09:04 AM
END OF

## Question 4-9

The following 2 ECGs were recorded during a treadmill test on a young woman studied for palpitations. She had a structurally normal heart and the resting ECG was entirely normal. The first ECG (**Figure 4-9A**) caught the onset and the second (**Figure 4-9B**) captured the termination of a tachycardia although the 2 ECGs are not quite continuous. The tachycardia is alarming, even though it terminated spontaneously.

The tachycardia is most probably:

1. Torsades de pointes
2. VT
3. AFL with 1:1 AV conduction
4. Need more data

Figure 4-9A

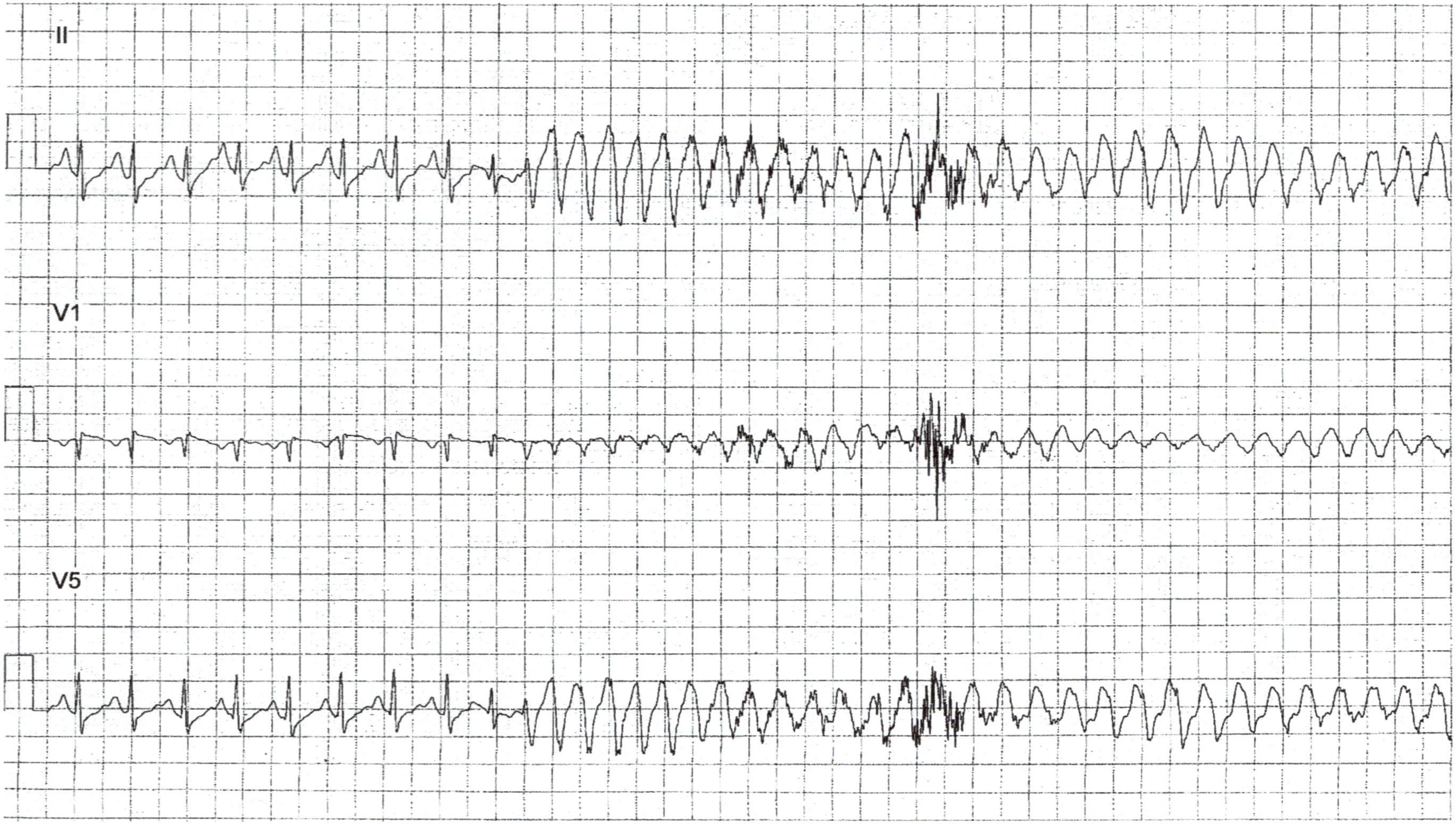

Figure 4-9B

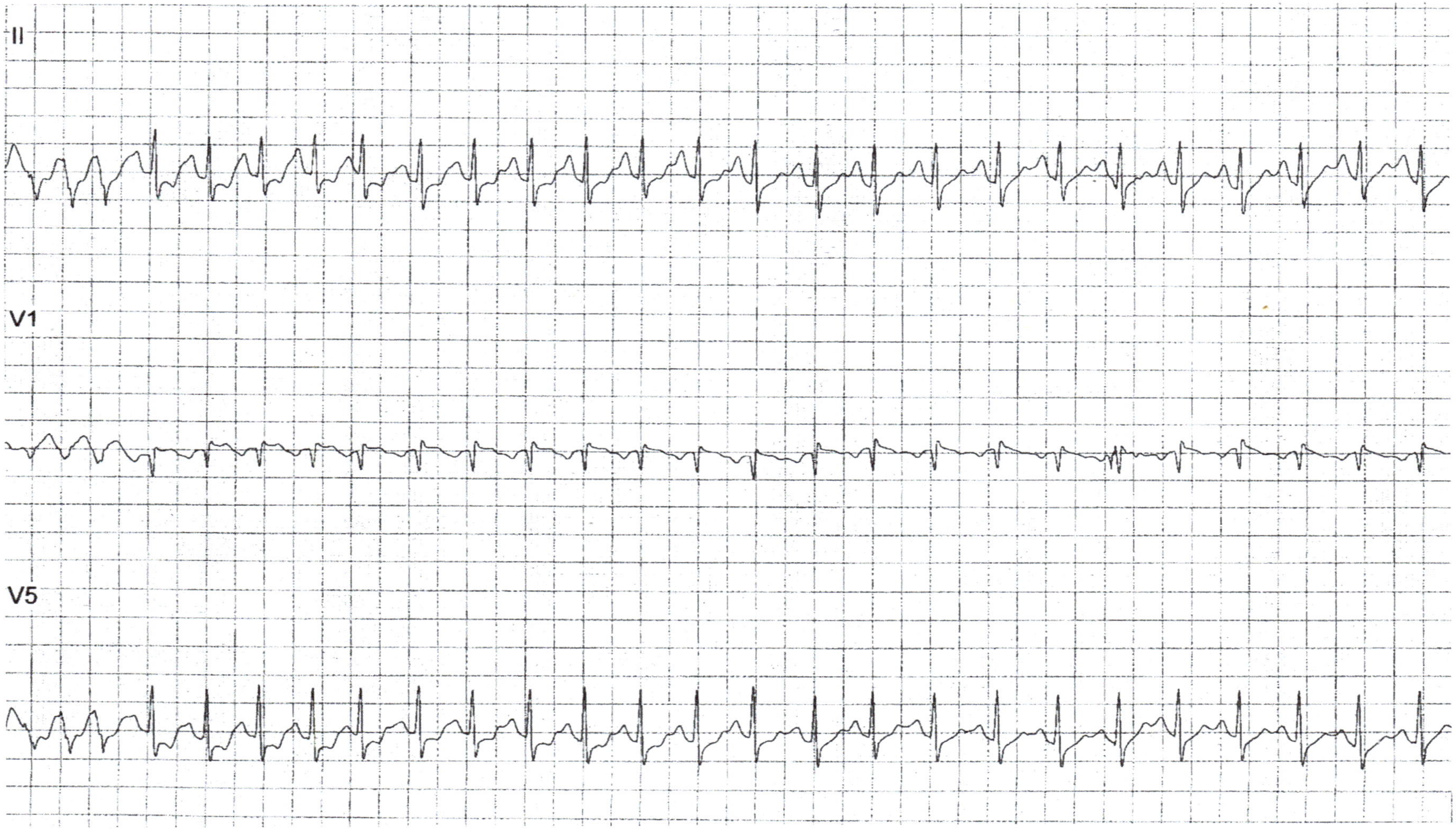

## Answer

The "reflex" answer is VT because it is very fast and slightly polymorphic (VT was the diagnosis on referral by an experienced clinical cardiologist). It has morphology consistent with torsades de pointes, but "torsades" generally refers to VT in the specific context of QT prolongation, and this is clearly not the case.

The tachycardia can be divided into 3 distinct zones with 2 "transition" areas. This is a relatively "clean" tracing, free of significant artifact, and we are indeed fortunate to have the onset and termination, since just looking at the "middle zone" of the tachycardia provides little clue to the mechanism.

The CL is slightly irregular; around 200 ms.

**Figure 4-9C** is a magnification of the onset of tachycardia. Magnification of important areas is frequently essential to evaluate more subtle observations and measurements and are used elsewhere in this book.

Figure 4-9C begins with 2 sinus cycles (**small squares**) followed by a cycle that is a little premature. The QRS is relatively normal, although admittedly a little "transitional" (potentially fusion or "incomplete" bundle branch block).

The first 2 P waves in sinus rhythm are quite prominent but a P wave is not seen where it would be expected in front of the third QRS. It is replaced by another deflection (**circles**) also distorting the ST segment, best explained as a PAC fusing with the expected sinus beat. The subsequent diastolic interval is also deformed arguably by a second PAC. The second WCT QRS is also again potentially fused, with one component from the normal QRS and one from the WCT, but also potentially incomplete bundle branch block.

In a nutshell, it would be problematic for VT to begin with a PAC unless it was a "coincidence."

**Figure 4-9D** shows the termination of the WCT, with sinus

Figure 4-9C

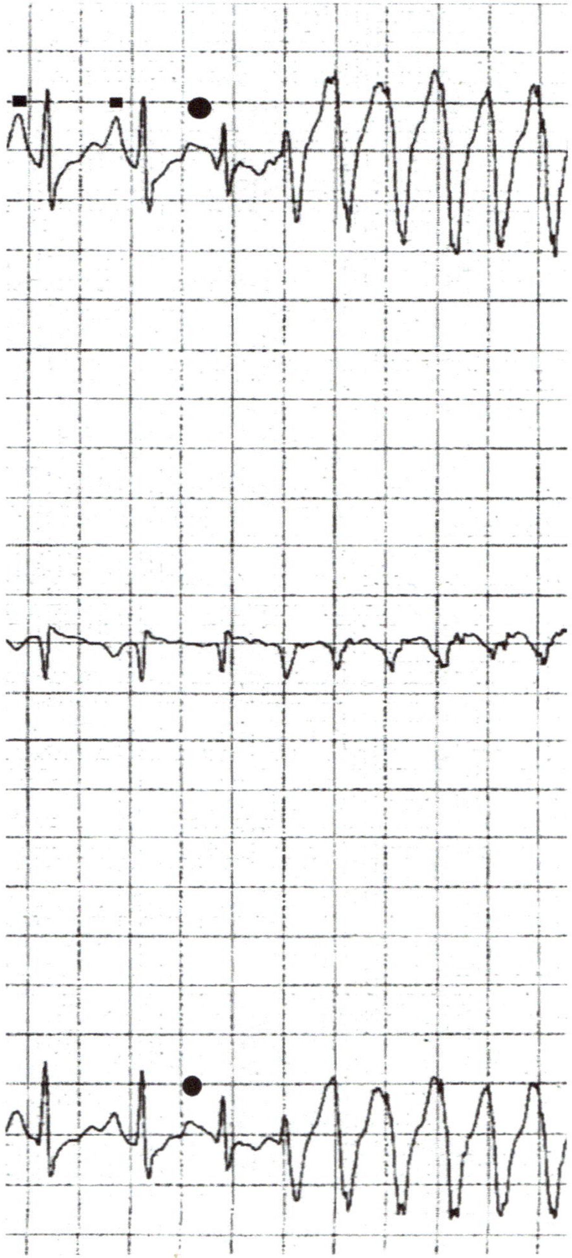

Figure 4-9D

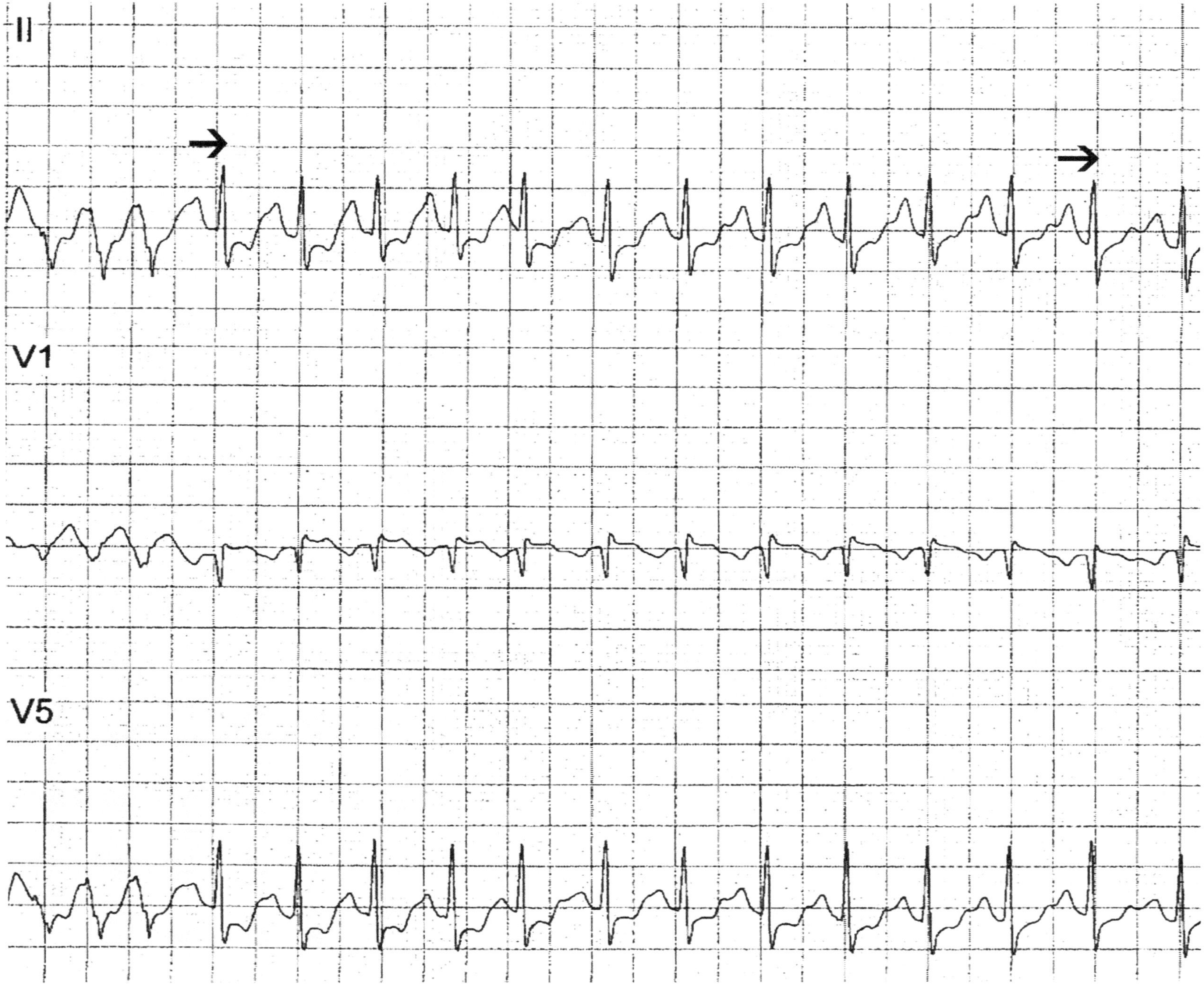

tachycardia appearing after the break (fourth beat). The horizontal arrows indicate the PR interval of the first sinus beat closely coupled to the last WCT beat. *This PR interval is unchanged from the subsequent PR intervals during sinus tachycardia.* One would reasonably (although not infallibly) expect such a closely coupled cycle to exhibit a slightly longer PR interval if the WCT were VT due to almost universally observed concealed conduction into the AV node early after VT cessation, even if there was no overt VA conduction (author's observation). Thus, neither the onset nor the termination favors VT.

This tracing teaches a systematic approach: breaking the tracing into distinct zones with careful measurements and asking what would expect during each from a specific hypothesis. Some options are more physiologically compelling based on the observations in spite of the "reflex" diagnosis of polymorphous VT.

A diagnosis of VT is not impossible here, but would require initiation by a very closely coupled PAC in the presence of "enhanced" AV node conduction (the PR interval of the initiating 2 PACs is very short). In addition, a closely coupled normal QRS beat at the termination of the wide QRS tachycardia (WCT) conducts with a short PR interval—the same PR interval seen in the subsequent sinus tachycardia beats. In general, one might expect some PR prolongation of such a closely coupled beat after the last beat of VT, and this does not happen.

The diagnosis of AFL with aberrancy or preexcitation explains the tracings with the fewest assumptions. We note that aberrancy patterns even without preexcitation can be quite unusual at such rapid rates as seen in AFL with 1:1 conduction.

The patient remained asymptomatic on β-blocker therapy after refusing EP study initially. Subsequent EP study showed neither inducible VT nor preexcitation although AV node conduction was brisk. She has remained well on β-blockers.

Figure 4-10A

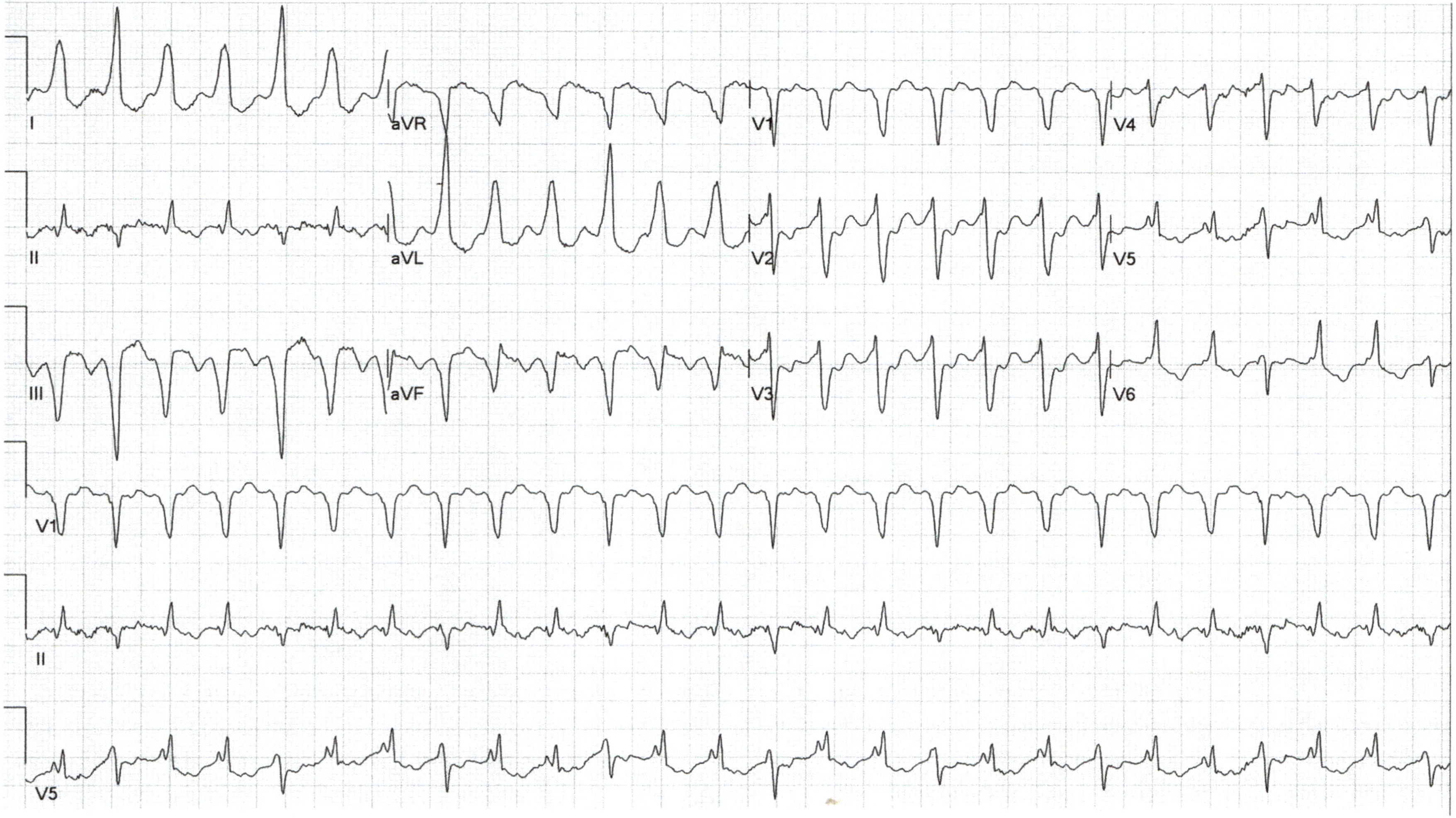

## Question 4-10

The WCT shown in **Figure 4-10A** is most probably:

1. VT
2. AFL with 2:1 block
3. AT
4. AVN reentry

## Answer

The wording of the question suggests that there is no absolute or "smoking gun" proof of mechanism in this difficult tracing. The final "truth" is not known, but the tracing provides a useful exercise in learning an approach.

One sees a LBBB-0type tachycardia, but the QRS morphology here is *atypical* with QS in $V_1$ and minimal change in a small initial R wave from $V_2$ up to $V_6$. This is more compatible with VT than aberrant conduction.

WCT resembles a right posteroseptal or right paraseptal preexcitation pattern (LBBB, inferior Q waves), but one would expect taller R waves across the precordial leads if this were a preexcitation pattern. Thus, we have a WCT with what would be an "atypical" LBB pattern, and our best answer would be VT.

A careful delineation of the limits of ventricular activation (i.e., the interval from the first onset of the QRS to the termination, **grey zone** in **Figure 4-10B**) shows a sharp deflection well seen in leads 2 and $V_5$ (**arrow**) in diastole that is *presumptively* a P wave. There is some artifact in the tracing, but there appears to be one QRS for each P wave.

This causes some pause for reflection and makes one consider

Figure 4-10B

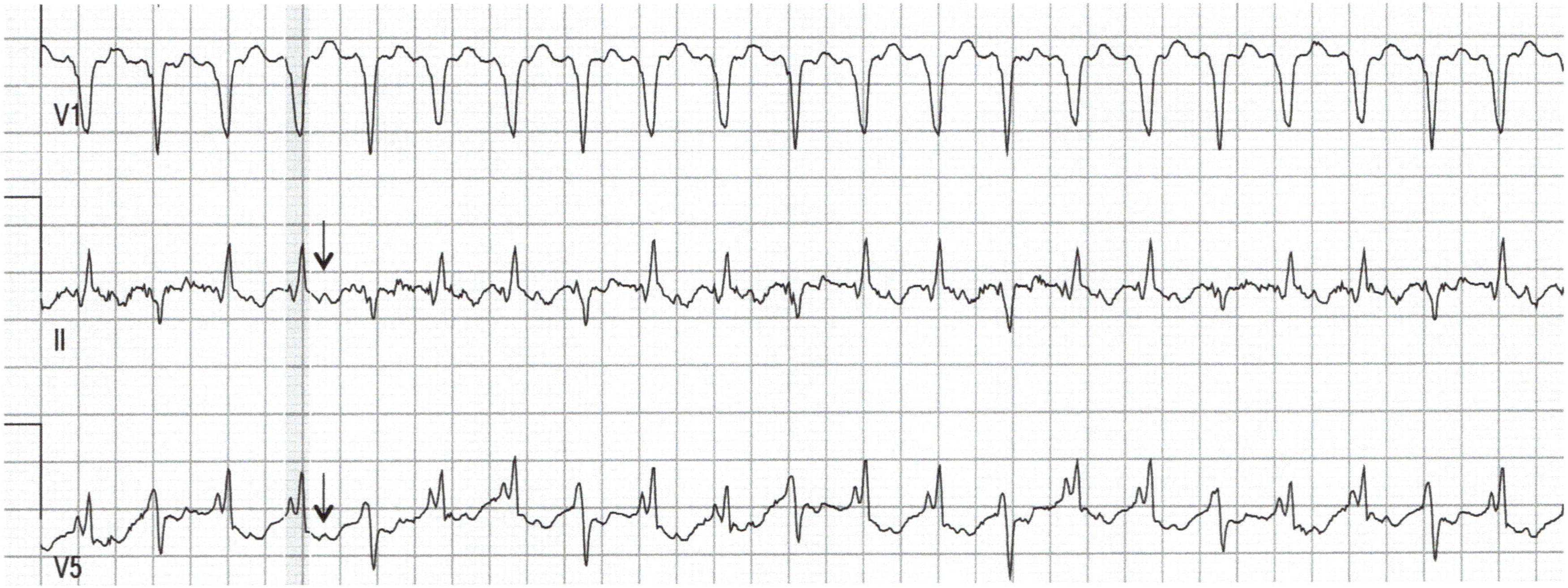

SVT. Whether the atrium is driving the ventricle or vice versa is not clear.

Finally, we observe that there is a repetitive pattern or "group beating" in that every third beat is different. Such "transition zones" are always worth a close look, and the area of interest has been amplified to measure accurately (**Figure 4-10C**).

We carefully indicate the onset of the QRS in this lead by a line for the 2 uniform cycles (beats 1, 2) and then continue to draw lines at the *same interval* to see if the irregular cycle perturbed the tachycardia. We see that the different QRS (beat 3) is not immediately preceded by a P wave, and its onset is *on time* with our line of the expected next QRS.

What happens subsequently? The next tachycardia beat 4 now begins *before* our line, earlier than where expected, and is followed by a P wave that also appears to be a little earlier. Thus, the different QRS beat *advanced (reset) the tachycardia.*

The change in ventricular activation of beat 3 influenced the tachycardia, implying that the ventricle is part of the tachycardia circuit. This *rules out AT and AVNRT,* which would not be influenced by a change in ventricular activation.



Figure 4-10C

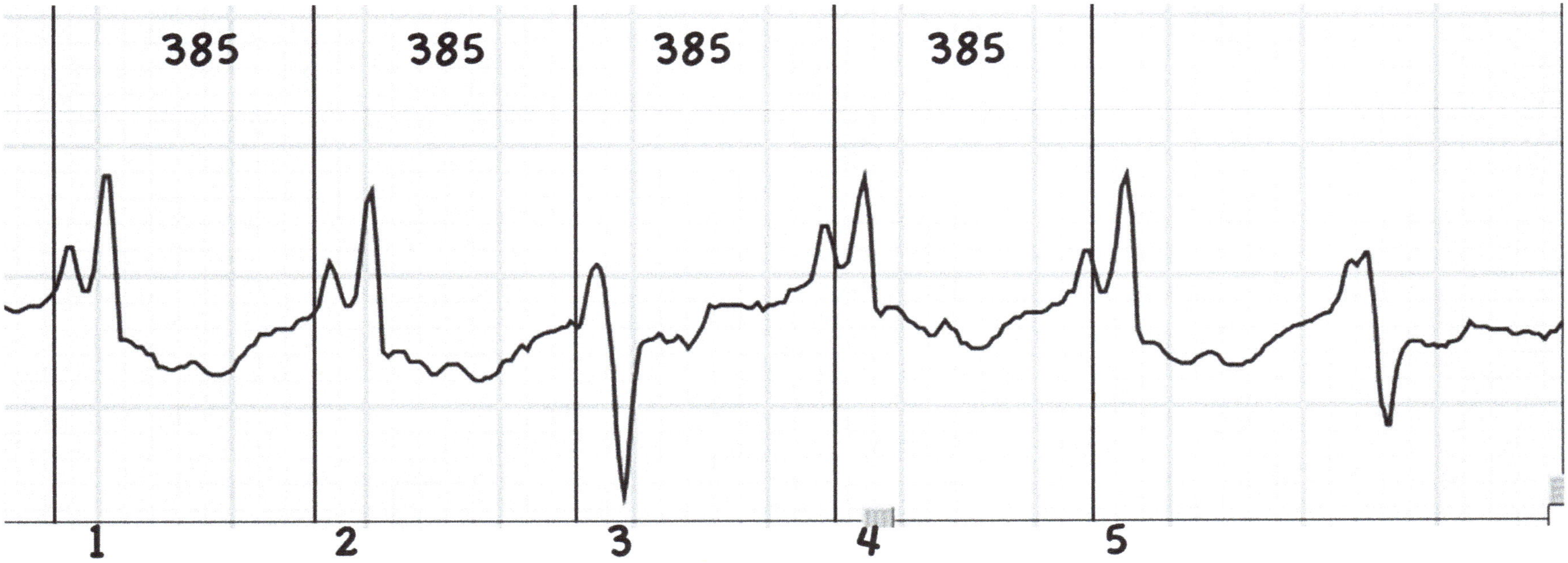

Our presumptive diagnosis to this point has been VT based on the QRS morphology. Is the above observation consistent with this diagnosis? A VT mechanism may be a "figure of 8" circuit with 2 circuits sharing the same slow-conduction zone. One circuit may be shorter or faster than the other. It is thus feasible that every third beat goes over the shorter circuit, which would explain the earlier arrival or "reset" of the next beat. Alternatively, it is also theoretically possible that every third beat is a late-coupled PVC during macroreentrant VT causing ventricular fusion and resetting the VT.

We have clearly ruled out AT and AVNRT or AFL, but any other conceivable explanation is theoretically possible as long as the ventricle is involved in the tachycardia mechanism. If the tachycardia were orthodromic AVRT over a left-lateral AP, a change from LBBB aberrancy to normal QRS or another PVC during tachycardia could result in earlier arrival of the retrograde

P and advance the tachycardia. The ventricle is, of course, part of the circuit in AV reentry. Thus, the reset of the tachycardia here could represent AVRT.

Our patient was an elderly gentleman with previous anterior and inferior myocardial infarction (MI) and never known to have SVT. Thus, VT is by far the higher probability answer in our context, especially related to the answering of our multiple-choice question where AV reentry is not given as an option.

This is a difficult tracing, and the "true" explanation is not known, since the patient never had electrophysiological assessment. However, in the end, it points out the value of careful measurement and thinking "electrophysiologically."

Figure 4-11A

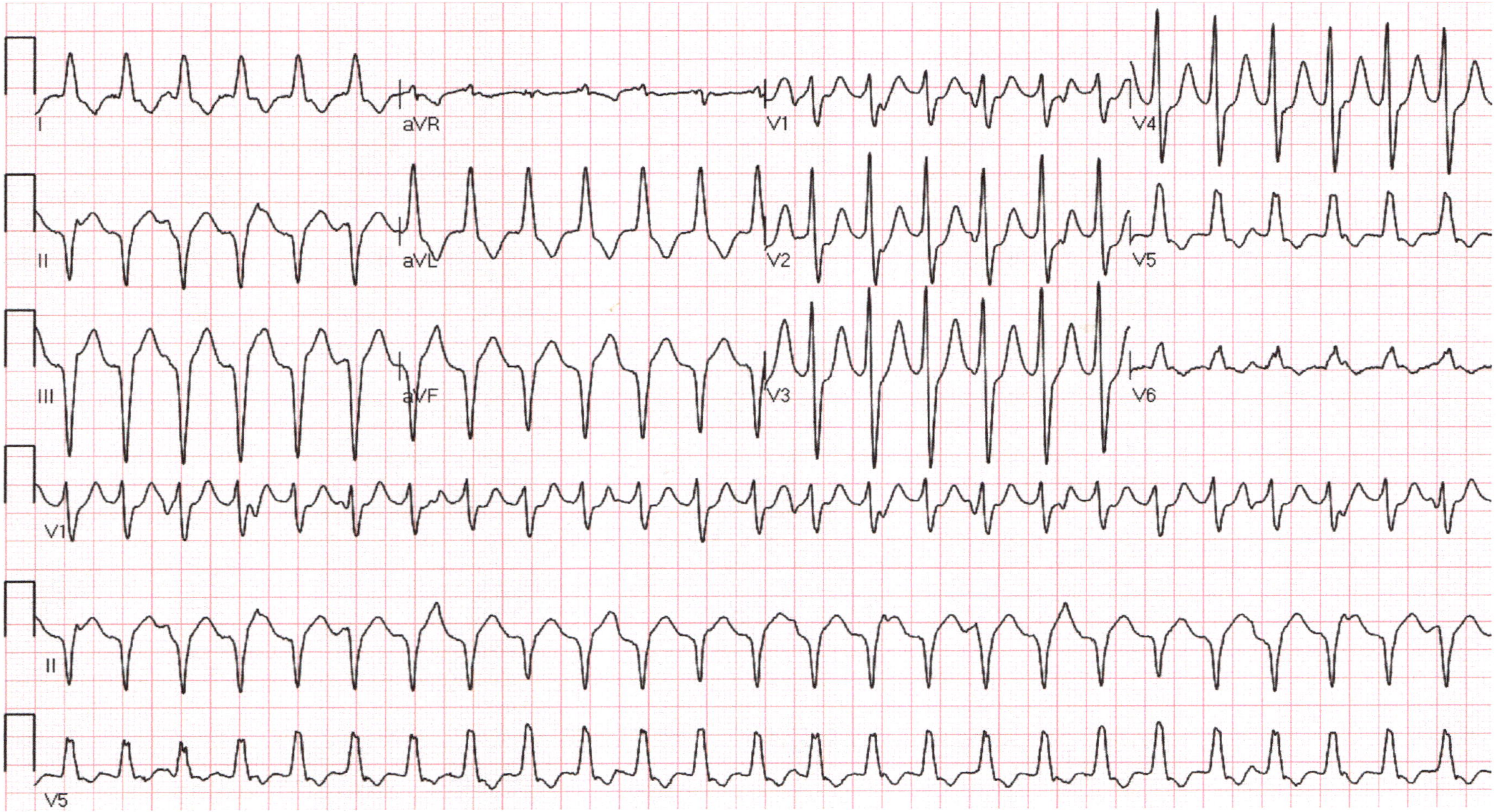

## Question 4-11

The ECG in **Figure 4-11A** is recorded from a 56-year-old man presenting with palpitations. The most likely tachycardia mechanism is:

1. VT
2. AVNRT
3. AVRT
4. Need more data

## Answer

This relatively "narrow" and stable regular WCT has left bundle branch block morphology with strongly superior axis. The morphology is a little atypical for LBBB, in that the initial R in $V_1$ is a little wider than "classical" and the R is higher than S in $V_2$, but otherwise, it is a "passable" LBBB pattern.

Such tachycardias are frequently misdiagnosed in the community (as was this one). The more experienced practitioner will carefully look for atrial activity in spite of the initial overall impression of SVT. Although *all* leads should be carefully examined, *the most productive lead is usually the one showing the smallest QRS*. Of course, the smaller P waves are often obscured in leads with the larger QRS complexes.

In this example, $V_1$ has a relatively small QRS, and indeed the P wave is relatively obvious (**blue dots** in **Figure 4-11B**). AV dissociation is evident with no discernable VA conduction. It is interesting that often only 1 or 2 of the 12 leads may convincingly show P waves in these WCT—a cautionary footnote when only 1 or 2 leads are available to make the diagnosis.

Relating to our question, AV reentry is clearly ruled out since the atrium is a necessary link in this tachycardia. It is more difficult to rule out AV nodal reentry, since the atrium is not a necessary component of the tachycardia circuit in AVNRT and AV dissociation during tachycardia is possible. However, the best answer to our question is still VT, since the question allows the element of probability to be considered—that is, which is "most likely"?

Figure 4-11B

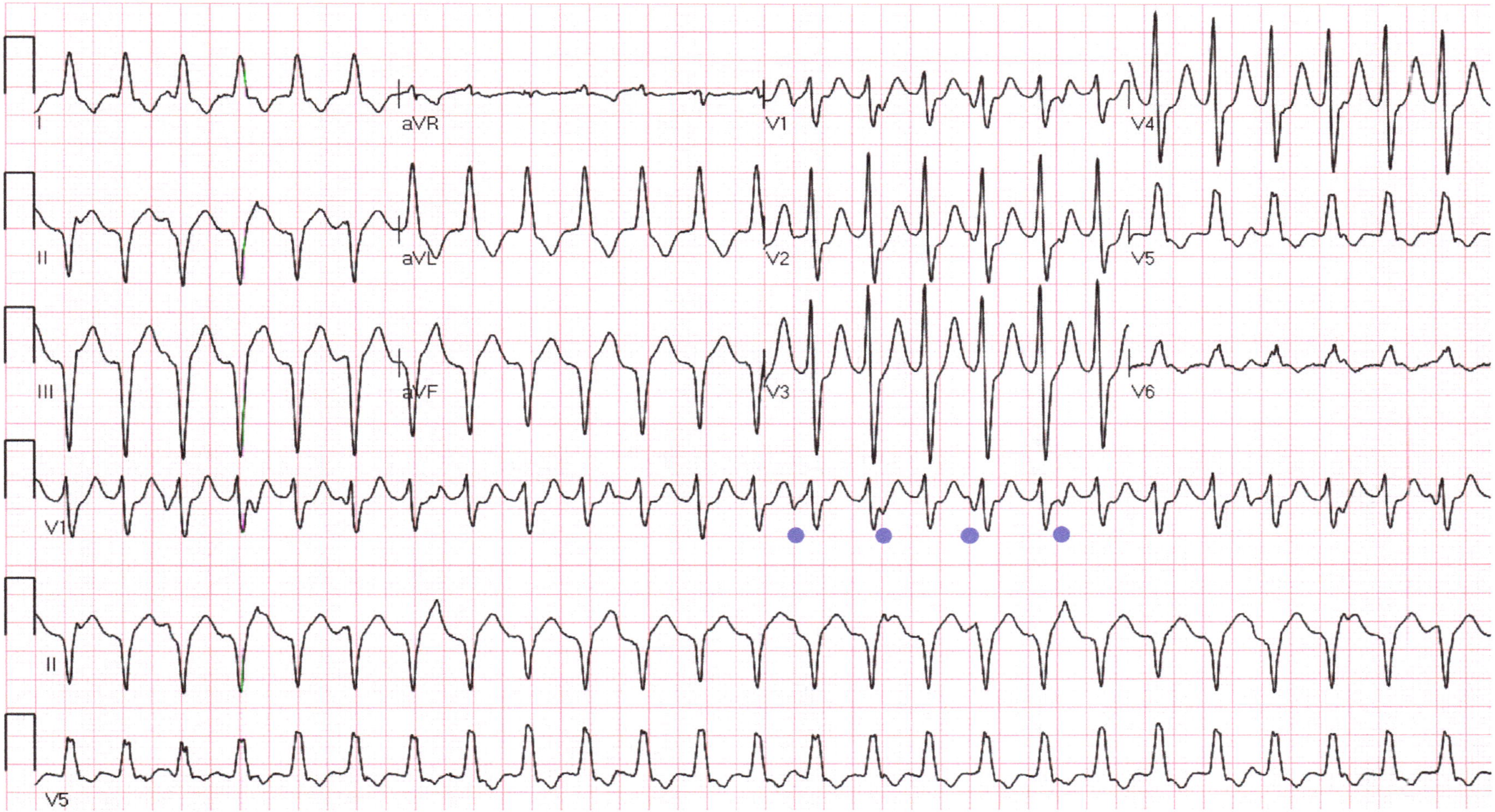

Figure 4-12

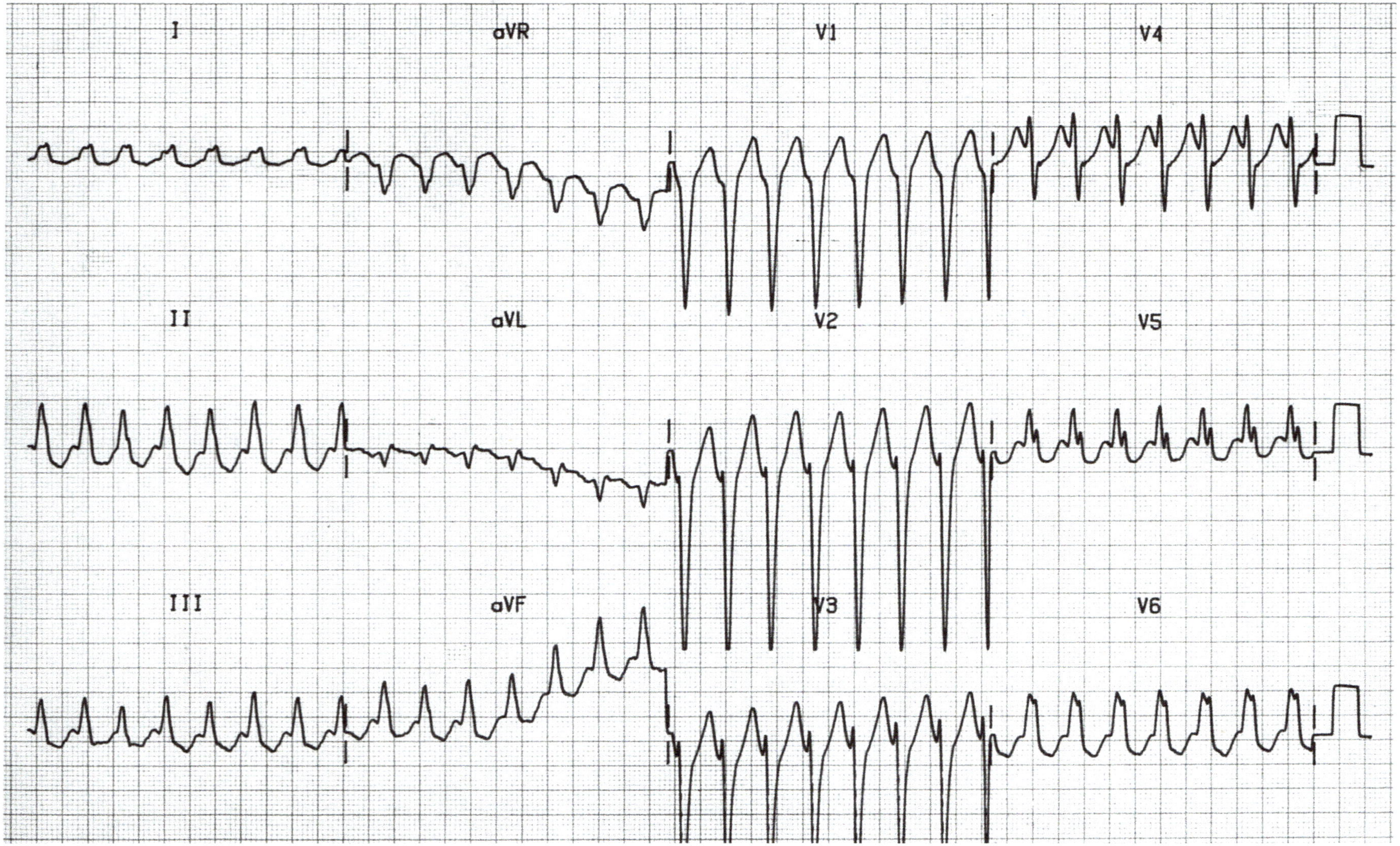


Question 4-12

## Question 4-12

The ECG in **Figure 4-12** is recorded from a 64-year-old woman who was previously well except for hypertension.

The tracing represents:

1. VT
2. SVT with aberrancy
3. Preexcited tachycardia
4. Need more data

## Answer

This tachycardia is perfectly regular with a CL of 340 ms. There is a little "bump" in the ST segment best seen in lead aVL, but P wave activity is not discernable with any certainty.

The most striking feature of the tachycardia is that the QRS has a very *typical* morphology for LBBB, and this puts SVT with LBBB aberrancy at the top of our list for differential diagnosis. It would be a passable QRS for preexcitation over an atriofascicular AP, although this would not be frequently observed in the setting of a hypertensive 64-year-old woman who previously was well. VT can't be completely ruled out entirely, but it would have to be a right ventricular VT breaking out near the RV apical region to give it this QRS morphology.

A word about exam strategy. The answer to the multiple choice as it is phrased would be Option 4, need more data. If the question included a word such as "probably," the respondent is being told that there is no absolutely unequivocal answer and is asked to consider *probability* in coming to a conclusion. In such a case, the correct answer would then be Option 2, that is, SVT with aberrancy.

This patient was subsequently proved to have AFL with 2:1 AV block. Adenosine would be useful to clarify this in an acute clinical setting.

Question 4-13

Figure 4-13A

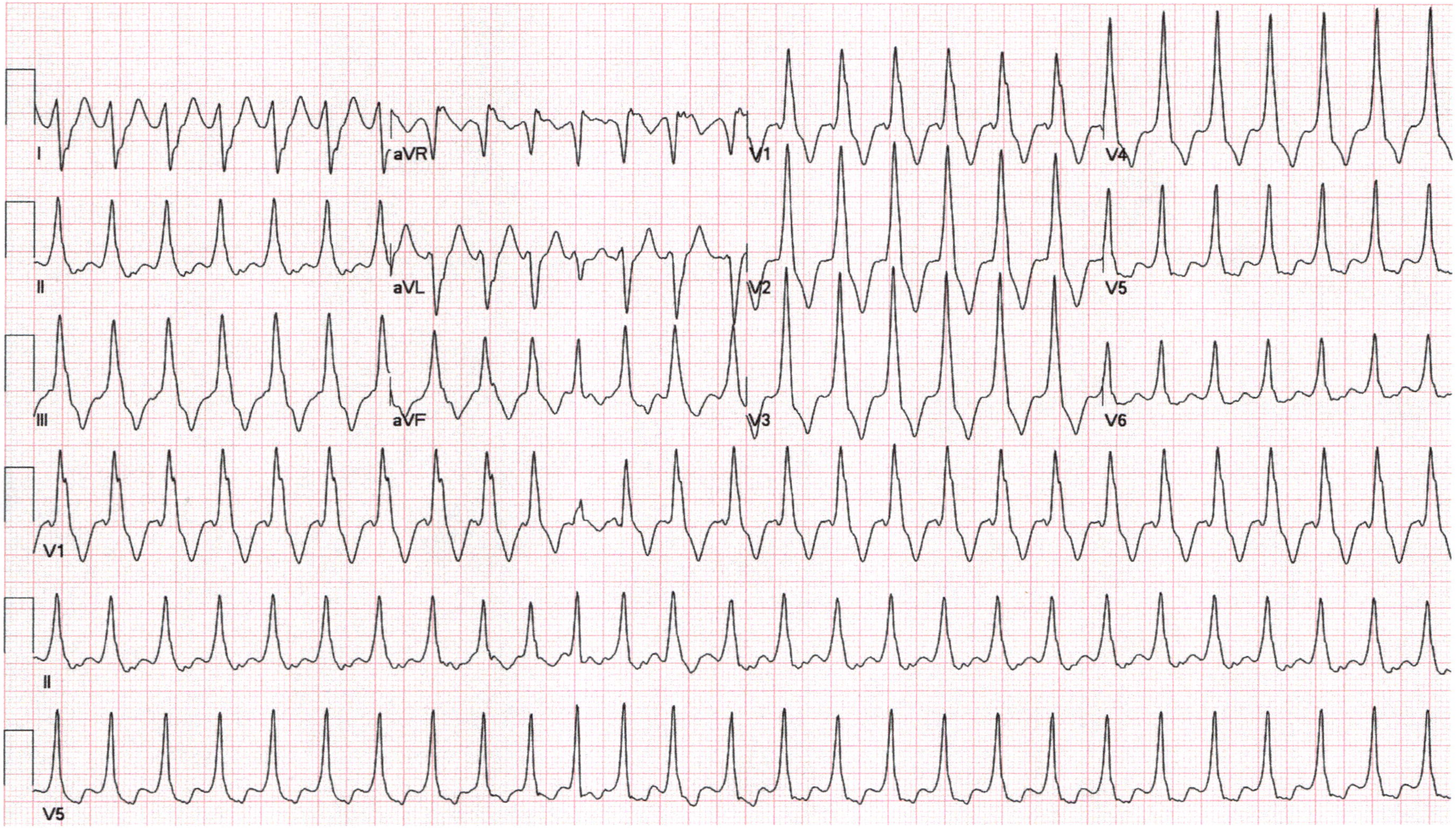

## Question 4-13

The tracing in **Figure 4-13A** is best interpreted as:

1. VT
2. SVT with aberrancy
3. Preexcited tachycardia
4. Need more data

## Answer

This ECG was interpreted as VT by a very experienced cardiologist. Was this wrong? Clearly, it is not compatible with bundle branch block aberration with inferior axis and precordial concordance. In addition, there is a narrower complex in the center of the tracing that our cardiologist called a "capture" beat.

However, the QRS morphology suggests that the ventricular rhythm is originating from the base of the left ventricle (positive concordance), so that this could also be a preexcited tachycardia. It is important to remember that the *preexcited tachycardia will have a ventricular origin at the insertion of the accessory pathway and will not be distinguishable from a VT focus coming from a comparable region.*

In this case, the patient had essentially a normal ECG except for a subtle delta wave, suggesting a left lateral AP. The tachycardia was subsequently reproduced in the electrophysiology (EP) lab and was antidromic tachycardia, conducting antegradely over the AP and retrogradely over the normal AV conduction system.

**Figure 4-13B** magnifies the rhythm strip before and after the putative capture beat (**blue dot**). The tachycardia is quite regular at the beginning, CL 376 ms. There is a suggestion of atrial activity (**blue lines**) in repolarization not seen clearly in all beats. However, the tachycardia starts to become a little irregular even before the "narrow" beat. This is compatible with a little flurry of ventricular ectopic activity. A PVC from the right ventricle would tend to "normalize" ventricular activation coming from the left ventricle (this has been aptly called "pseudo normalization").

The first WCT beat that comes a little early, 376 to 358 ms, is actually preceded by a P wave that is a little early. That is, the change in the QRS cycle is preceded by a change in the atrial cycle, a finding that excludes VT. This might be a late-coupled PVC (**blue dot**) fusing with the tachycardia and resetting the next cycle. The latter reflects good access of the PVC to the excitable gap of the circuit, compatible with our diagnosis of antidromic tachycardia. The following slight shortening of the QRS interval is again preceded by a similar shortening of the P-P interval.

This is admittedly a difficult tracing, which depends on subtle changes in the presence of atrial activity that is not absolutely clear. Nonetheless, it illustrates the approach to this type of tracing, and the explanation is compatible with the known diagnosis of antidromic tachycardia proven at EP study.

To be fair, the correct answer to our multiple-choice question should be Option 4, because we "need more data" than the ECG during tachycardia alone to be certain of what is happening.

Figure 4-13B

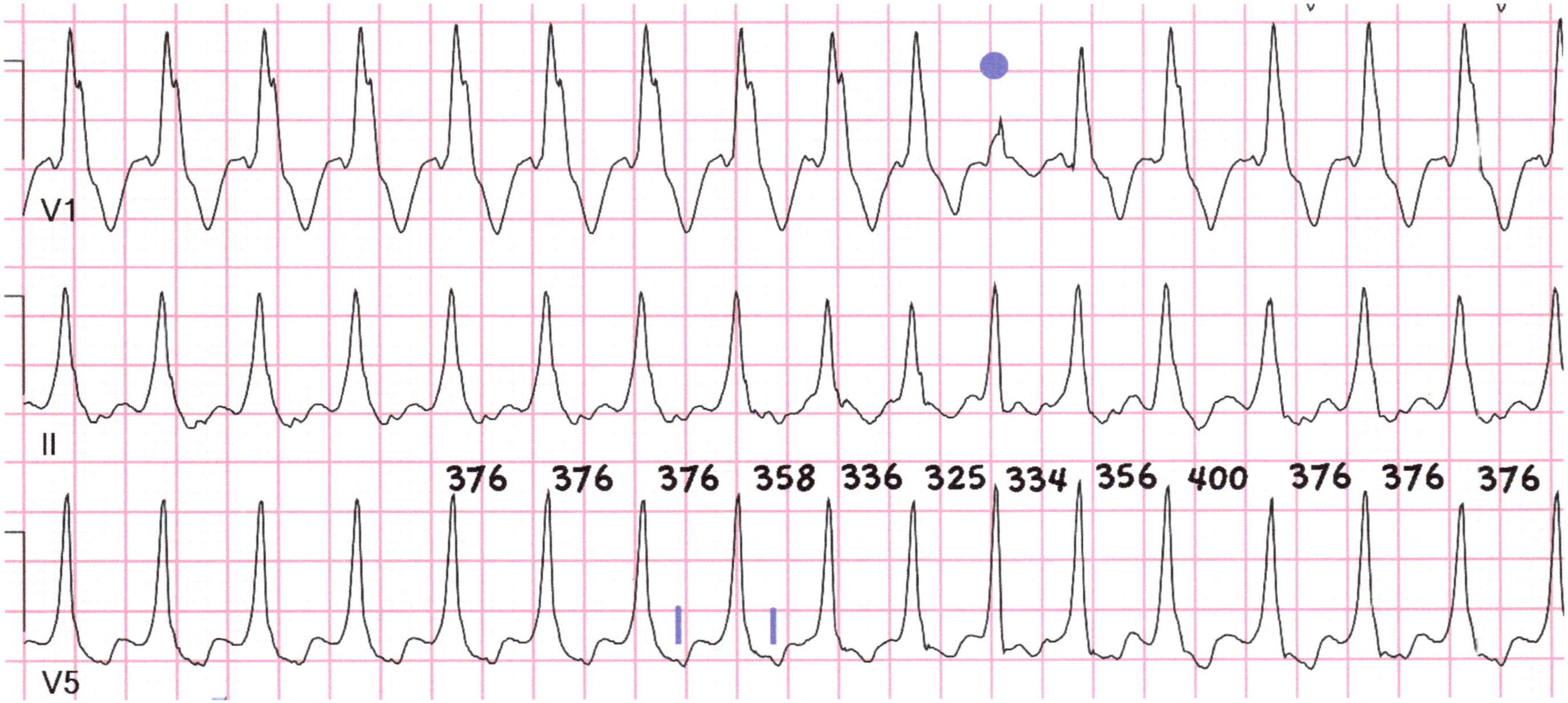

Figure 4-14A

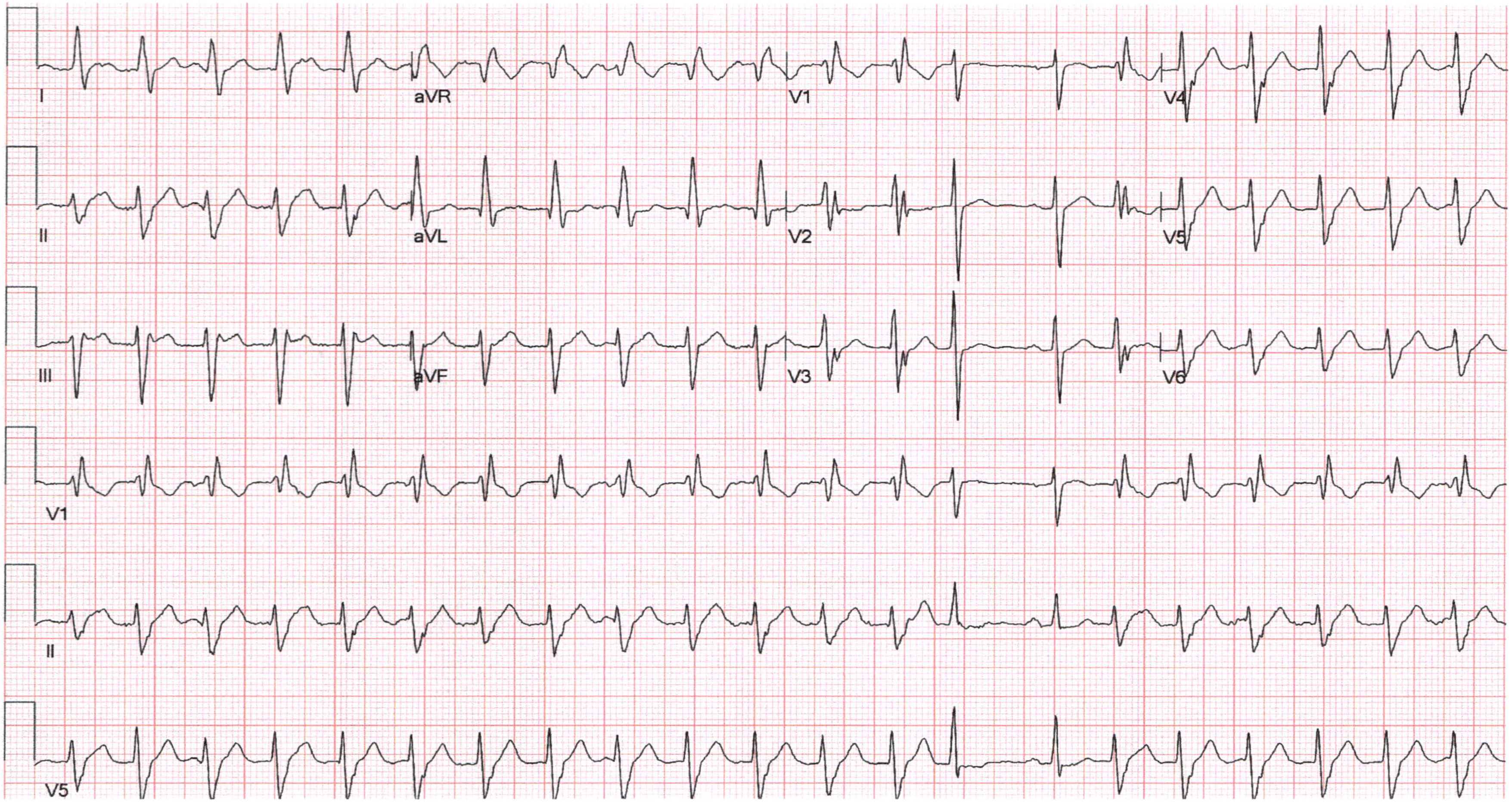

## Question 4-14

The individual whose ECG during palpitations is shown in **Figure 4-14A** has no known heart disease and a normal ECG during sinus rhythm.
The tracing illustrates:

1. VT
2. Preexcited tachycardia
3. AV reentry
4. AVNRT

## Answer

This WCT has RBBB morphology with left-axis deviation (see also **Question 4-1**). As I had pointed out previously, bifascicular block as aberrancy is very rare and favors VT unless the patient had previous left anterior hemiblock or bifascicular block. It is also not a QRS that is compatible with known accessory AV pathways. Knowing that the baseline ECG was normal, *this is almost certainly VT on the basis of QRS pattern alone.*

Atrial activity is hard to appreciate but reasonably seen during tachycardia in lead $V_1$ (**blue dots**) as shown in **Figure 4-14B**, which magnifies this lead and the leads immediately above and below. This is AV-dissociated. Termination with a narrow QRS is observed, and this is most probably a capture beat but also conceivably an AVN echo that terminates VT. The **red dots** indicate the P wave in sinus rhythm and that of the capture beat, and it is evident that the T wave of the last VT beat is taller than the rest, compatible with the sinus P wave "sitting" on the T wave.

Termination of VT by a capture beat is very rare, but we must remember that the mechanism of this type of idiopathic left ventricular VT is closely related to the His-Purkinje system with good access to it by supraventricular impulses, and both initiation and termination of this type of VT by atrial beats and SVT have been reported. One cannot, of course, entirely discount coincidental termination of the VT at the time of the capture beat.

Finally, we note that the interval preceding the first VT beat when it restarts is relatively free of artifact and has no suggestion of a preceding P wave (**red line**). Thus, the tachycardia begins with a PVC of the same morphology of the subsequent WCT, further proof that this is VT.

Figure 4-14B

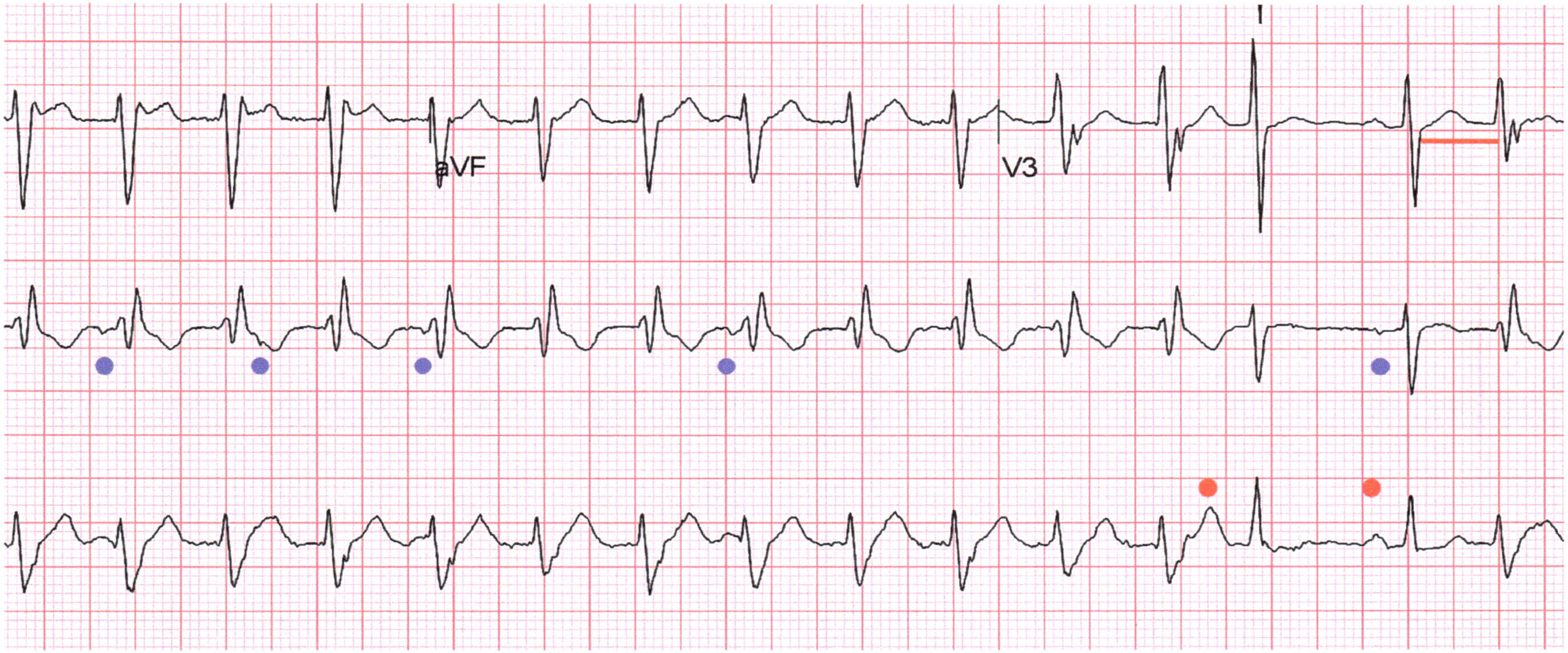

Question 4-15

Figure 4-15A

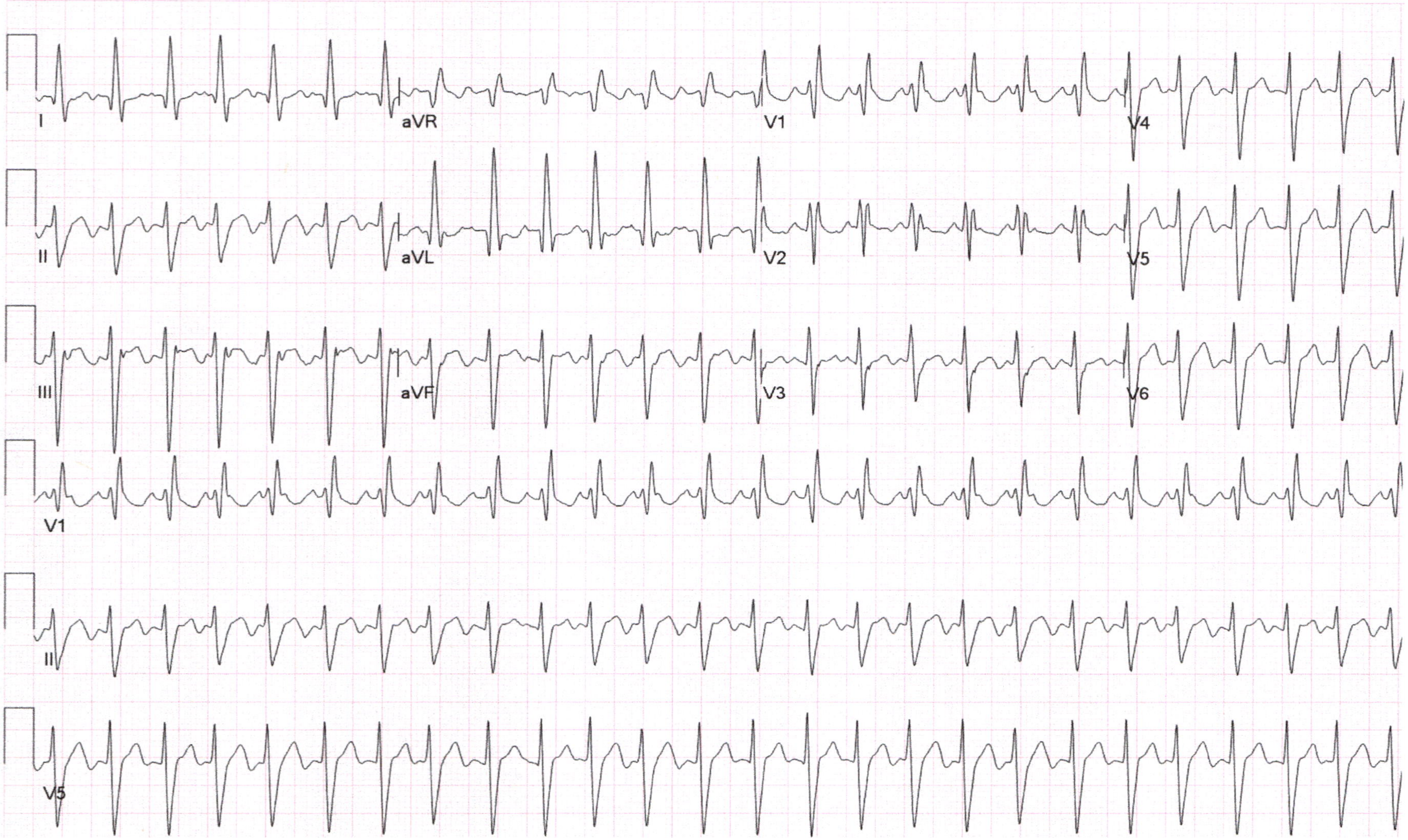

## Question 4-15

The tracing in **Figure 4-15A** is best interpreted as:

1. VT
2. AFL
3. AV reentry
4. AVNRT

## Answer

This WCT again has RBBB morphology with left-axis deviation (see also **Questions 4-1** and **4-14**).

Bifascicular block as an aberrancy pattern favors VT unless the patient had previous left anterior hemiblock or bifascicular block. A candidate P wave is seen in mid to late diastole (for example in lead $V_1$).

The exercise now is to "walk" through the P waves with calipers at *half the atrial CL* to search for a second, more subtle deflection that would indicate a second concealed P wave (usually near the QRS). In our example, this becomes obvious as seen in the magnified **Figure 4-15B**, where atrial activity is highlighted with **blue dots**. The ventricular rate is slightly variable so that the interval between the QRS and the second P wave varies a little. It is now clear that this is AFL. Of course, remember that a second P wave cannot be ruled out if the midpoint of the atrial cycle falls right into the QRS, where there is little chance of distinguishing it from the much larger QRS. Also, it is noted that indeed the baseline ECG (**Figure 4-15C**) showed a fixed RBBB and left anterior fascicular block (LAFB) pattern, as one would expect with the rarity of bifascicular block as an aberrancy pattern.

Figure 4-15B

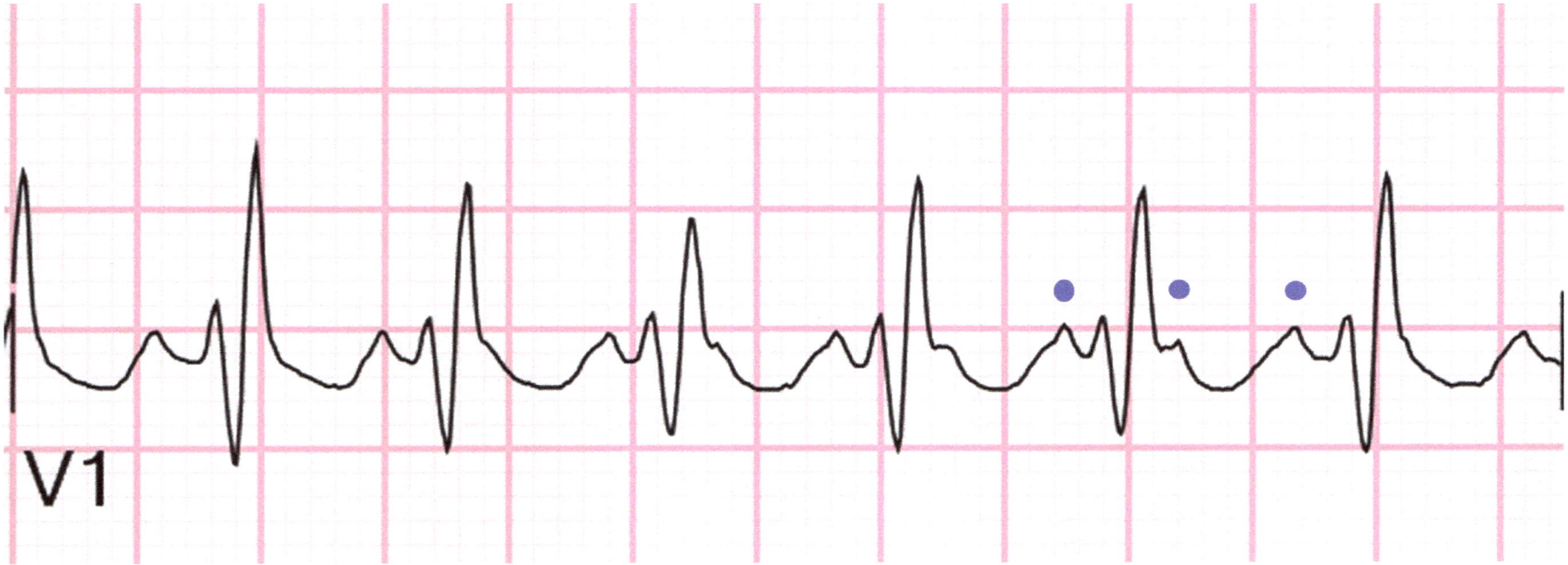

Figure 4-15C

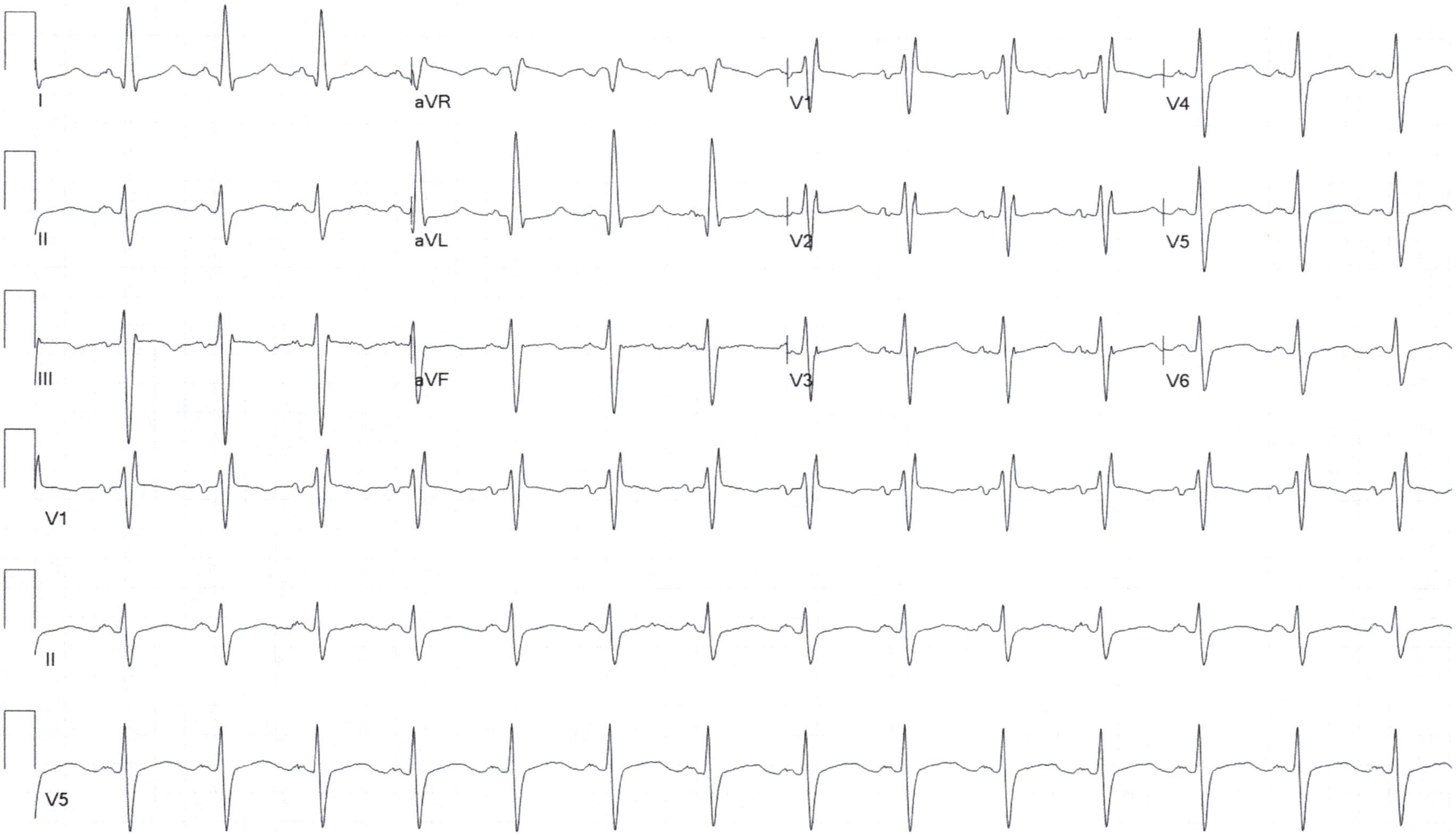

Question 4-16

Figure 4-16A

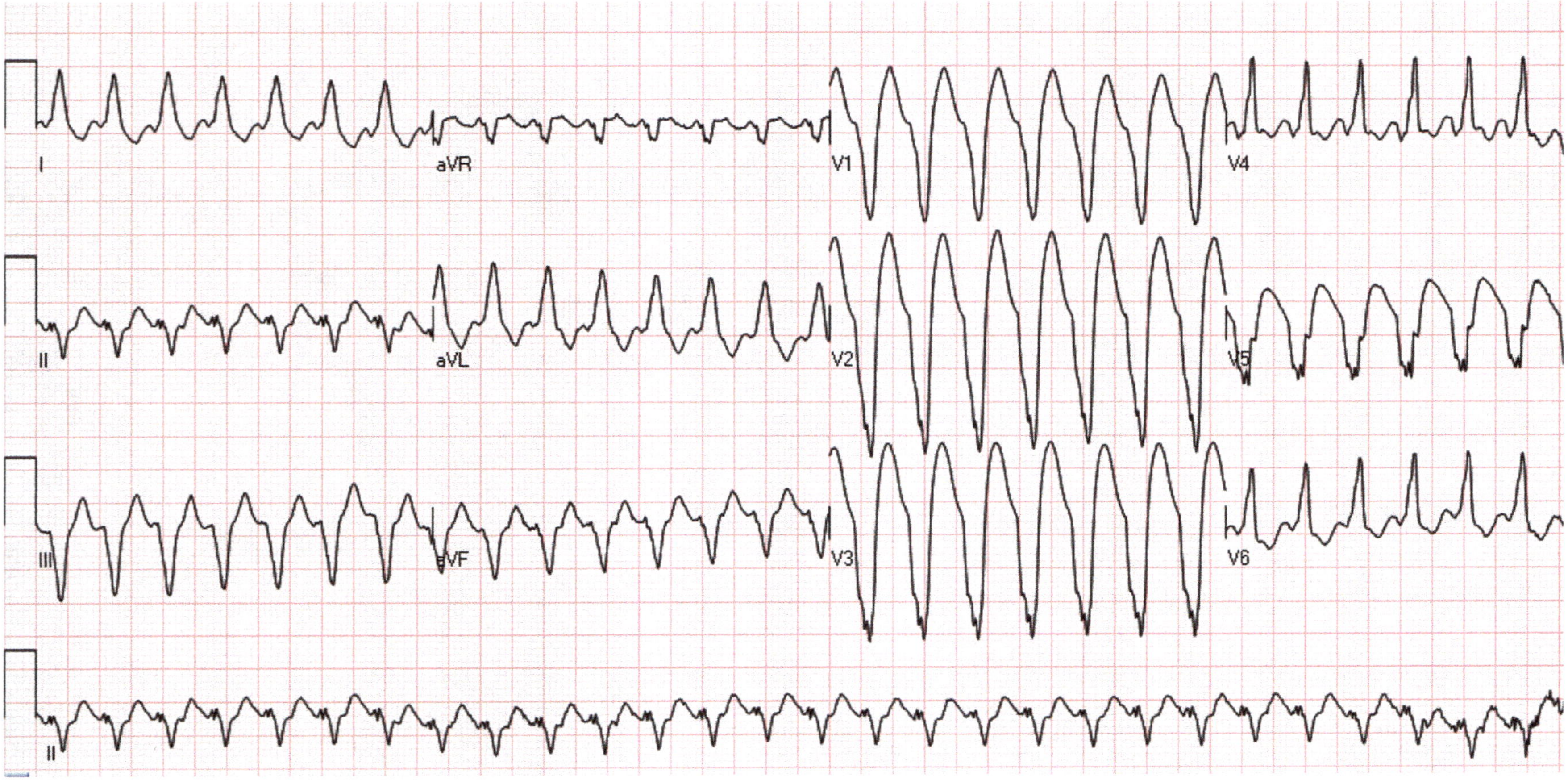

Figure 4-16B

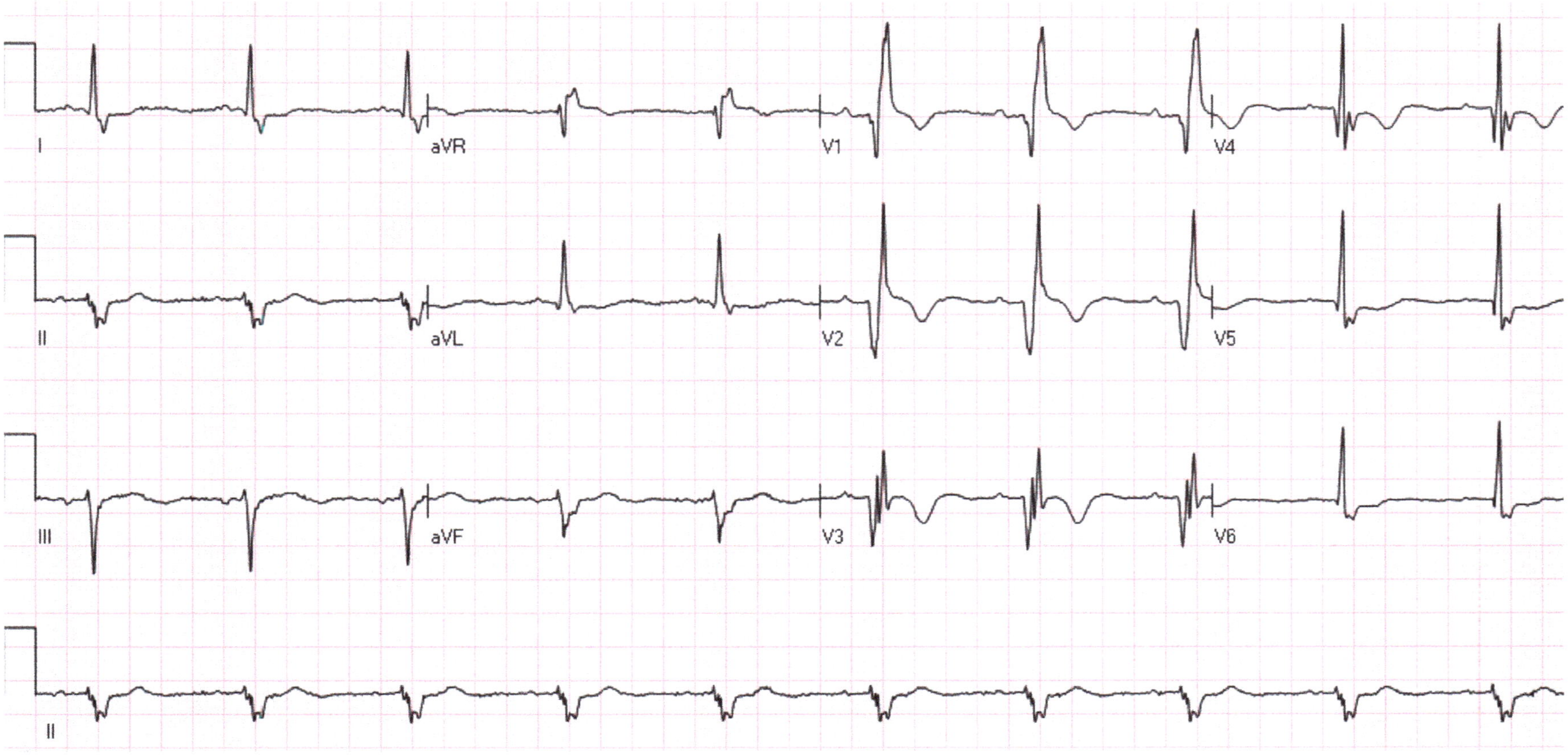




## Question 4-16

The tracings (**Figures 4-16A** and **4-16B**) are recorded from the same patient within a few minutes of each other. The WCT is best interpreted as:

1. Ventricular tachycardia
2. SVT with aberrancy
3. SVT with preexcitation
4. Need more data

## Answer

This WCT resembles left bundle branch block with left axis deviation. The QRS is not "typical" for LBBB, most notably in the anteroseptal leads with a broad QS complex and slow downslope of the initial Q wave. This strongly favors VT. Finding P waves with confidence is challenging.

However, the resting ECG is helpful and essentially verifies the diagnosis of VT. We note the pattern of anteroseptal MI that greatly enhances the probability of VT for the WCT. More importantly, we note the RBBB and left anterior hemiblock bifascicular block pattern at a relatively modest heart rate. One would consider it extremely unlikely that the right bundle would conduct at the rate of the WCT to allow an SVT with LBBB. This is a very useful concept presented elsewhere and emphasizes the value of the baseline ECG.

In fact, ***any*** QRS that would be ***different*** from a baseline bundle branch pattern (in this case, RBBB and LAFB) would in all probability be VT.

Figure 4-17A

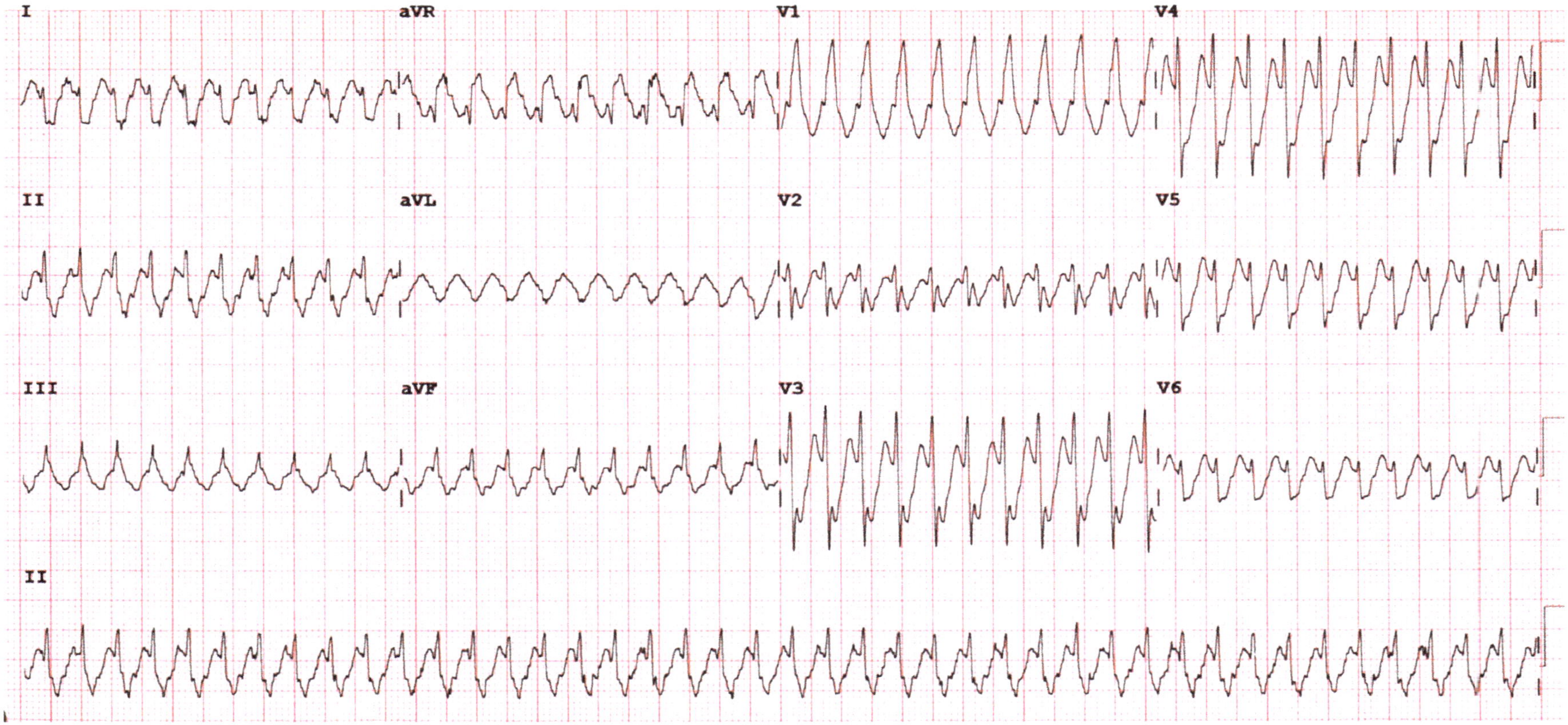




## Question 4-17

The tracing (**Figure 4-17A**) is best interpreted as:

1. Ventricular tachycardia
2. SVT with aberrancy
3. Preexcited tachycardia
4. Need more data

## Answer

This WCT of CL approximately 230 ms has right bundle branch block morphology with extreme right axis deviation. The R waves in lead $V_2$ diminish suddenly, recover a little in $V_3$ and $V_4$ and lose amplitude again in $V_5$ and $V_6$. Atrial activity is certainly not clearly evident. The patient has no known heart disease and his baseline ECG shown in **Figure 4-17B** is unequivocally normal.

One can reasonably only go by QRS appearance in this example. It is very far from a "perfect" RBBB pattern and this would favor VT. In addition, it is not a usual preexcitation pattern.

No arrhythmia was inducible at electrophysiologic study. However, the AV nodal refractory period was quite short so that our *presumptive diagnosis was atrial flutter with 1-to-1 conduction*. There has been no recurrence over 6 months after empirical tricuspid-caval ablation, although this is admittedly not definitive.

Some very bizarre and difficult to explain aberration patterns can be seen at such rapid heart rates even in patients with no apparent heart disease. Flutter with 1-to-1 conduction must remain in the differential diagnosis even when the QRS morphology suggests VT. Adenosine given during the tachycardia in Figure 4-17A may have been diagnostic, but unfortunately was not done.

Figure 4-17B

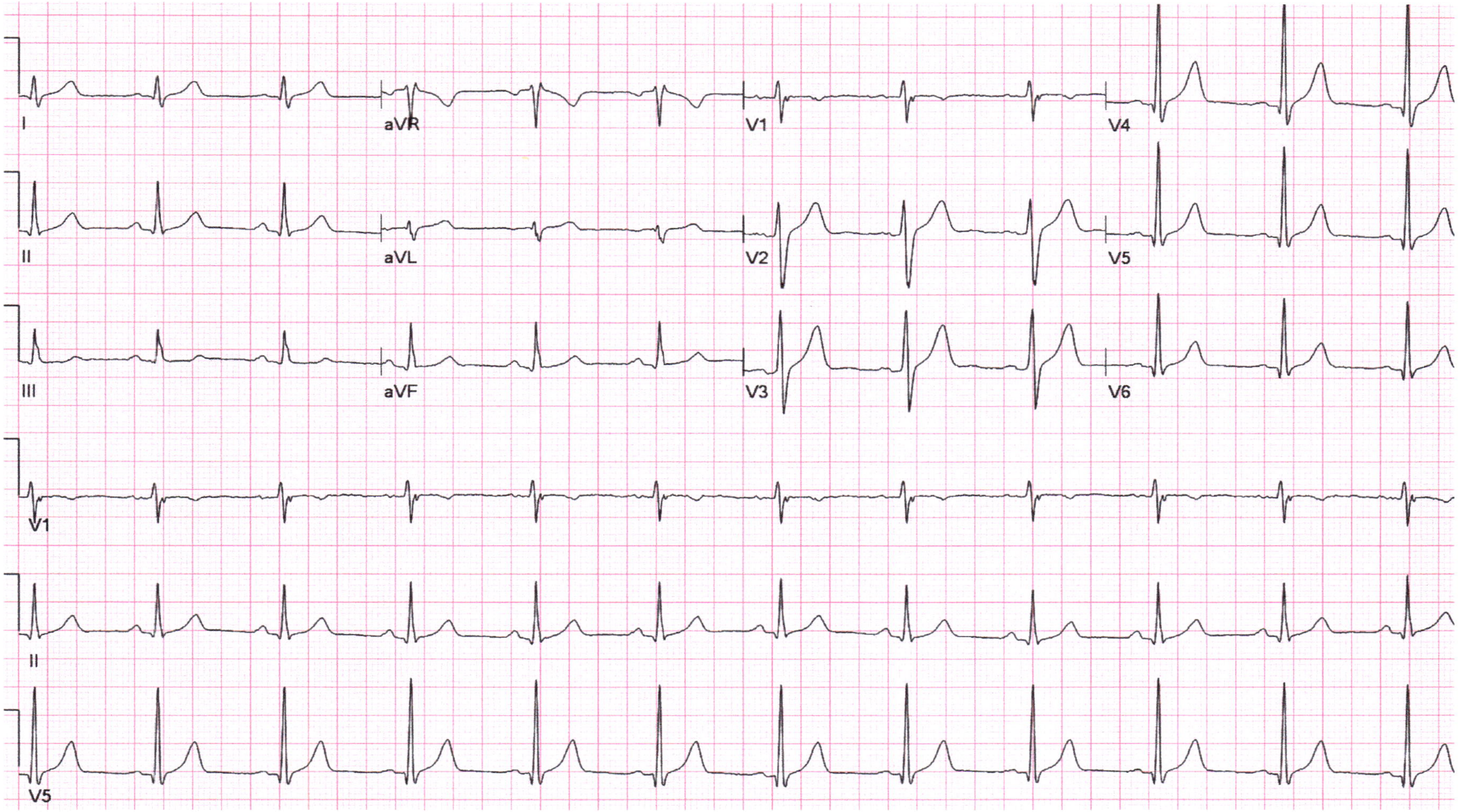

# Chapter 5

## The Rhythm Strip

Figure 5-1

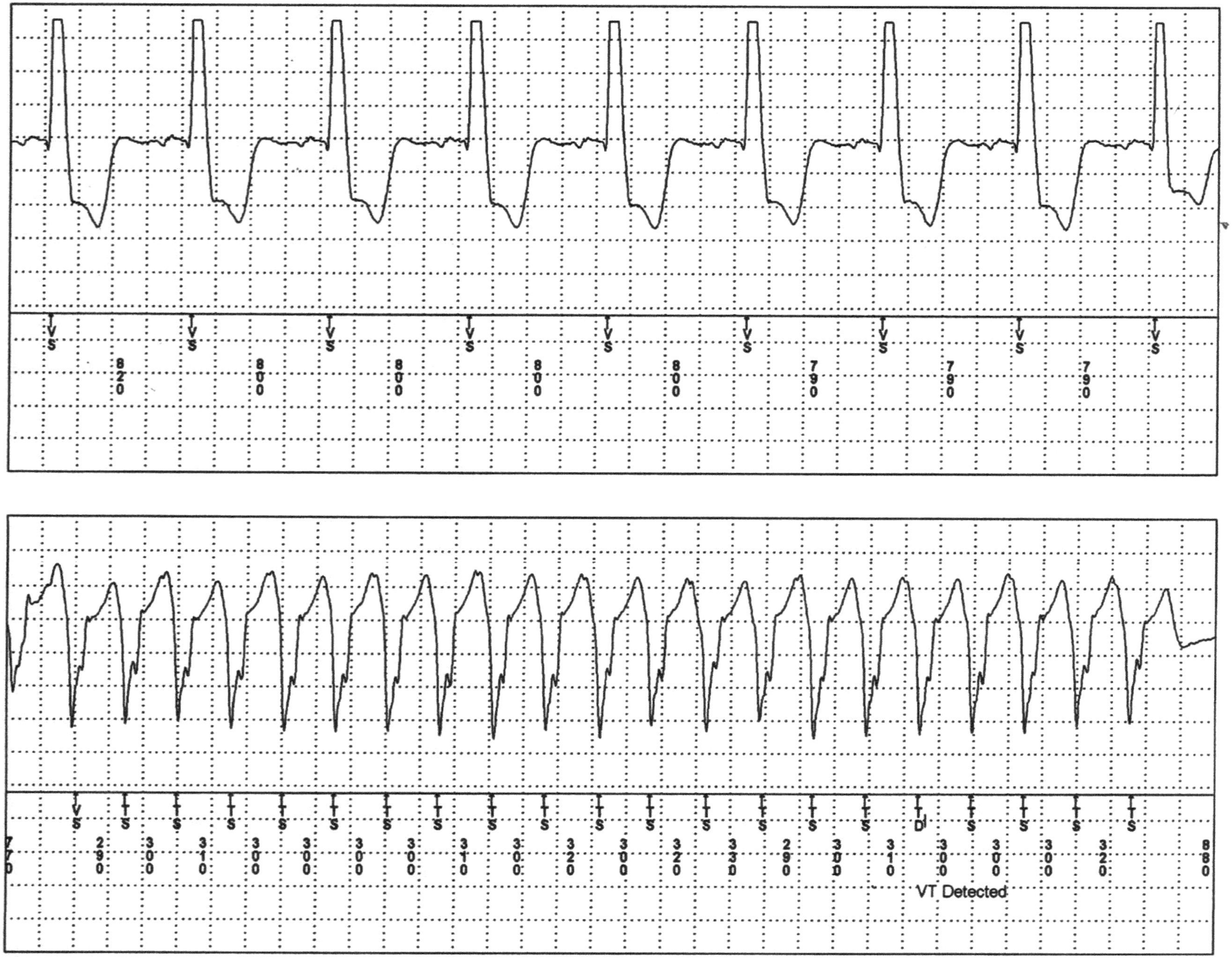
VS VS VS VS VS VS VS VS VS
820 800 800 800 800 790 790 790
VS TS TS TS TS TS TS TS TS TS TS TS TS TS TS TS TS TS TD TS TS TS TS TS
770 290 300 310 300 300 300 300 310 300 320 300 320 330 290 300 310 300 300 300 320 880
VT Detected

## Question 5-1

**Figure 5-1** shows a monitor recording (from an implantable loop recorder) of asymptomatic tachycardia. The most likely tachycardia mechanism is:

1. Ventricular tachycardia (VT)
2. Supraventricular tachycardia (SVT) with aberrancy
3. Atrial flutter (AFL)
4. Need more data

## Answer

The baseline rhythm is sinus with a wide QRS, and left bundle branch block (LBBB) was noted on the 12-lead ECG. We don't see the onset of this wide complex tachycardia (WCT) at a cycle length (CL) of approximately 300 ms. The strip is quite "clean" of artifact, and there is a notch at the top of every second T wave suggestive of a P wave. This would suggest VT with 2:1 retrograde conduction.

We further note that the baseline sinus rhythm at a relatively slow rate has a QRS with bundle branch block (LBBB on the full ECG). This would make it unlikely that a rapid SVT with right bundle branch block (RBBB) would emerge. This again strongly favors VT, which was the case in this instance.

In fact, *any tachycardia with QRS different from the bundle branch block pattern in the baseline rhythm is almost invariably VT.* My frequent teaching colleague Dr. Martin Green originally pointed out this observation to me—I often call it the "Green rule." I have, however, seen an exception to this rule in a patient with bundle branch block and an accessory pathway (AP) not apparent in sinus rhythm who developed a preexcited SVT.

Figure 5-2

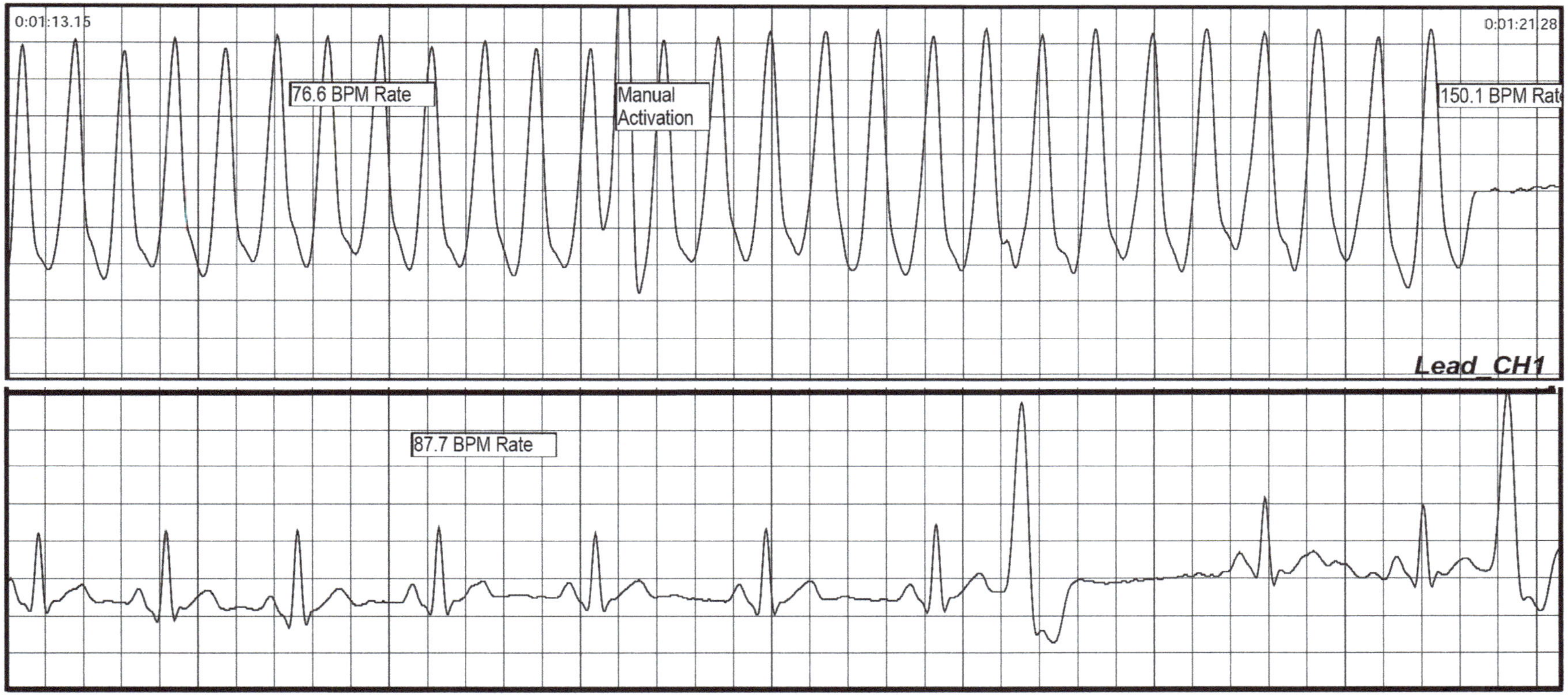


## Question 5-2

The mechanism of the WCT shown in **Figure 5-2** is:

1. VT
2. SVT with aberrancy
3. AFL with 1:1 AV conduction
4. Need more data

## Answer

The diagnosis of the WCT in the upper strip is challenging. P waves can't be seen with any confidence, and a single lead doesn't allow use of 12-lead QRS morphology criteria. The tachycardia onset, often very valuable diagnostically, is not available. It is likely that few would offer a confident diagnosis looking at this WCT.

The real clue to the puzzle comes from the lower strip, which shows 2 single extrasystoles. Neither is preceded by atrial activity, and each is followed by a negative deflection in the early ST segment—very suggestive of retrograde P waves. *These are clearly ventricular, and since the WCT has identical QRS morphology, the tachycardia is in all reasonable likelihood ventricular*—as was subsequently proven to be in this case.

The diagnosis of isolated extrasystoles is often more straightforward, and looking for any identical to the WCT in question can be very valuable.

Figure 5-3A

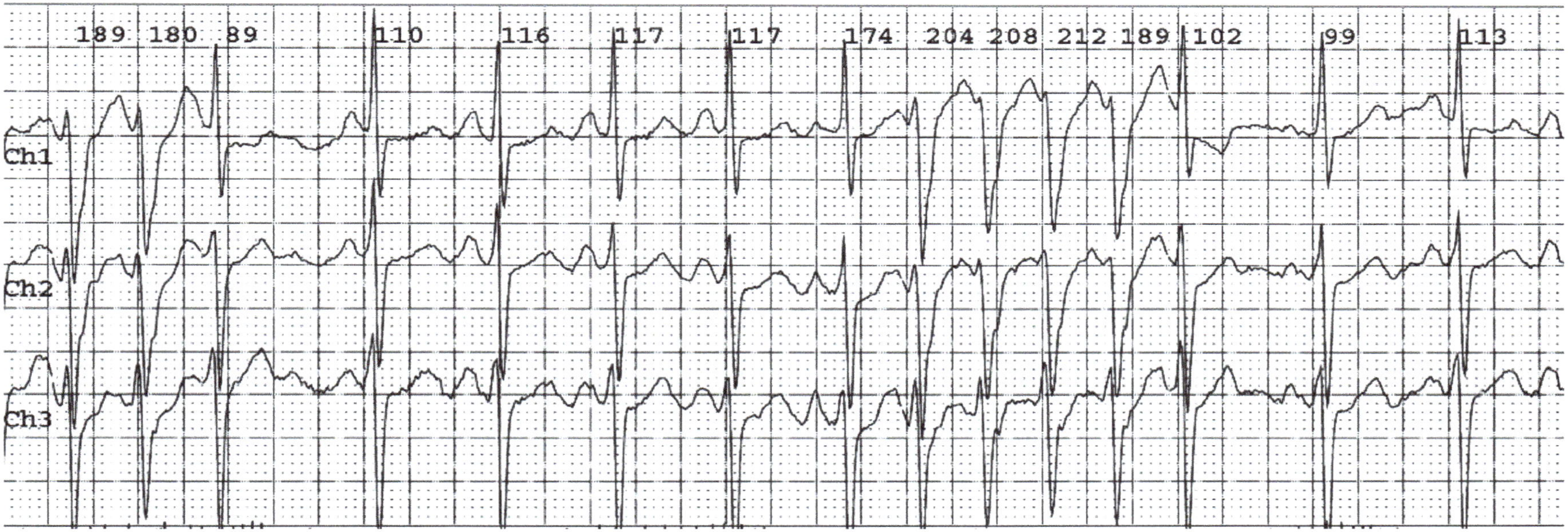


Question 5-3

## Question 5-3

The mechanism of the WCT shown in **Figure 5-3A** is:

1. VT
2. SVT with aberrancy
3. Preexcited SVT
4. Need more information

## Answer

This WCT allows us to examine both the onset and the termination of the tachycardia (**Figure 5-3B, arrows**). We see that the first beat of WCT is preceded by deformation of the P wave, best explained by a premature atrial contraction (PAC). VT initiation preceded by a PAC would be extremely coincidental.

The last beat of the tachycardia normalizes *without change* in the preceding CL. This makes VT very unlikely, since concealed retrograde conduction to the AV node during VT is almost universal, even in the absence of overt retrograde atrial conduction, and this would be expected to delay any supraventricular impulse arriving after the last QRS of VT.

In addition, a coincidental capture beat with such exact timing that *also terminated the VT* or arrived exactly at the spontaneous termination would be difficult to imagine. Note that we see this happen twice on our short strip, suggesting that a bundle branch is part of the circuit of this SVT. In this scenario, resolution of LBBB in AVRT over a left pathway would result in a shorter VA interval and termination of tachycardia if the AVN refractory period was reached.

Figure 5-3B

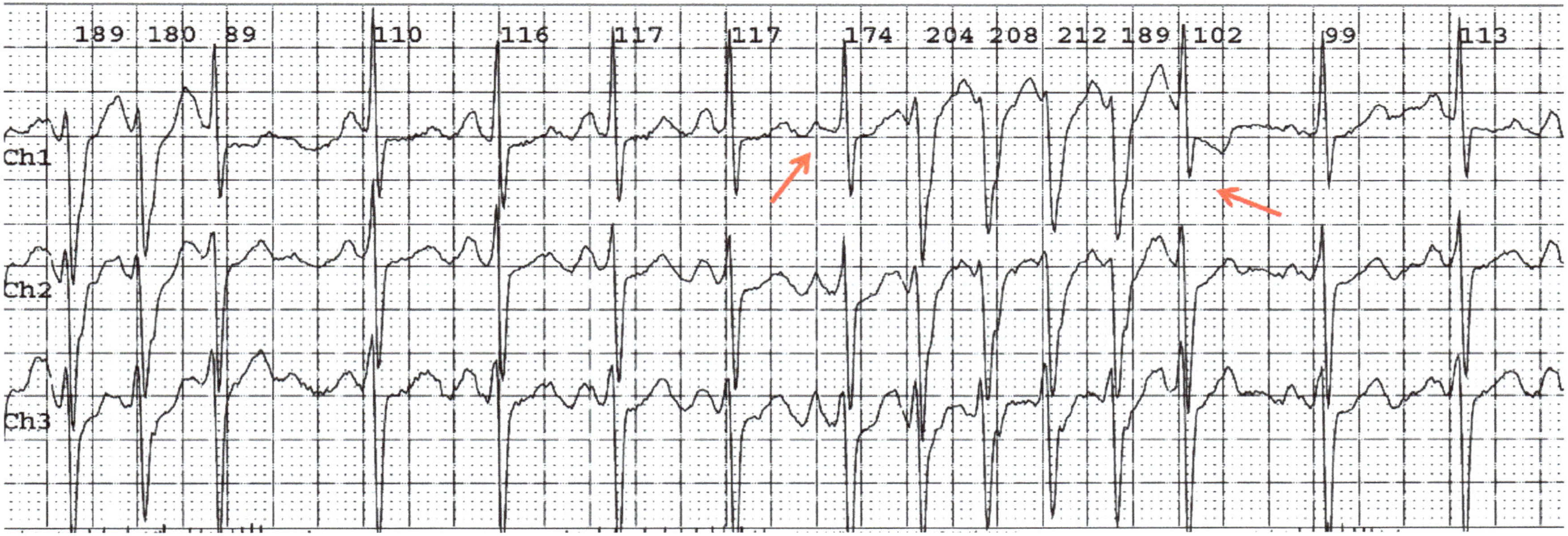
189 180 89 110 116 117 117 174 204 208 212 189 102 99 113
Ch1
Ch2
Ch3

Figure 5-4A

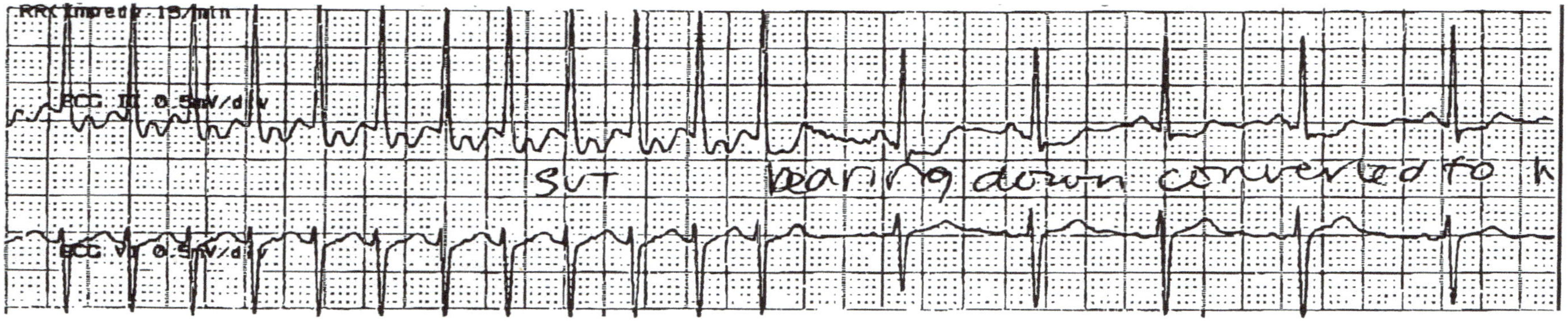


Figure 5-4B

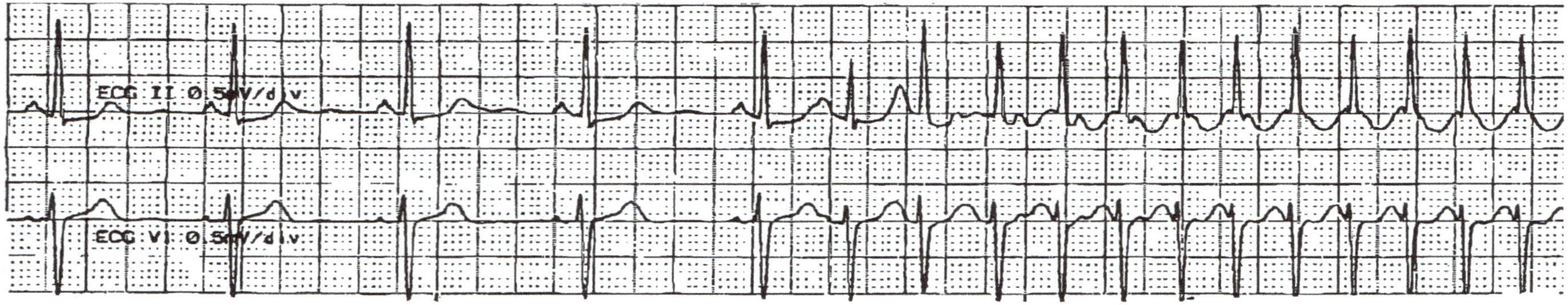

## Question 5-4

The most likely tachycardia mechanism for the tracings shown in **Figures 5-4A** and **5-4B** is:

1. Atrial tachycardia (AT)
2. Atrioventricular nodal reentrant tachycardia (AVNRT)
3. Atrioventricular reentrant tachycardia (AVRT)
4. Need more data

## Answer

This patient, a 54-year-old woman, was referred for recurrent "short-RP tachycardia, probably AVNRT." The tachycardia was observed to terminate after "bearing down" (Figure 5-4A). This initial diagnosis is certainly reasonable, although generally such a tachycardia would terminate in the anterograde slow pathway (i.e., last event being a retrograde P wave) with vagal stimulation.

The tachycardia recurred shortly after (Figure 5-4B), and the onset tells a more complete story. The SVT begins with a couple of PACs and seems established by the third beat. The RP interval, similar to that in Figure 5-4A, shortens progressively and disappears in the QRS as the tachycardia speeds up slightly, making the diagnosis of AT obvious.

The designation of "short RP" is merely an ECG descriptor and doesn't mean that conduction is proceeding from QRS to P. Did the referring doctor look at the upper tracing and make up his mind too early? AT may terminate with vagal maneuvers, or the termination may have been coincidental.

Figure 5-5A

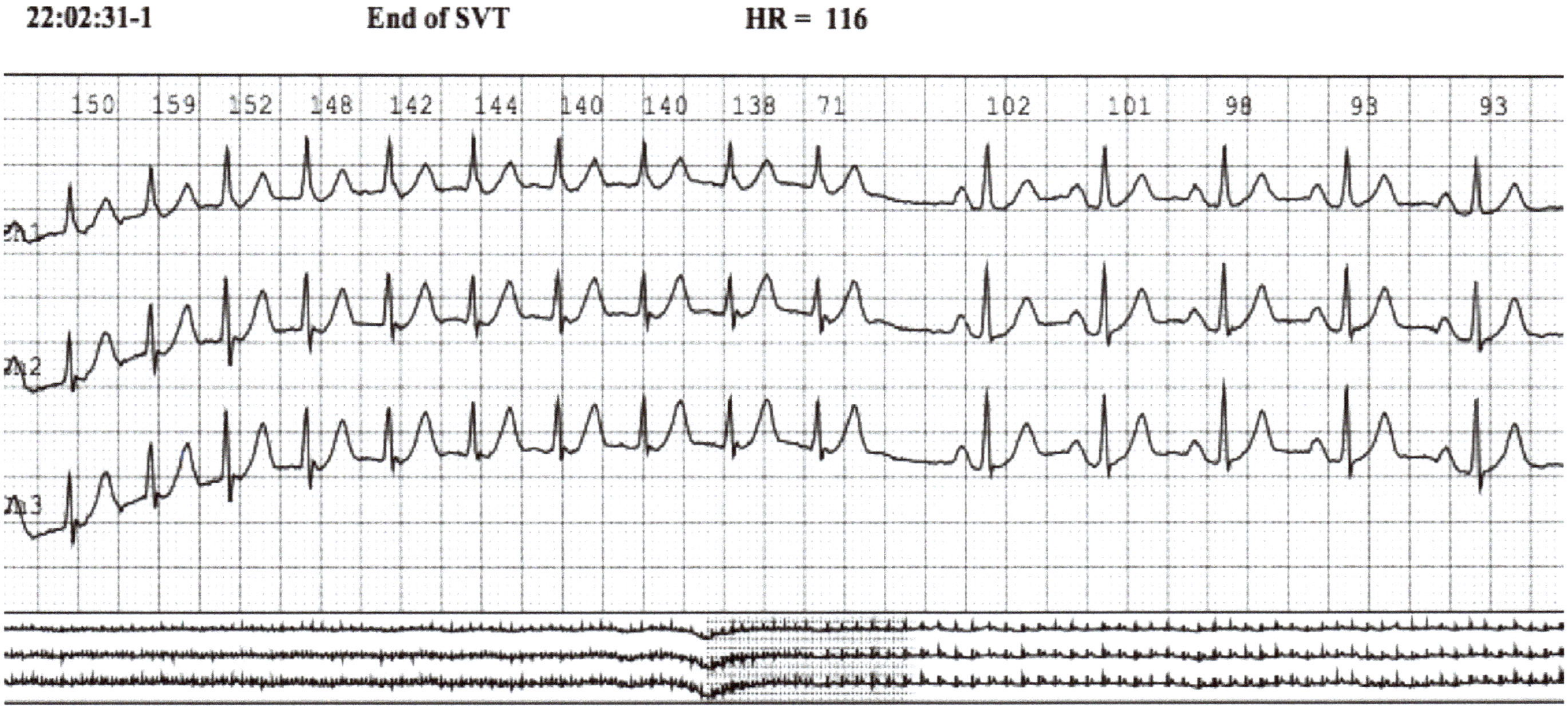


## Question 5-5

The mechanism of SVT shown in **Figure 5-5A** is:

1. AT
2. AVNRT
3. AVRT
4. Need more data

## Answer

The key to this diagnosis is the identification of P waves. The tracing is quite free of artifact, facilitating the identification of more subtle points. The P waves are not immediately obvious. The most useful step is a careful "side-by-side" comparison of the tachycardia beat and the sinus beat, which in this tracing is conveniently facilitated by them being adjacent to each other.

The **blue arrows** in **Figure 5-5B** highlight the difference between the 2, and a small deflection after the QRS during SVT, but not present in sinus rhythm, is most probably the missing P wave.

The tachycardia ends with a P wave. This virtually rules out AT, since of course it would be very coincidental if AV block occurred at the exact cycle that AT terminated. The PR interval during tachycardia is very long, reflecting conduction over a slow AV nodal pathway. The VA interval (or RP interval) is too short to be AV reentry.

The P wave in this clean record can only be "hiding" at the end of the QRS during tachycardia and not elsewhere, noting that the ST segment and T wave are identical in sinus rhythm and tachycardia.

Thus, the correct answer here is Option 2, AVNRT.

Figure 5-5B

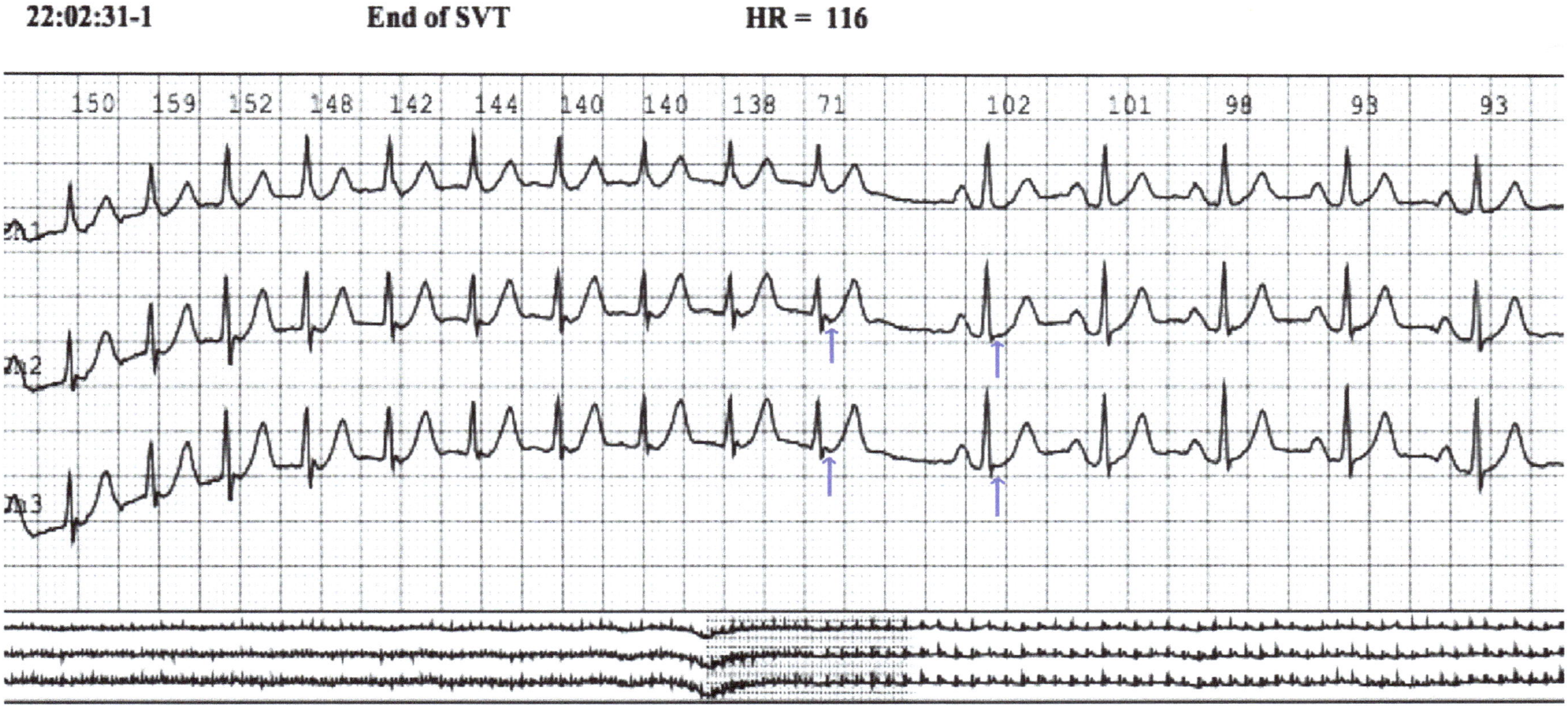
22:02:31-1
End of SVT
HR = 116
150
159
152
148
142
144
140
140
138
71
102
101
98
93
93

Figure 5-6A

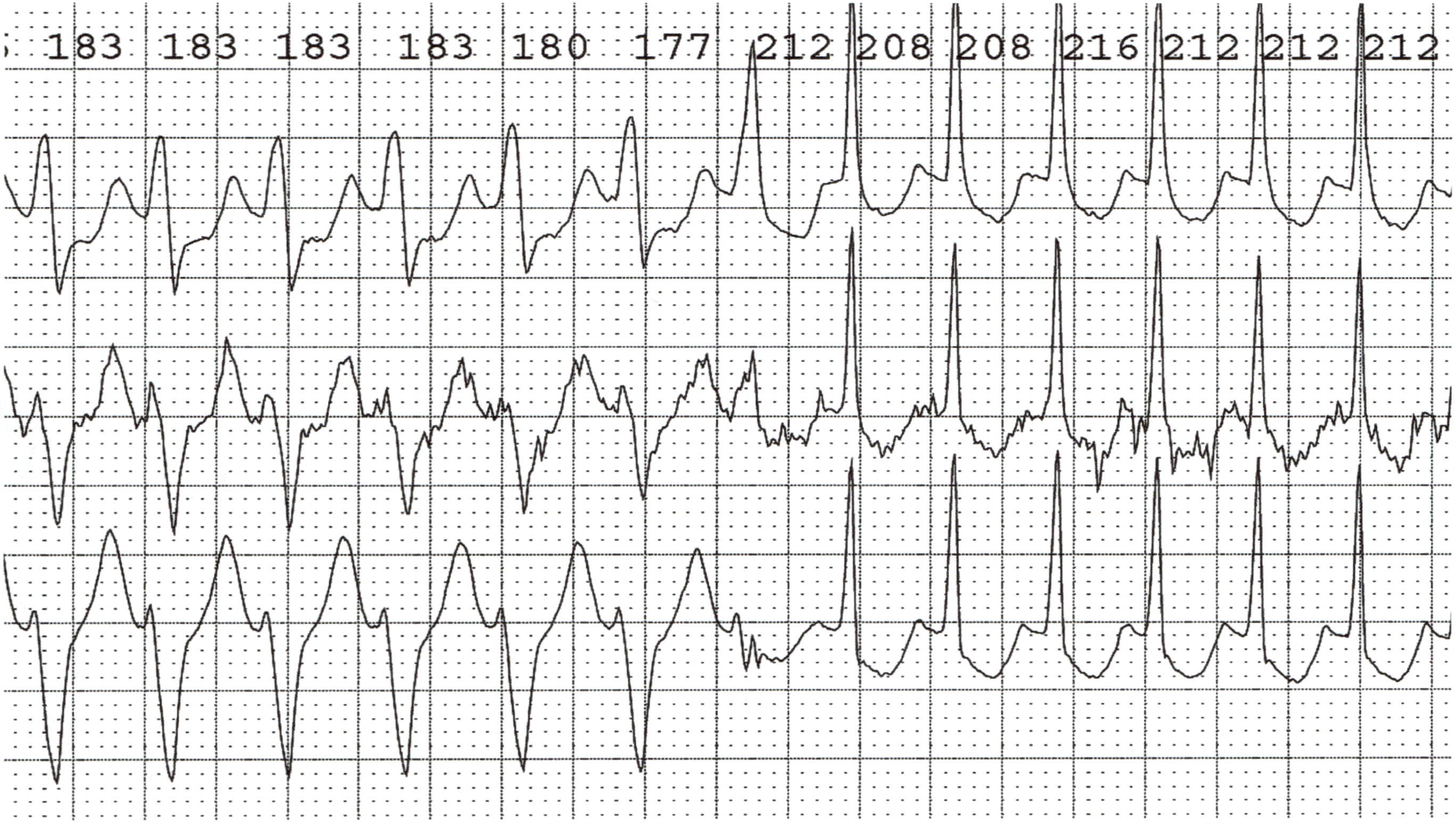

## Question 5-6

Question 5-6

The tachycardia mechanism in **Figure 5-6A** is:

1. AT
2. AVNRT
3. AVRT
4. VT and SVT

## Answer

The numbers at the top of this 3-channel rhythm strip show instantaneous heart rate for the cycle indicated (i.e., inverse of CL). One hardly needs to measure anything to establish the "big picture." A WCT is interrupted by a "different" QRS most compatible with a premature ventricular contraction (PVC) and turns into a narrow SVT, slightly faster than the WCT.

We first ask ourselves if this is all one tachycardia or 2 different tachycardias. In general, it is far more likely that it is one tachycardia, just on the basis of prevalence. For example, if we concluded that the WCT were VT, we would have to postulate that a very late-coupled PVC not only stopped the VT but initiated an SVT on the same beat—not impossible, but less plausible.

If we hypothesize that it is all one mechanism with a rate change in the tachycardia, the answer is easy. *Any tachycardia that changes rate purely on the basis of a change in QRS, from a bundle branch block pattern to normal,* **must** *incorporate the involved bundle branch in its mechanism.*

The WCT here had a LBBB pattern (seen on 12-lead ECG, not shown). Our case is therefore well and simply explained by AVRT over a left AP with and without LBBB aberration. The smaller circuit size during normal QRS (i.e., distal LBB to the left AP) becomes longer with development of LBBB (reflecting the extra time to get from the RBB to the left AP).

Obviously, neither AT nor AVNRT would incur a rate change in the event of any bundle branch block.

We can be a little more certain by making some measurements (**Figure 5-6B**). Although subtle, P wave activity is visible during both tachycardias (**black arrows**). The VA interval during WCT is longer than that during narrow QRS tachycardia, again explicable by AVRT over a left AP.

We see further that the PVC that initiates the change has its initial portion "on time" (**asterisks**) and with the same morphology as the WCT. Thus, it is a very compelling fusion beat between the PVC and the WCT. Finally, this fusion beat advances the next P wave (338 to 307 ms) *and the next QRS*. This is, of course, analogous to the "His-refractory PVC" fusion, indicating that the His had to be refractory. This PVC advances the next P wave, proving the presence of the AP in the tachycardia.

It seems intuitively obvious that a late PVC that gets into the circuit must have good access to the "excitable gap" of the circuit, explicable by a left PVC near a left AP. We can also look at this as "fusion with reset," which is the hallmark of a macroreentrant arrhythmia that AVRT represents.

To be very clear and simple, there is *no* chance that a late PVC such as this would influence AT or AVNRT.

Figure 5-6B

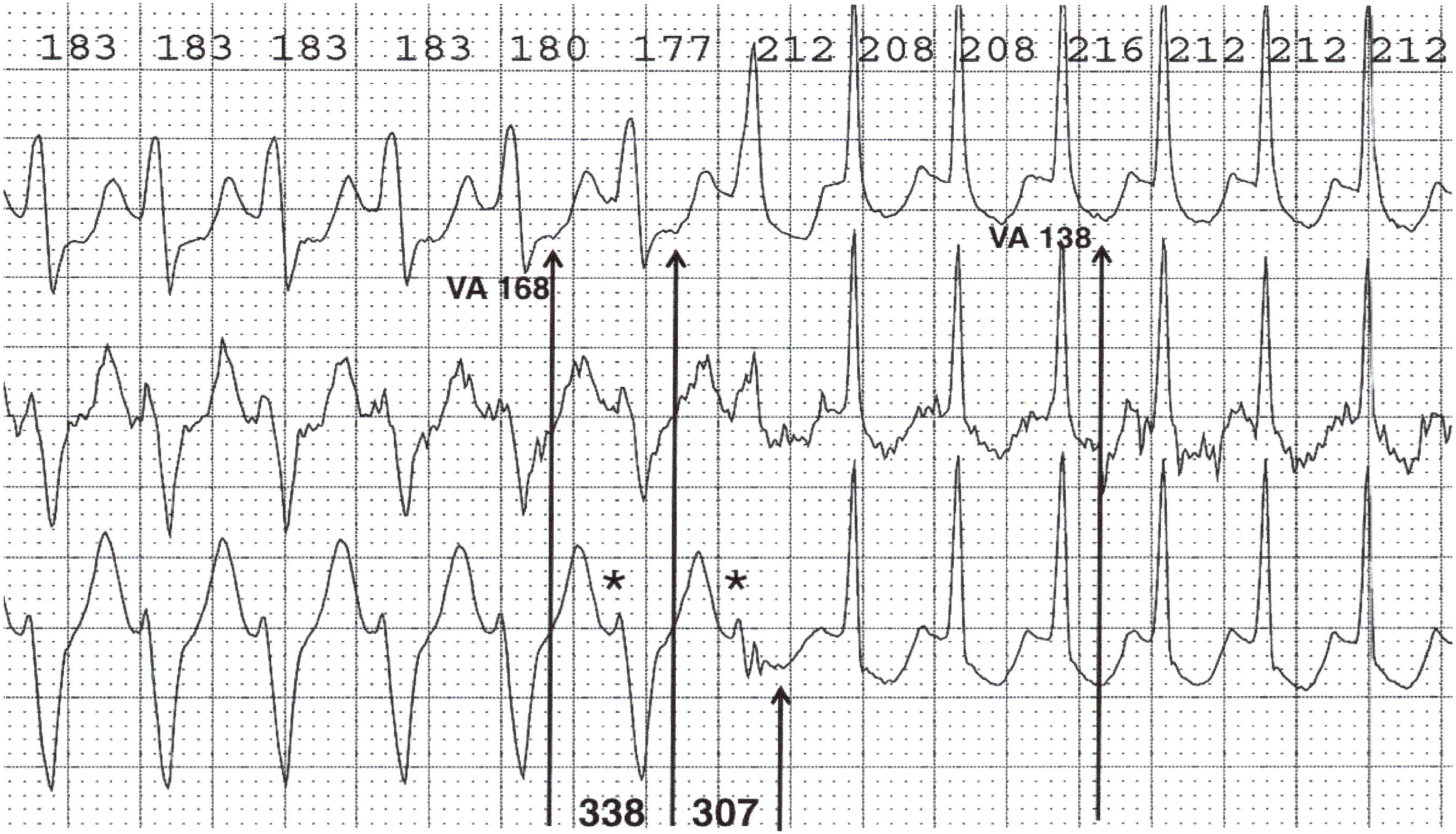
183
183
183
183
180
177
212
208
208
216
212
212
212
VA 168
VA 138
*
*
338
307

Figure 5-7A

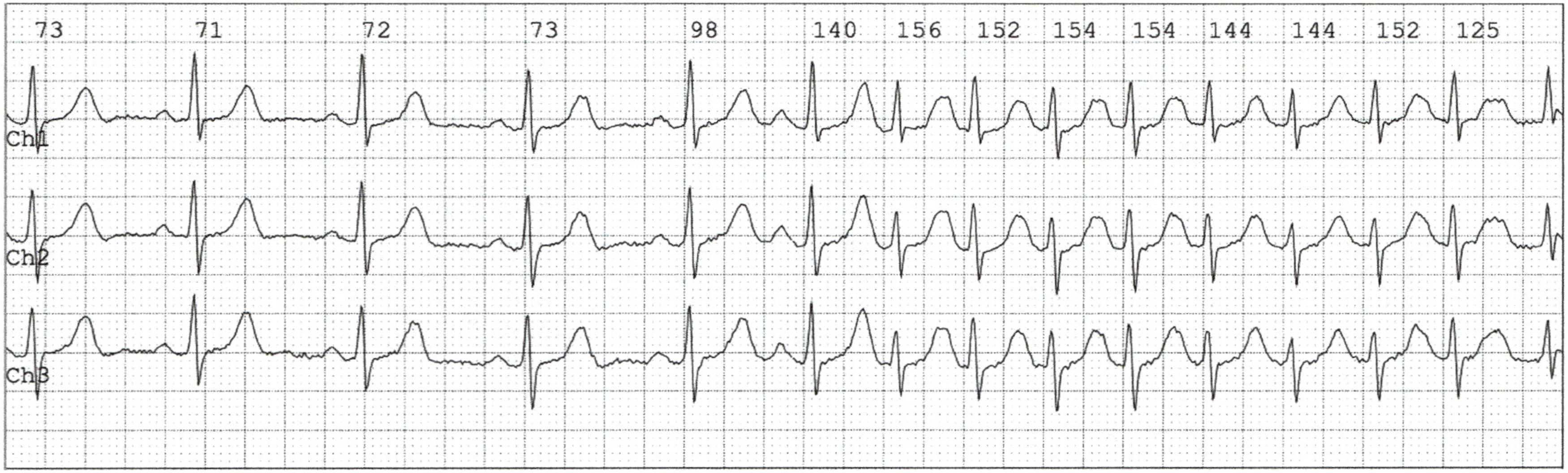

## Question 5-7

Question 5-7

The mechanism of SVT in the ECG shown in **Figure 5-7A** is:

1. AT
2. AVNRT
3. AVRT
4. Junctional tachycardia (JT)

## Answer

**Figure 5-7A** depicts the onset of a narrow QRS tachycardia identical to sinus, clearly SVT. Atrial activity is not easily evident during tachycardia.

The tachycardia begins with 2 PACs (**asterisks** in **Figure 5-7B**), the second of which manifests as distortion of the T wave—that is, a taller T wave in this case, appreciated after careful comparison with the T wave of the sinus beats. There is *no* prolongation of the PR interval with these 2 PACs, PR prolongation being almost universally required for onset of junctional reentrant tachycardia, AVNRT or AVRT. (However, note that the permanent form of junctional reciprocating tachycardia- (PJRT-) type of SVT—as described by the late Philippe Coumel—can begin by sinus acceleration without precedent ectopy or PR prolongation.)

A second important observation is the vector of the P wave during tachycardia. Although we are not sure of the exact ECG leads, the tachycardia P is in the same direction as the sinus P wave and is most probably "high-to-low," essentially ruling out AVNRT and AVRT. Careful inspection of the T waves during tachycardia (i.e., the last 3 cycles, horizontal bars) shows a slight variability of the T wave, most compatible with variability of the tachycardia cycle length (TCL) causing variable ECG summation (electrocardiographic "fusion") of P and T.

Figure 5-7B

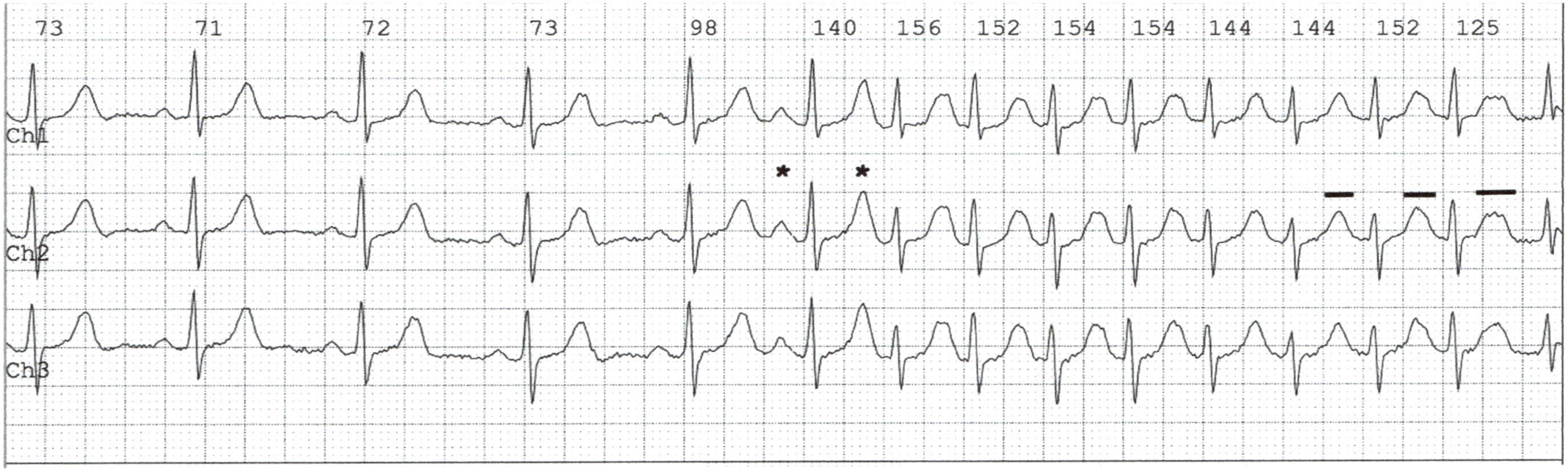

Figure 5-8A

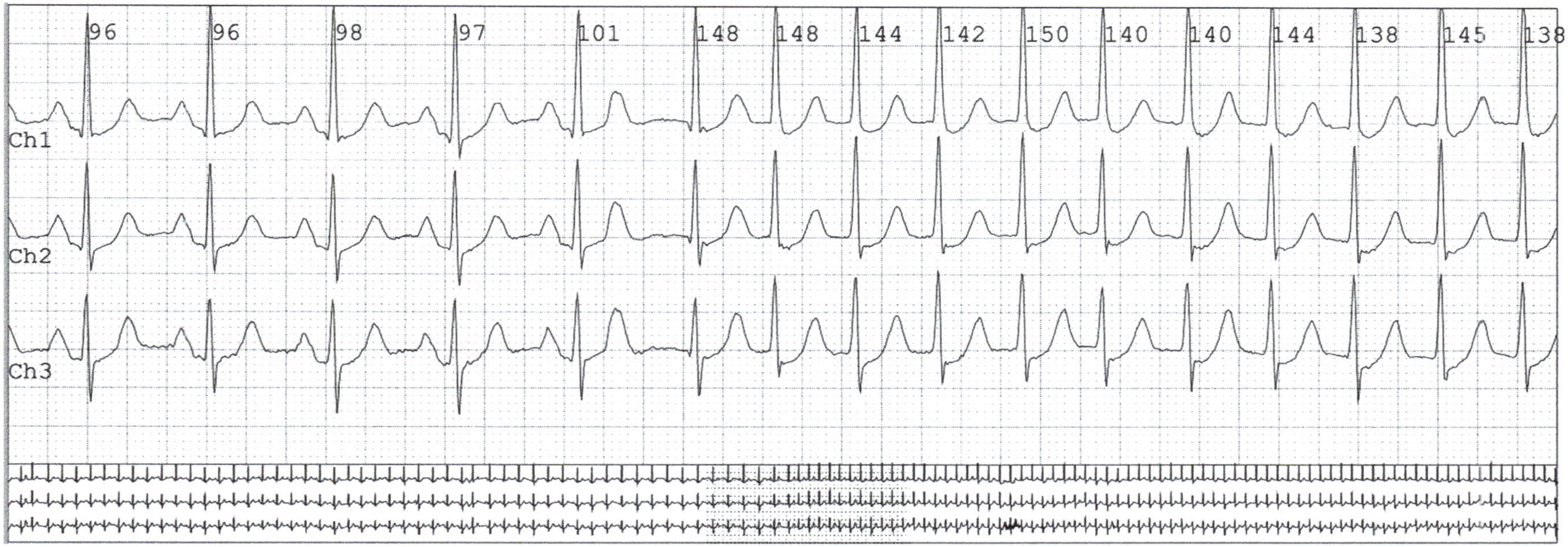


## Question 5-8

This 58-year-old man has recurrent tachycardia represented by the figure. The mechanism of SVT in the ECG shown in **Figure 5-8A** is:

1. AT
2. AVNRT
3. AVRT
4. JT

Question 5-8

## Answer

Figure 5-8A depicts the onset of a narrow QRS tachycardia (QRS identical to sinus)—clearly SVT. Atrial activity is not immediately obvious during tachycardia.

The tachycardia begins with a PAC (**asterisk** in **Figure 5-8B**) that distorts the T wave, that is, creating a taller T wave in this case, *appreciated after careful comparison with the T wave of the last sinus beat.*

There is now *marked* prolongation of the PR interval (**horizontal line**) indicating conduction over a slow AV nodal pathway. This is most probably AVNRT, although AVRT may also involve anterograde conduction over a slow anterograde AV node pathway. It could theoretically also be junctional tachycardia after the PAC blocks in the AV node, although this would be at least statistically much less likely.

A second observation comes from a careful search for atrial activity during SVT (see **Question 5-5**), and in particular, comparison of the terminal QRS complex of tachycardia versus sinus rhythm (**open circles**). A subtle change during SVT, best appreciated by a direct "side-by-side" comparison of the complexes in sinus rhythm vs. tachycardia, suggests the presence of atrial activity at the end of the QRS during tachycardia, and this tracing now is most compatible with AVNRT. Of course, such a short RP interval rules out AVRT.

*It is also worth repeating that a P wave that's not obvious "hides" best within a QRS or merges with the T wave.*

Figure 5-8B

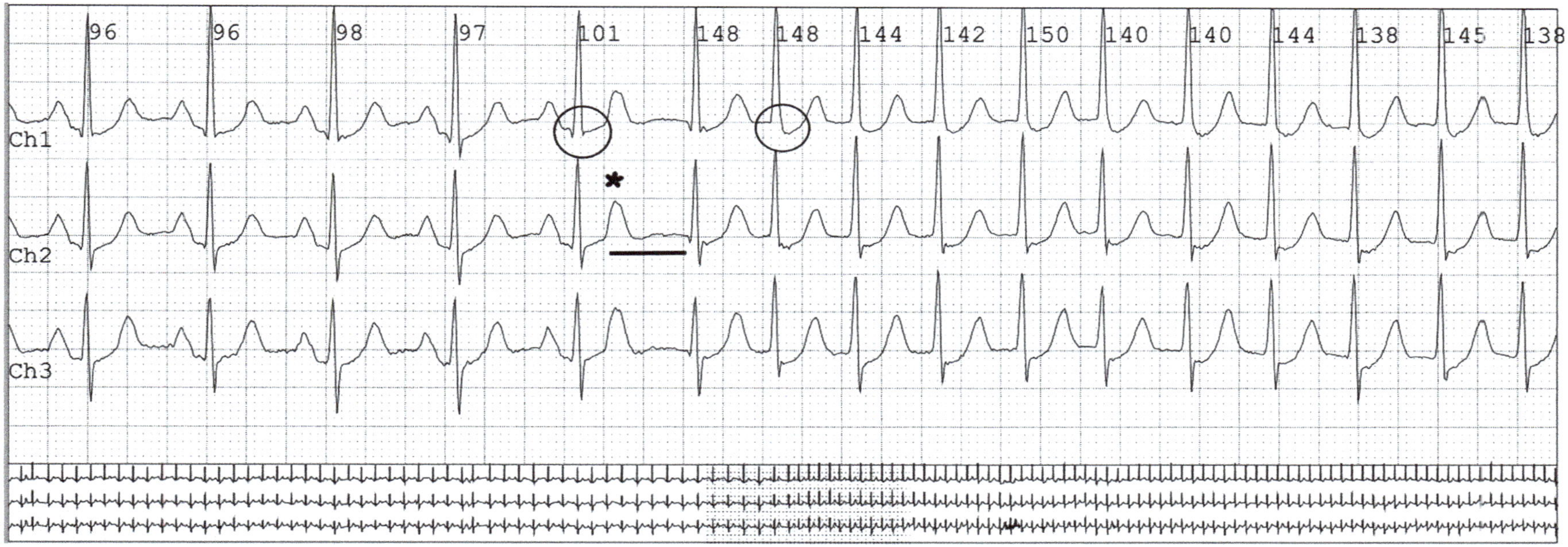
96
96
98
97
101
148
148
144
142
150
140
140
144
138
145
138
Ch1
Ch2
Ch3
*

Figure 5-9A

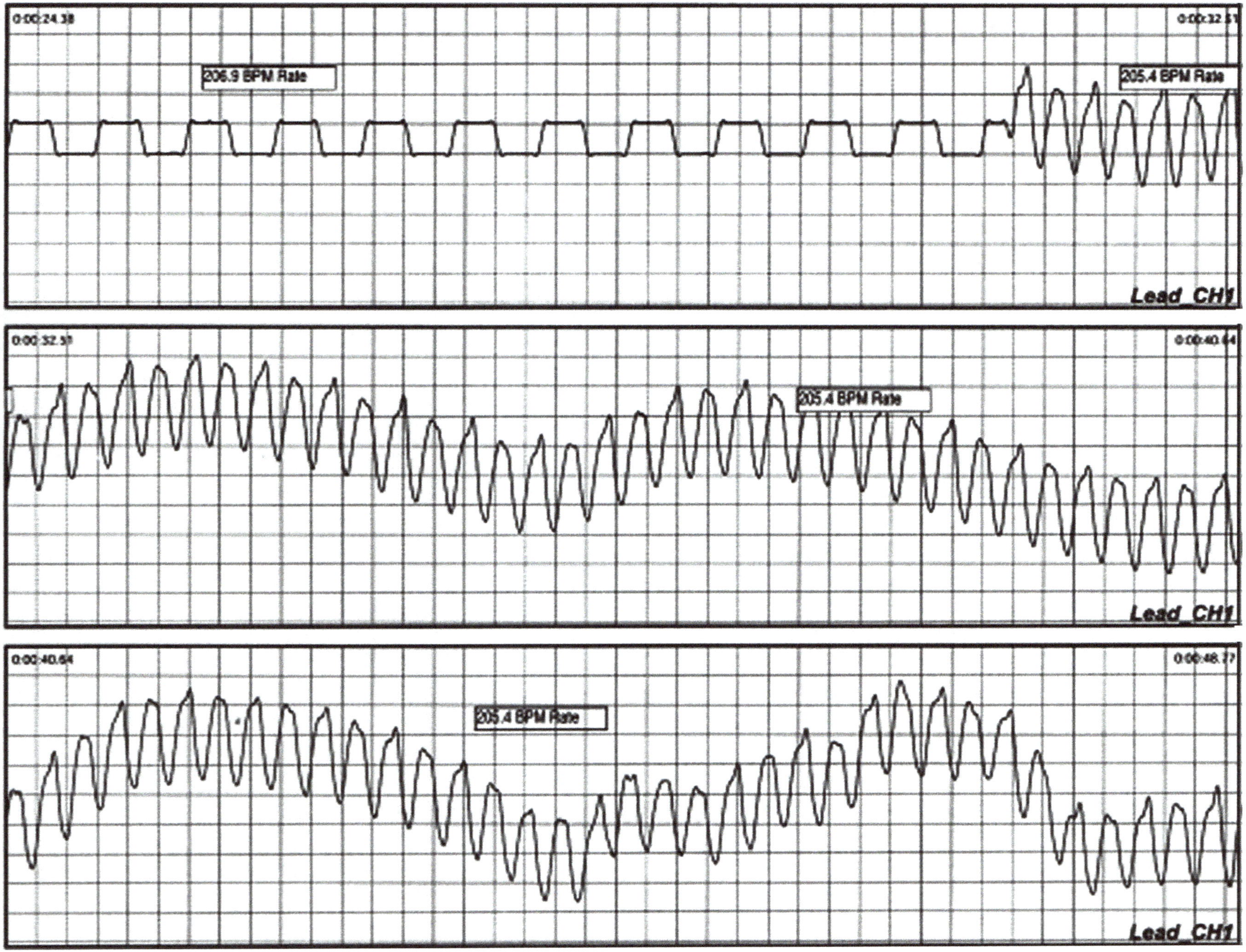
0:00:24.38
206.9 BPM Rate
0:00:32.51
205.4 BPM Rate
Lead_CH1
0:00:32.51
205.4 BPM Rate
0:00:40.64
Lead_CH1
0:00:40.64
205.4 BPM Rate
0:00:48.77
Lead_CH1

## Question 5-9

A 38-year-old man without known heart disease was monitored for palpitations, as shown in **Figure 5-9A**. The mechanism of tachycardia is:

1. VT
2. AFL with aberrancy
3. Antidromic tachycardia
4. Need more data

## Answer

It does not take a long time to throw in the towel on this rhythm strip. The patient was remarkably well during this tachycardia, but that is, of course, not helpful diagnostically. It is well known that the patient could be in extremis during SVT and relatively asymptomatic during VT. Any of the multiple-choice options are viable, and we clearly need more data.

The needed information is forthcoming a short time later in **Figure 5-9B**, which reveals the diagnosis as AFL, in this case with aberrancy. Even a 12-lead ECG might not help here as there is virtually no chance of seeing atrial activity. In addition, aberrancy at this heart rate can have bizarre and difficult to explain aberration patterns suggestive of VT. Fortuitous observation of higher-grade AV block came to the rescue in this instance.

Figure 5-9B

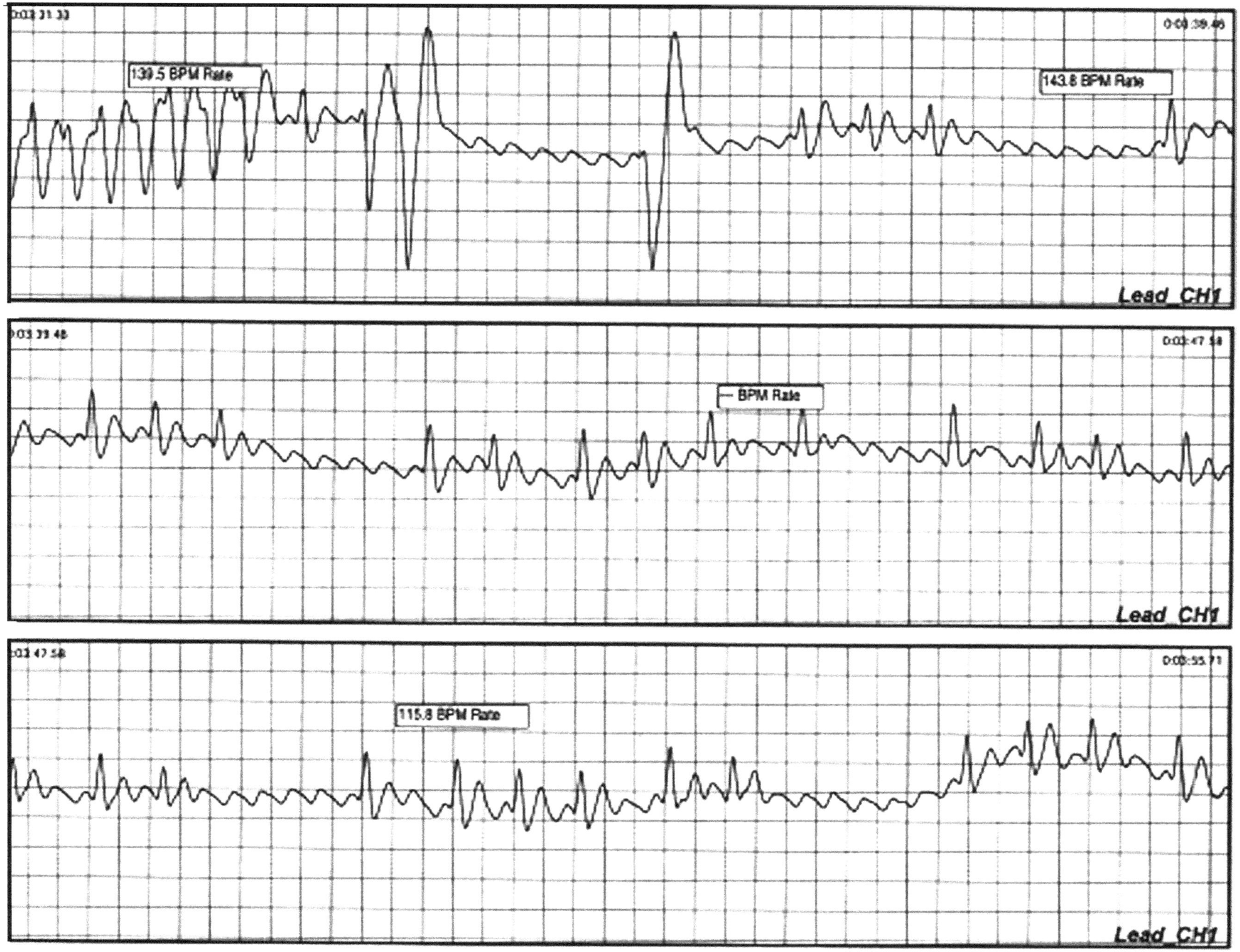
139.5 BPM Rate
143.8 BPM Rate
Lead_CH1
BPM Rate
Lead_CH1
115.8 BPM Rate
Lead_CH1

Figure 5-10A

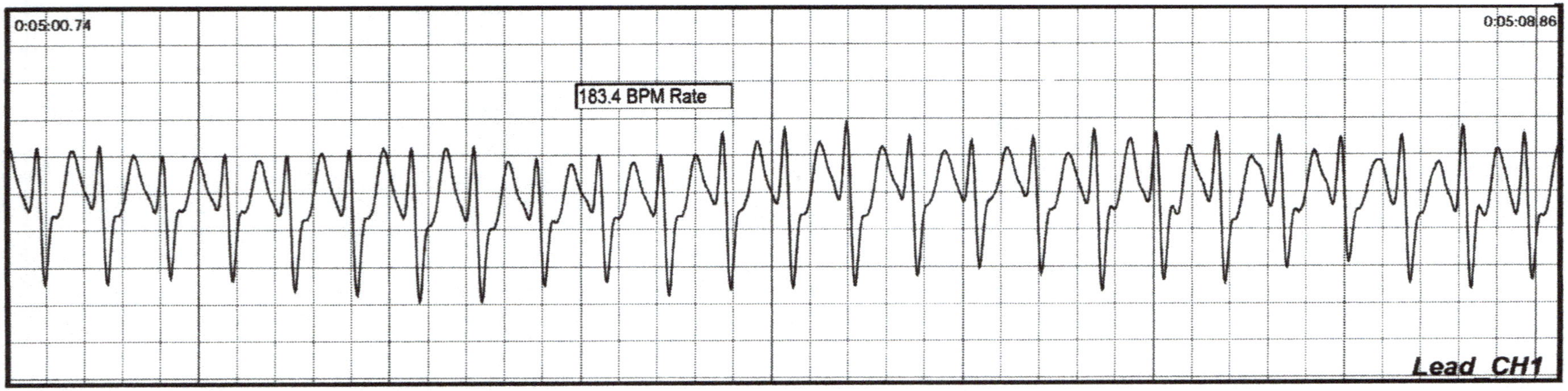

## Question 5-10

The QRS in the monitored strip shown in **Figure 5-10A** is identical to that seen in normal sinus rhythm (not shown).
The mechanism of tachycardia is:

1. AT
2. AVNRT
3. AVRT
4. Need more data

## Answer

This is a "clean" strip with minimal artifact, but there is no evident atrial activity on initial inspection of this record, a regular SVT at 180 beats per minute (bpm). A little notch continuous with the end of the QRS may suggest a P wave, but it is subtle and would be a tenuous call. A careful inspection of each T wave is more rewarding. The last 5 or 6 complexes show a subtle but distinct variability of the T wave shape best explained by a slightly inconstant "merger" (electrocardiographic fusion) of the T wave and subsequent P wave.

This becomes more apparent on inspection of an earlier segment of this tachycardia. The P waves are much more distinct at the beginning of **Figure 5-10B** and merge with the T wave with slight acceleration of the atrial rate. The best answer to our multiple question is AT. It could also reasonably be sinus tachycardia, but this would be a poor choice, as it is always wise to pick one of the options given in a multiple-choice question!

Figure 5-10B

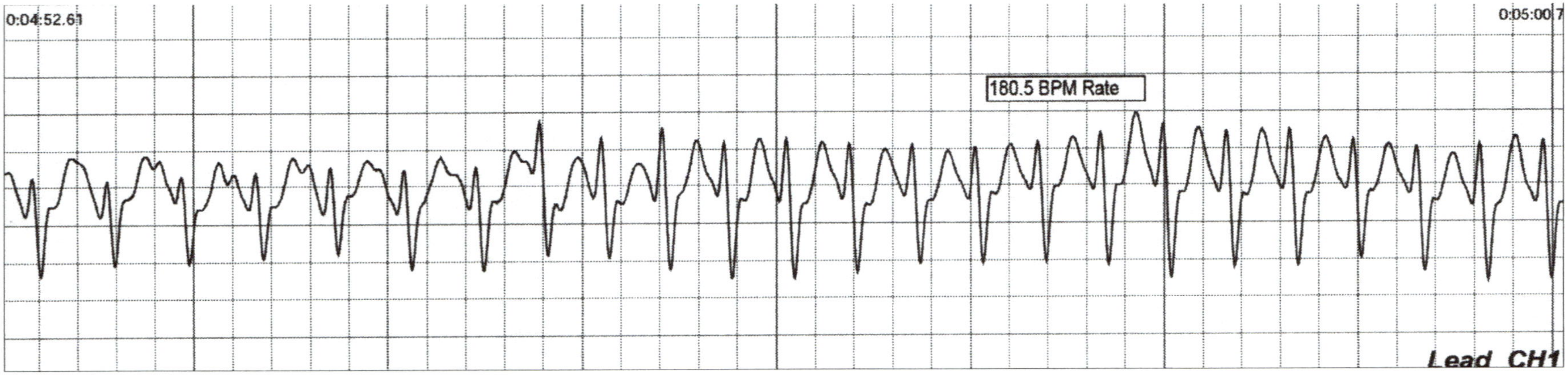

Figure 5-11

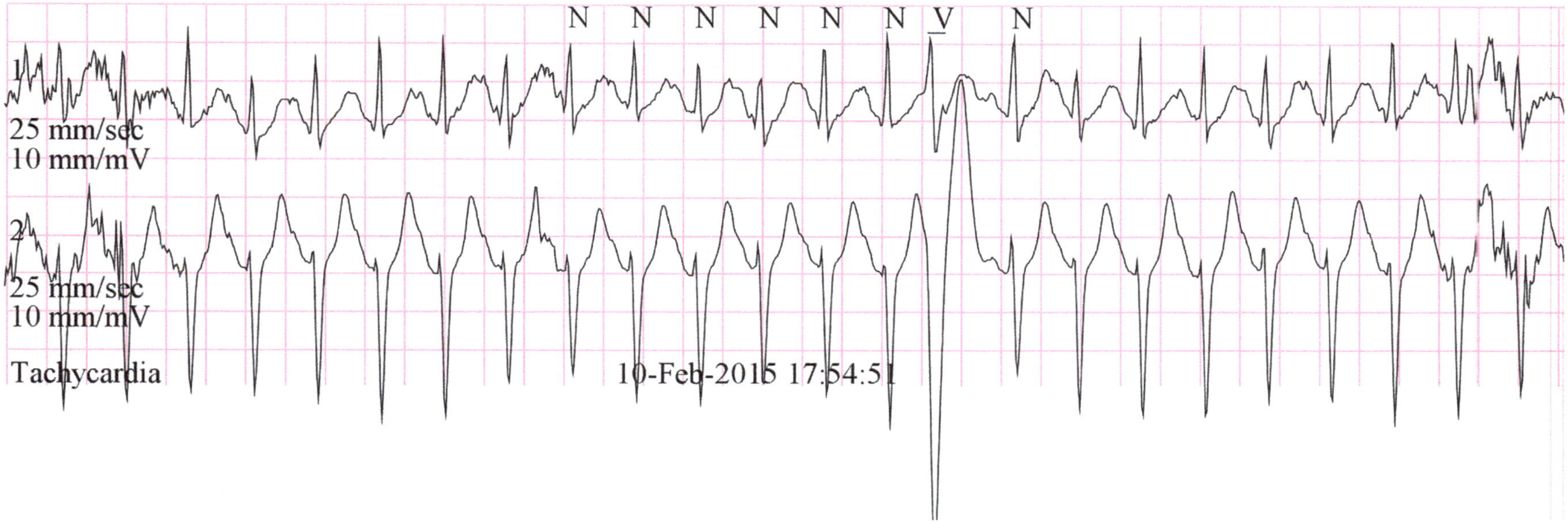




## Question 5-11

The QRS in the monitored strip shown in **Figure 5-11** is identical to that seen in normal sinus rhythm (not shown). The indication for monitoring was palpitations, but the patient was asymptomatic during the event.

The mechanism of tachycardia is:

1. AT
2. Sinus tachycardia (ST)
3. AVNRT
4. AVRT

## Answer

There is little hope of identifying P waves with confidence on most of this strip. However, the experienced electrocardiographer will immediately focus on the "gap" after the ectopic beat—most likely a PVC. An upright P wave in both the monitored frontal leads becomes obvious, and comparison with the sinus P wave elsewhere in the recording (not shown) shows it to be identical.

A subtle notch on the downslope of the T wave then becomes more evident and credible as the probable P wave during tachycardia (i.e., the "notch to QRS onset" is comparable to the "P to QRS onset" after the PVC).

Putting all our information together, this is probably ST, although we can't rigidly exclude AT. This should not be a complicated tracing for the reader but illustrates the value of looking for "irregularity" (in this case the diastolic "gap" after the PVC) in the monotony of the ongoing tachycardia.

Figure 5-12A

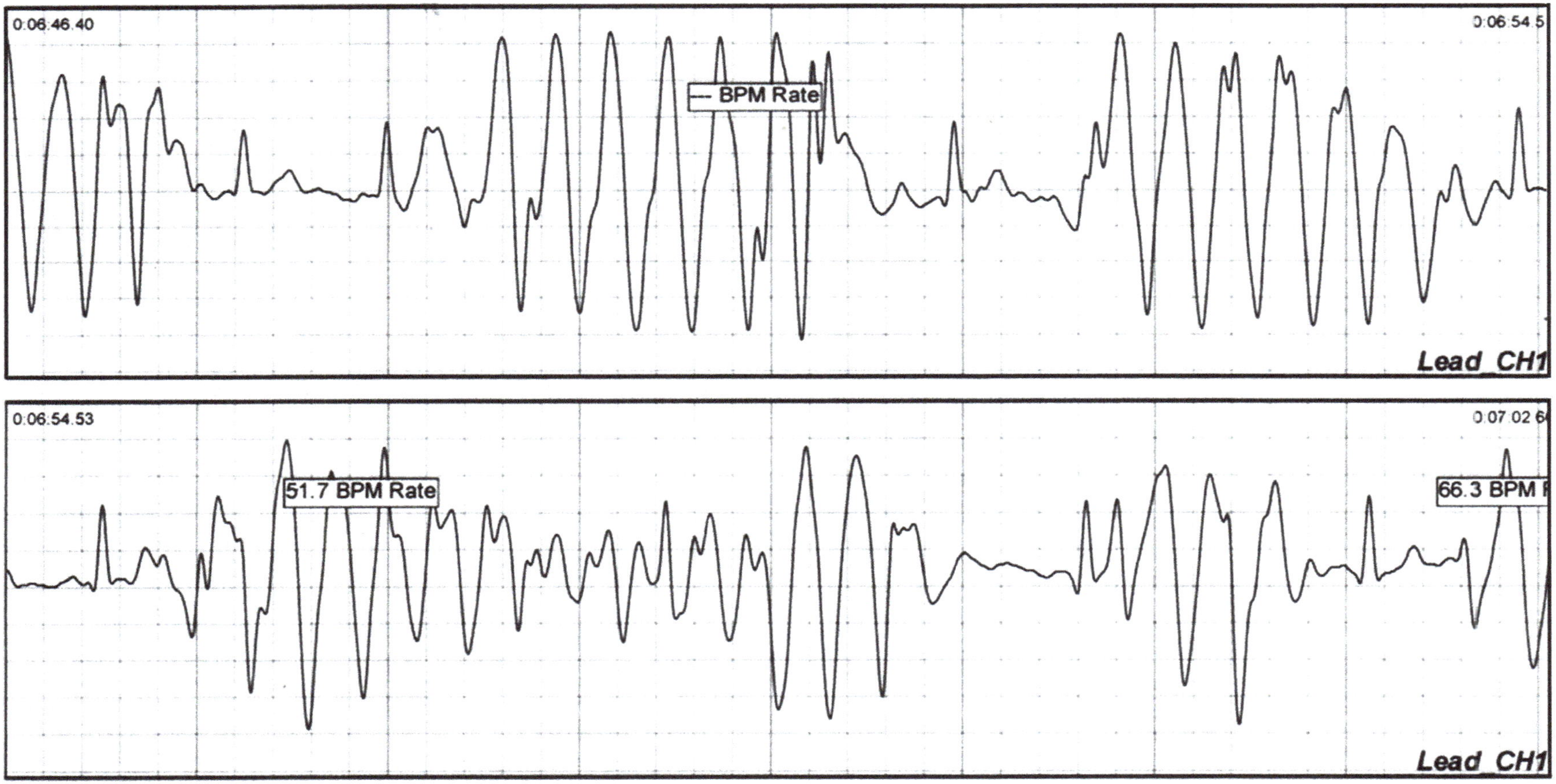


## Question 5-12

The strips in **Figure 5-12A** generated an urgent referral to the arrhythmia service. They are not continuous. The mechanism of tachycardia is:

1. Polymorphic VT
2. Torsades de pointes
3. Preexcited AF
4. Other

## Answer

The immediate clue that something is amiss is the wandering baseline and baseline noise. One is fortunate to identify 2 consecutive normal QRS complexes at the onset of strip 1 (Figure 5-12A).

One can then set calipers to this cycle and trace through the recording (**dots** in **Figure 5-12B**), after which the underlying sinus rhythm becomes apparent. *Another critical clue to the presence of artifact masquerading as arrhythmia is the presence of non-physiological intervals.* The **blue dots** identify such intervals. The first blue dot indicates a normal QRS followed within 100 ms by a sharp "pseudo" QRS. Such a short refractory period would not be physiologic (unless one were a chipmunk). This is an absolute "smoking gun" that indicates the presence of artifact.

To summarize, useful features to identify artifact pseudoarrhythmia include the presence of a wandering baseline and baseline noise and non-physiologic phenomena. If at least 2 normal QRS complexes are present, the calipers can be set to this interval looking for the underlying rhythm.

Figure 5-12B

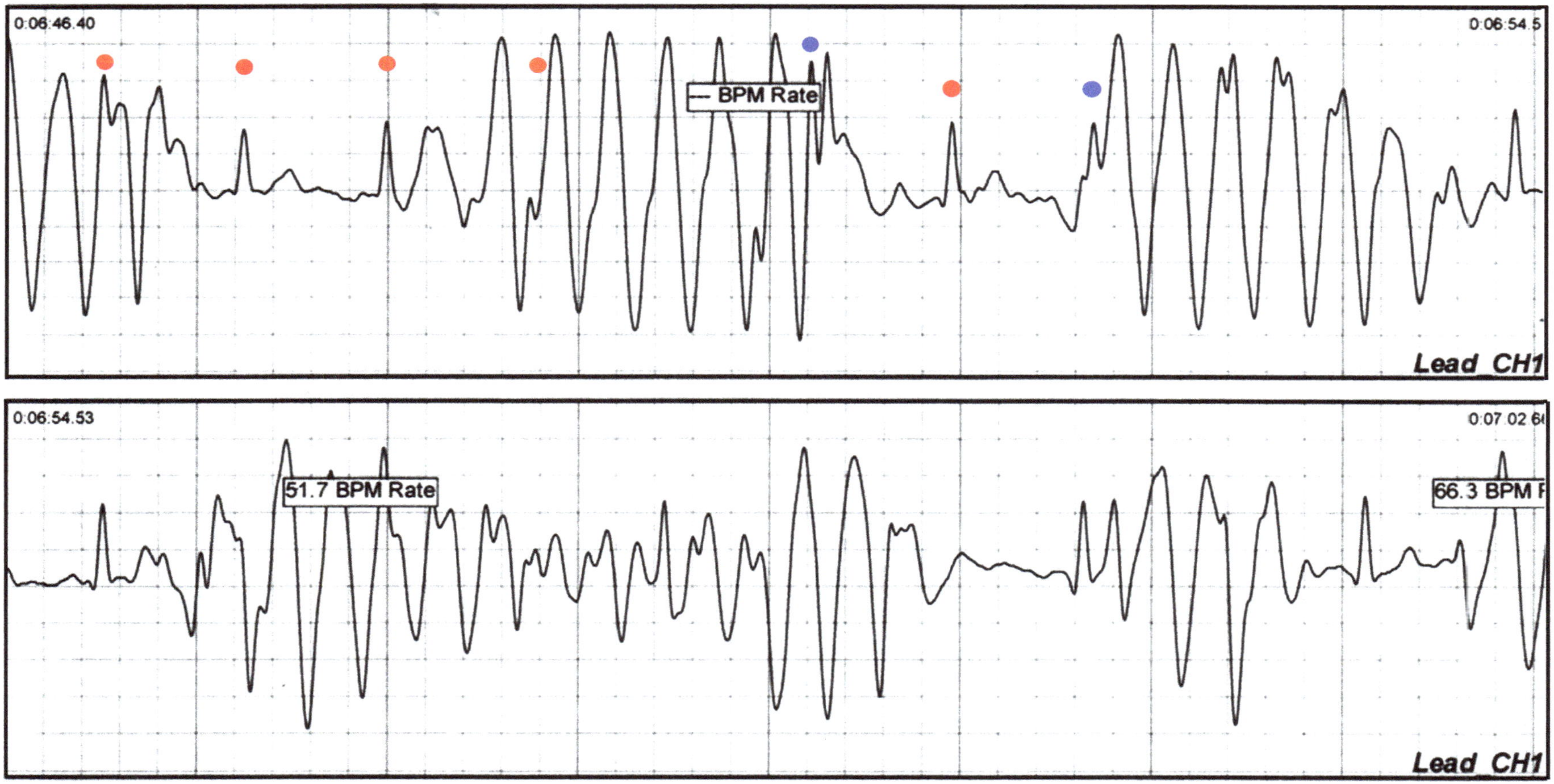
0:06:46.40
0:06:54.5
BPM Rate
Lead CH1
0:06:54.53
0:07 02 6
51.7 BPM Rate
66.3 BPM
Lead CH1

Question 5-13

Figure 5-13A

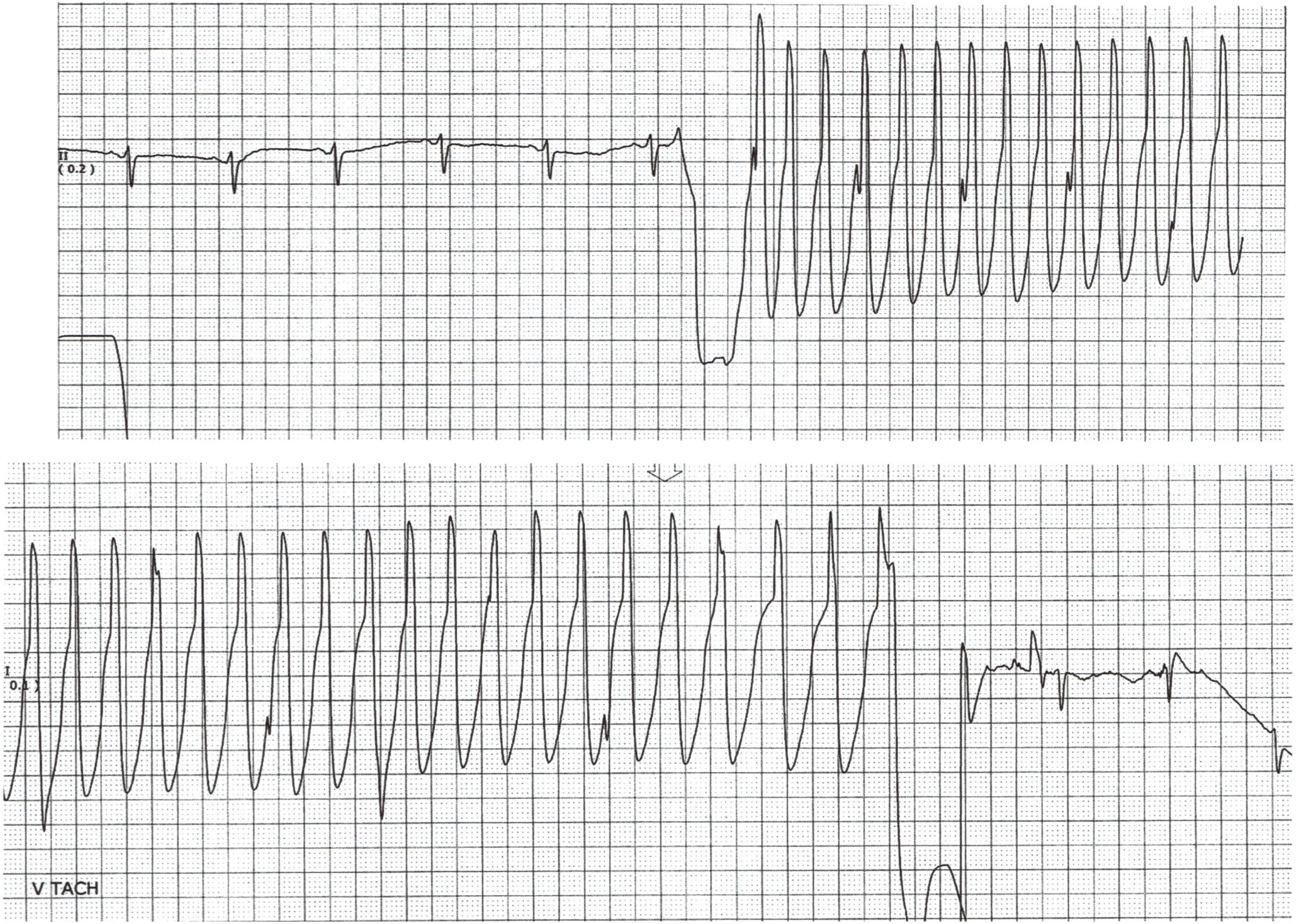

## Question 5-13

The strips in **Figure 5-13A** are not continuous. The patient was asleep at the time the tracings were obtained. The mechanism of tachycardia is:

1. VT
2. AFL
3. Preexcited AT
4. Other

## Answer

This is—or appears to be—a regular WCT interrupting sinus rhythm. Applying the principles described in **Question 5-12**, there should be absolutely no doubt that this is a pseudo tachycardia related to artifact. As discussed in that question, the baseline is unstable with large vacillations (**red arrows** in **Figure 5-13B**). When one sets calipers on a sinus cycle and traces through the recording (**dots** in **Figure 5-13B**), the underlying sinus rhythm becomes apparent. The **blue arrow** indicates a sinus beat following closely after an apparent PVC. It is virtually impossible for a normal QRS capture beat to follow a PVC so closely. A high index of suspicion for artifact and pseudo tachycardia will be very rewarding.

Figure 5-13B

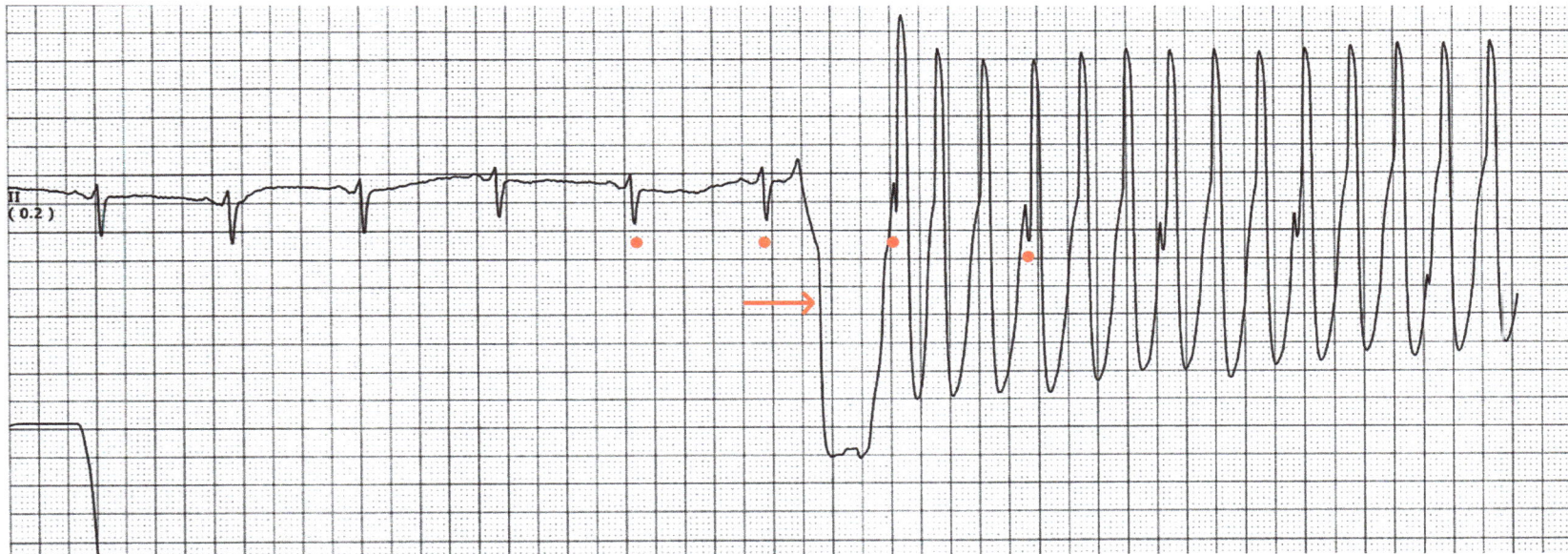

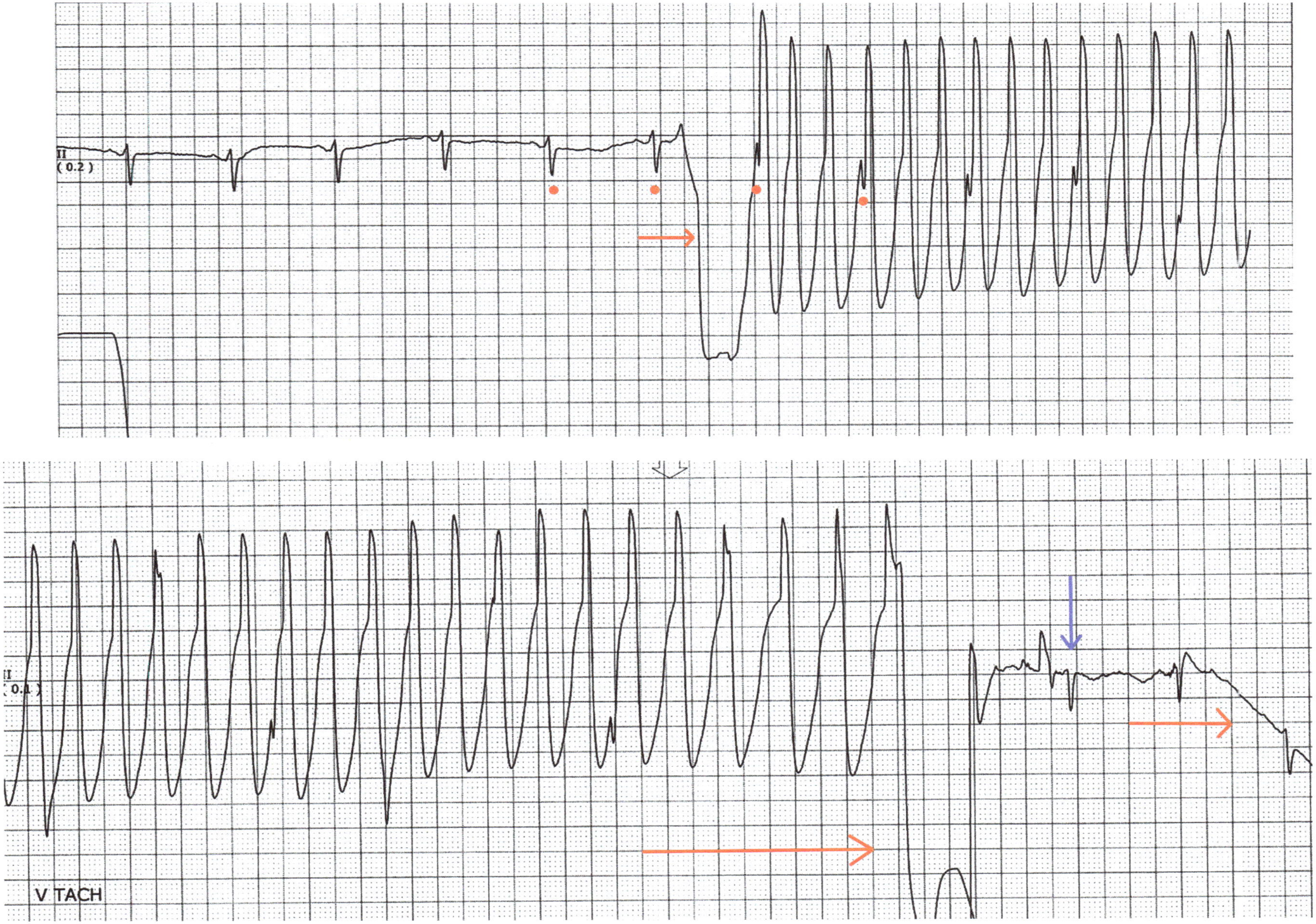

Figure 5-14A

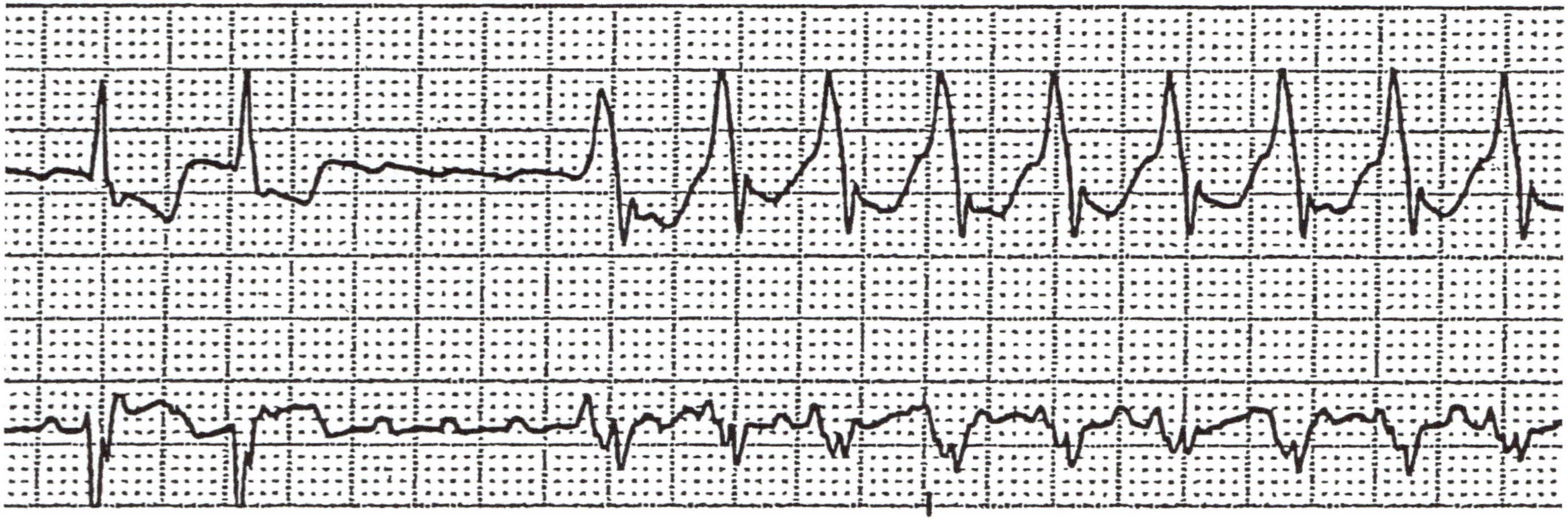

## Question 5-14

The wide QRS tachycardia shown in **Figure 5-14A** is most probably:

1. VT
2. AFL with aberrancy
3. Preexcited tachycardia
4. Insufficient data

## Answer

**Question 5-14** is meant as a contrast to **Question 5-15**, which is superficially similar. In both, we have evident P waves, and AFL is clearly present. The WCT starts with a wide QRS beat after a relatively long pause, militating against tachycardia-dependent aberrancy (**Figure 5-14B**). The WCT is relatively regular, and careful observation shows that the P waves are dissociated from the QRS complexes. The WCT CL is *not* a multiple of the AFL CL. This can only be VT.

Figure 5-14B

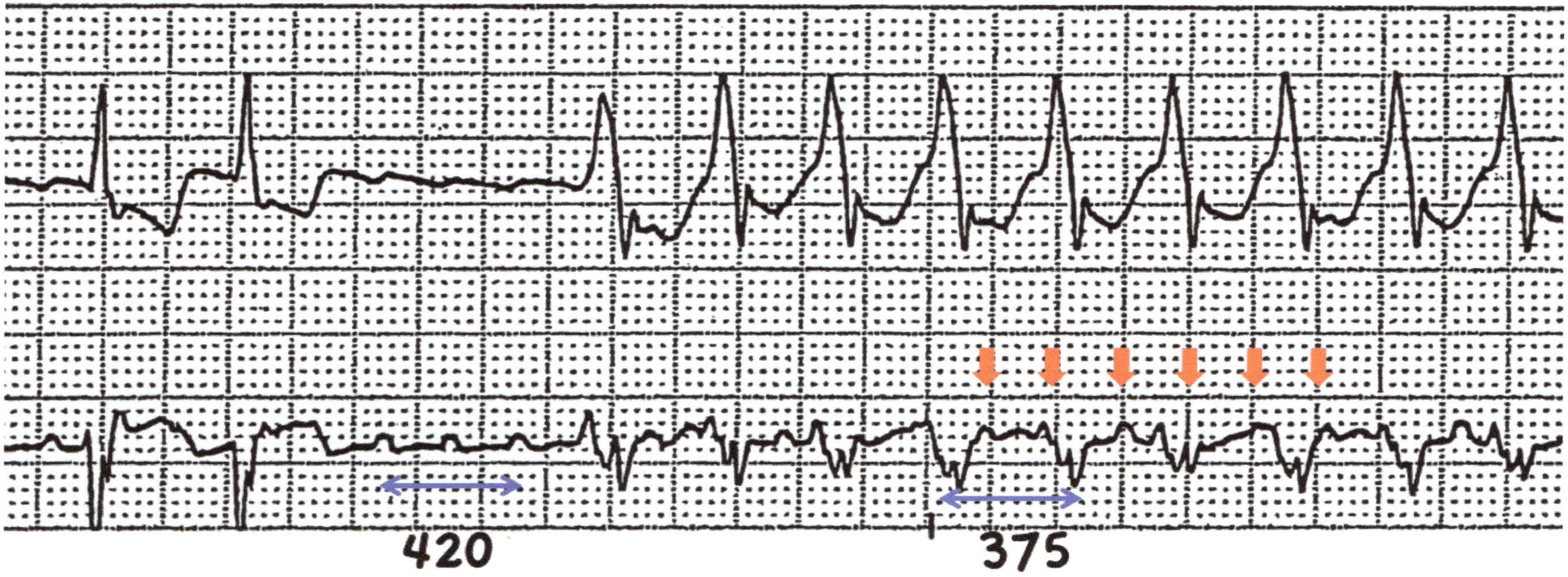

Figure 5-15A

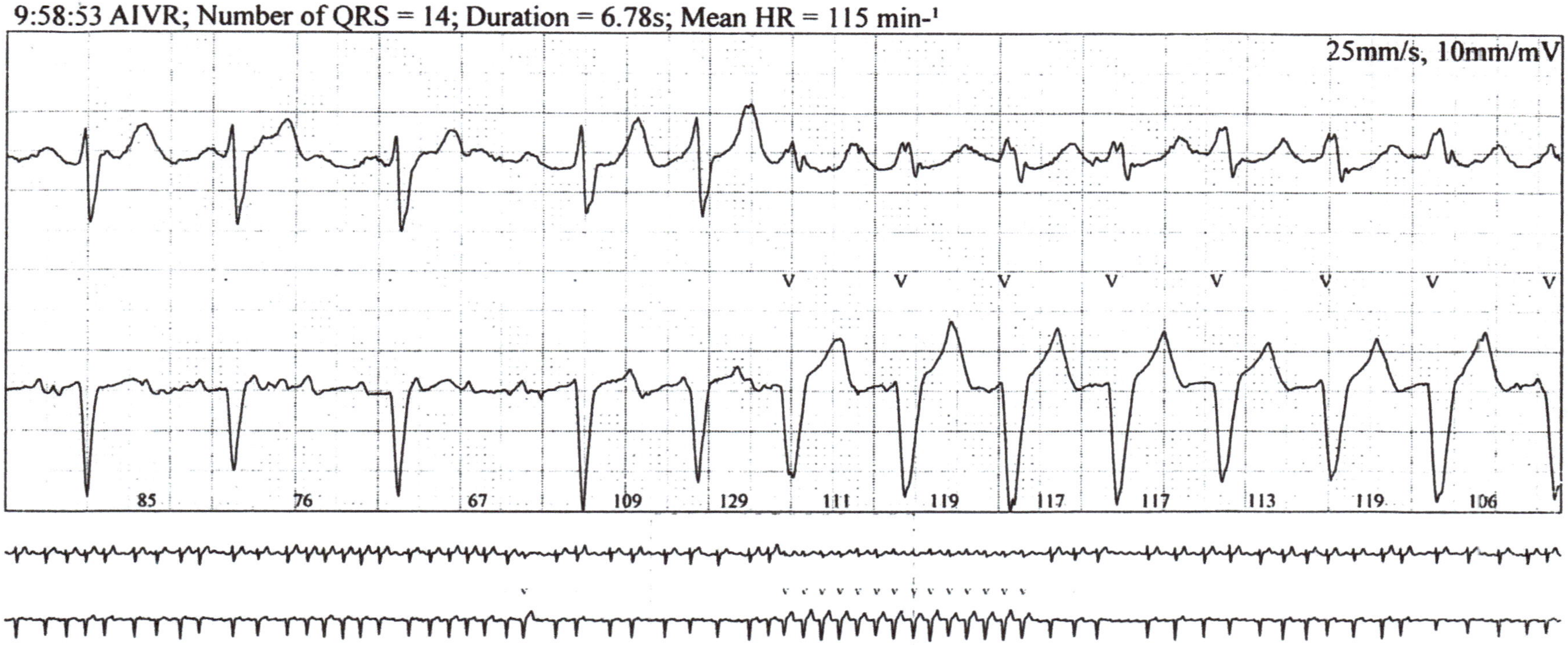


## Question 5-15

The wide QRS tachycardia shown in **Figure 5-15A** is most probably:

1. VT
2. AFL with aberrancy
3. Preexcited tachycardia
4. Insufficient data

## Answer

This is a somewhat irregular rhythm, but atrial activity is readily apparent at the tracing onset in the lower strip with CL about 250 ms—that is, AFL.

The WCT (lead locations unknown) has a relatively sudden onset of a faster ventricular rate, supporting a rationale for rate-related bundle branch block, hence AFL with aberrancy. The P waves are not well seen during the WCT.

We note that the CL of the WCT (**Figure 5-15B**) is predominately a multiple of the flutter CL. Unless a coexistent VT has such a CL by chance, this is excellent support for a diagnosis of AFL with aberrancy. Preexcitation is unlikely statistically but also because the onset of the WCT has a very rapid downstroke (lower channel), more in keeping with early engagement of the His-Purkinje conduction system.

Figure 5-15B

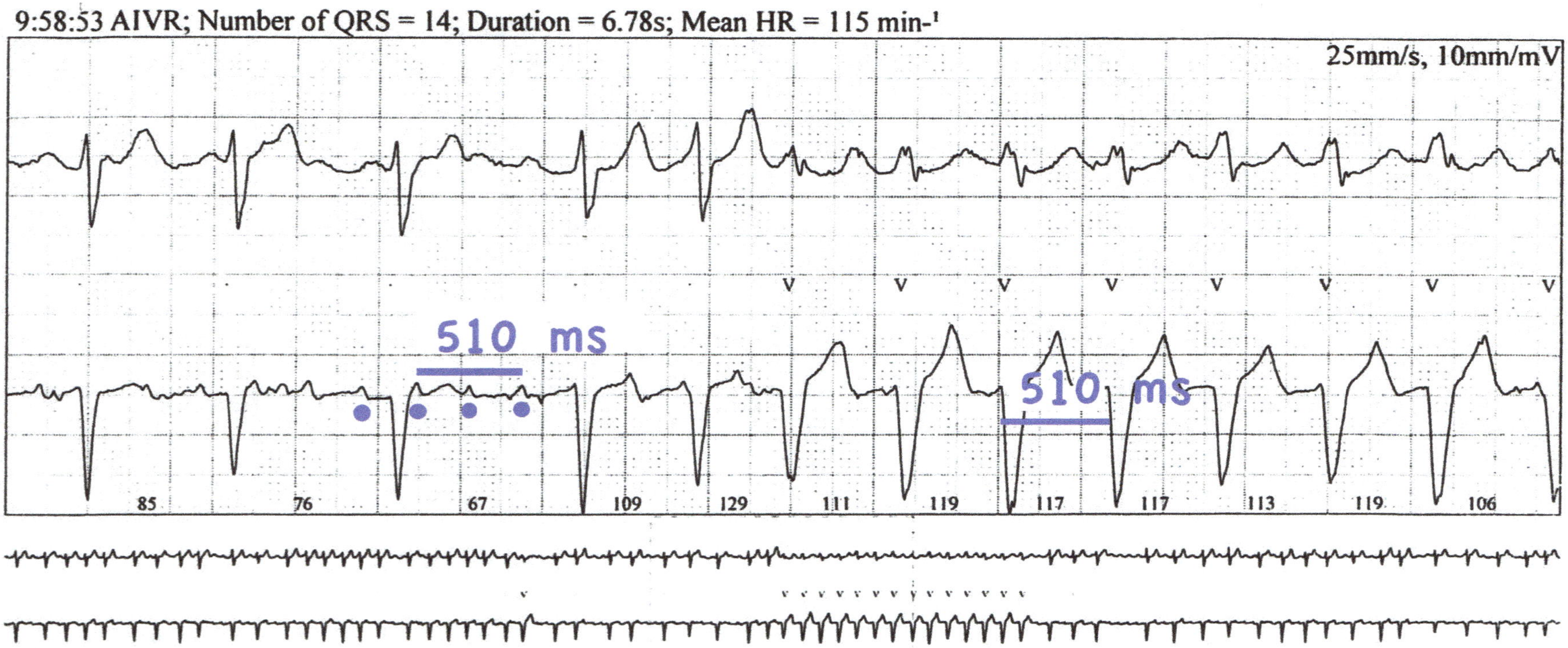

# Chapter 6

## The Irregular Tachycardia

Figure 6-1A

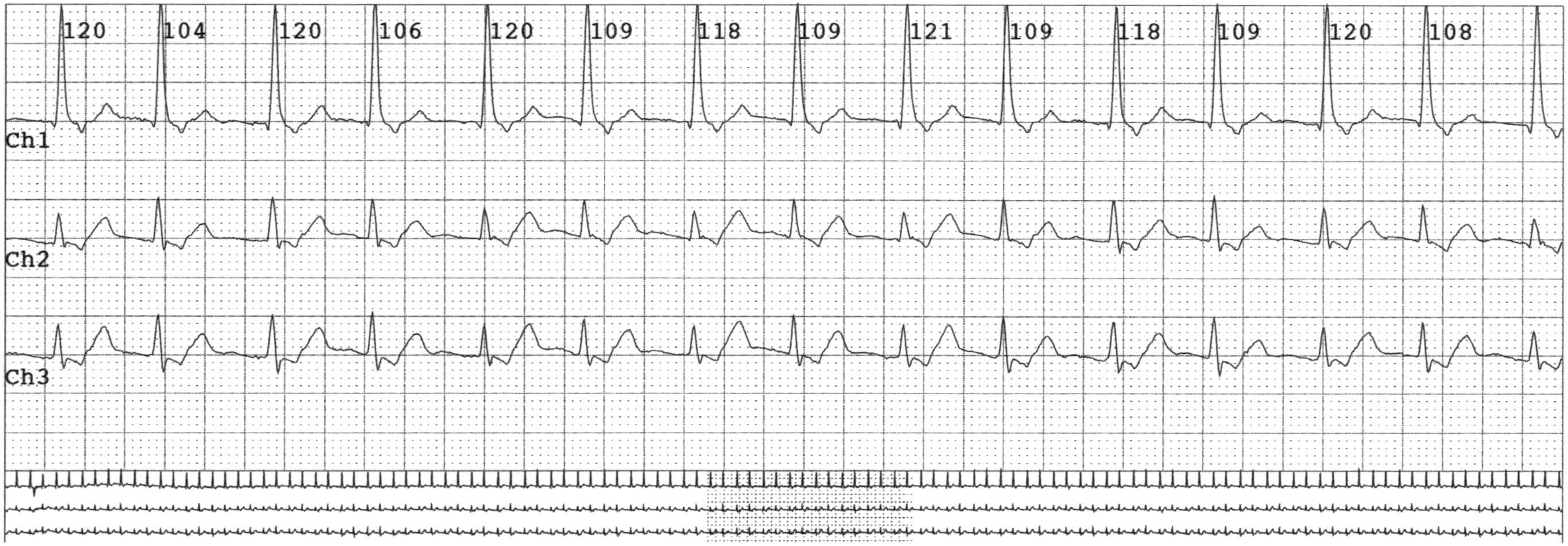
120
104
120
106
120
109
118
109
121
109
118
109
120
108
Ch1
Ch2
Ch3

## Question 6-1

The patient is a 44-year-old woman monitored for "palpitations." Based on the tracing shown in **Figure 6-1A**, the tachycardia mechanism is most probably:

1. Atrial tachycardia (AT)
2. Atrioventricular nodal reentrant tachycardia (AVNRT)
3. Atrioventricular reentrant tachycardia (AVRT)
4. Junctional tachycardia (JT)

## Answer

This tachycardia is somewhat irregular and was initially diagnosed as atrial fibrillation (AF). Nonetheless, a distinct deflection in the ST segment is a likely P wave candidate (**red arrow**, **Figure 6-1B**). We focus on the first part of the tracing and will use the irregularity to assist us.

We notice that each change in cycle length (CL) is reflected in the QRS first—that is, the change in the V-V interval (**black dots**) precedes the change in the P-P interval (**blue dots**). Another way of looking at this is that the QRS-P interval is constant during CL variation (that is, "linked" to the QRS), while the P to QRS interval varies. *This cannot be AT.*

CL variation, or "wobble" as I have called it, is a very valuable finding and well worth looking for. The principle, simply put, is that *the cause ("site") of sudden CL change can't be "downstream" from the initially observed site of change.* An AT is ruled out if the QRS moves before the P wave and vice versa.

With a very long PR interval (slow pathway) and a very short (QRS-P interval), this is most probably AVNRT.

Figure 6-1B

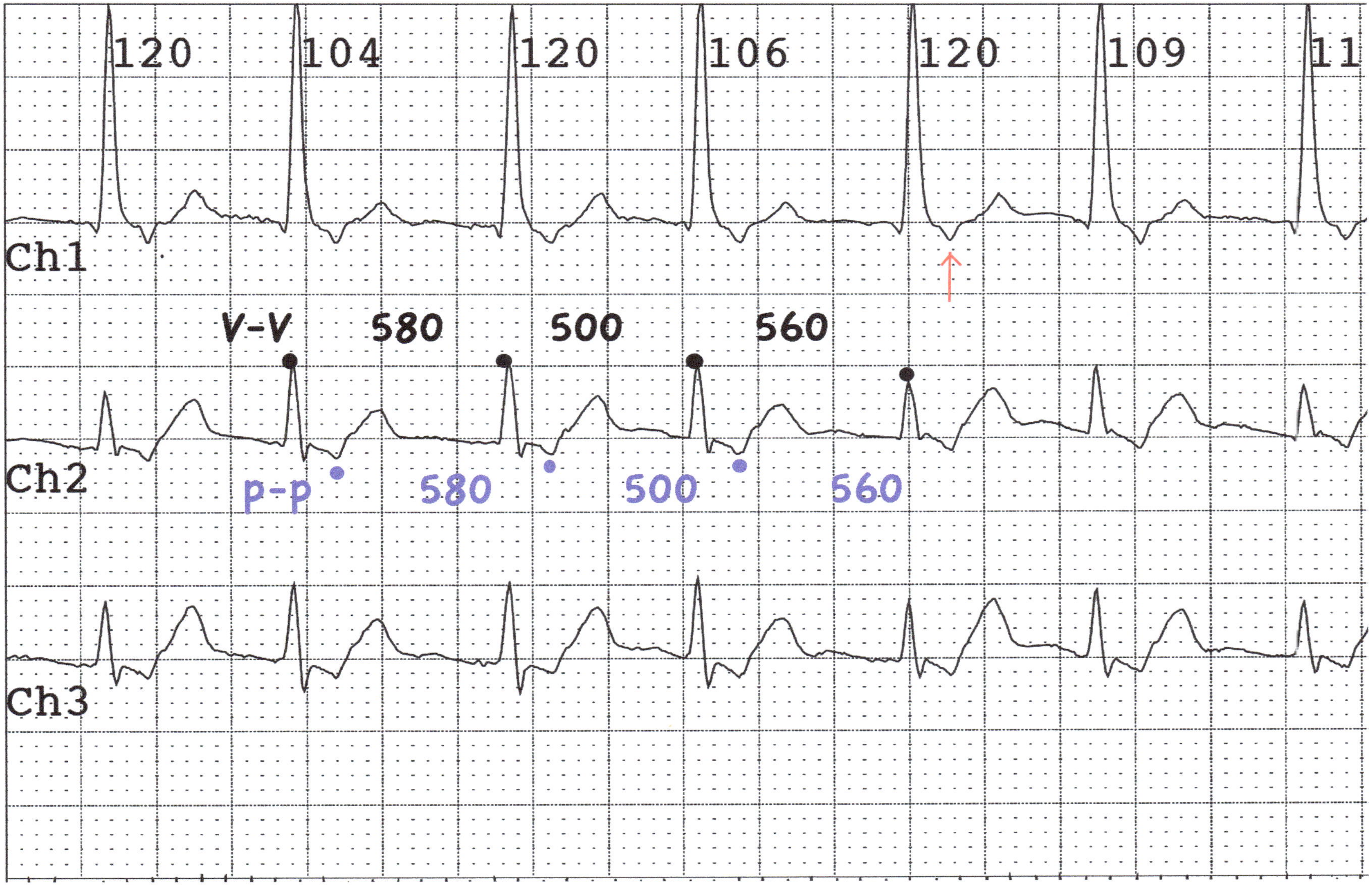
120
104
120
106
120
109
11
Ch1
V-V
580
500
560
Ch2
p-p
580
500
560
Ch3

Figure 6-2A

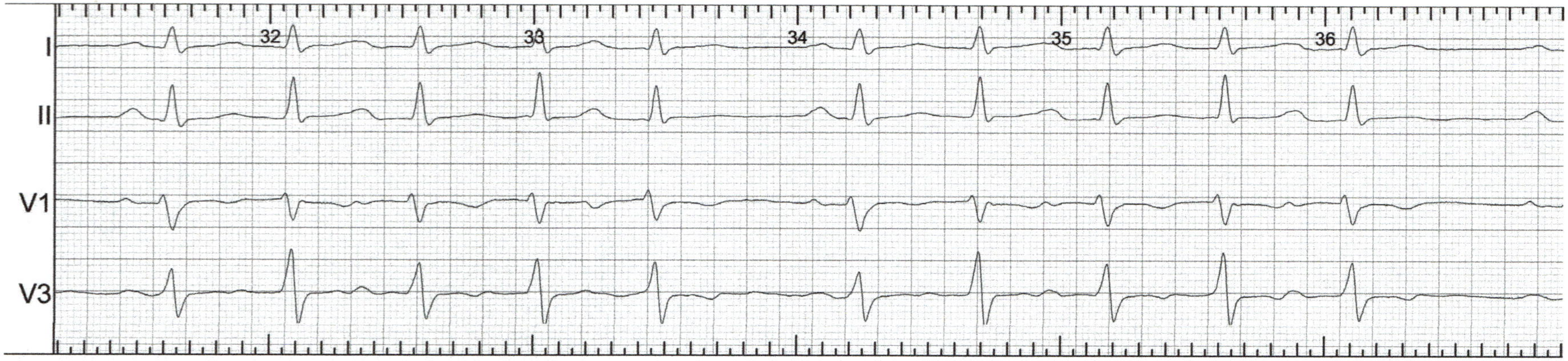

## Question 6-2

The ECG in **Figure 6-2A** illustrates:

1. Non-sustained AF
2. Non-sustained AVNRT
3. Junctional extrasystoles
4. Sinus rhythm

## Answer

The rhythm above was consistent for many minutes, with beats occurring in "groups" of 5 separated by a short pause (2 identical groups in a row illustrated in the tracing). It is slightly irregular.

*The key to the tracing is the identification of P waves*, which are most prominent in lead 2 and annotated in **Figure 6-2B**, which also adds a high right atrial (HRA) electrogram with lines to the QRS to facilitate identification of P waves and their relationship to the QRS.

It is thus obvious that the rhythm is sinus, and the sinus rhythm is regular. The first beat in the group is a sinus QRS and is followed by a second QRS not preceded by a P wave. The third QRS is again preceded by a P wave, but we note the PR interval is now longer—and this QRS, in turn, is followed by another QRS without a preceding P wave, now with a longer interval after the preceding QRS. The third P wave again has a longer PR but is not followed this time by a second QRS. The pattern then repeats itself.

This is clearly sinus rhythm (Option 4), but with 2 QRS complexes for each sinus cycle. The data fit well with the hypothesis that each P goes both over a "fast" AV node pathway and a "slow" AV node pathway. The slow pathway is blocked after the third sinus beat after prolongation of the PR interval.

PR prolongation is also occurring in the fast pathway (shorter PR interval), but it seems that block in the slow pathway allows the fast pathway to recover sufficiently to allow conduction over the fast pathway in the second sequence and start the sequence again. This sequence is probably easier to appreciate visually than verbally, by inspection of Figure 6-2B.

This type of tachycardia has been referred to as "non-reentrant" AV nodal tachycardia. It comes into the differential diagnosis of a supraventricular tachycardia (SVT), sustained or non-sustained, and usually a little irregular. The key is the identification of P waves, which will show that there in not a P wave for every QRS complex. Aberrant conduction of the second QRS may also give the impression of fixed, coupled premature ventricular contractions (PVCs) or non-sustained ventricular tachycardia (VT).

An alternate explanation is theoretically possible in our example: namely, frequent junctional extrasystoles. This would have to involve more assumptions about the variable timing of the extrasystoles relative to the preceding QRS and is less plausible here. Slow pathway ablation in this patient eliminated the problem.

*Acknowledgments:* The tracing was provided compliments of Dr. S. Modi.

Figure 6-2B

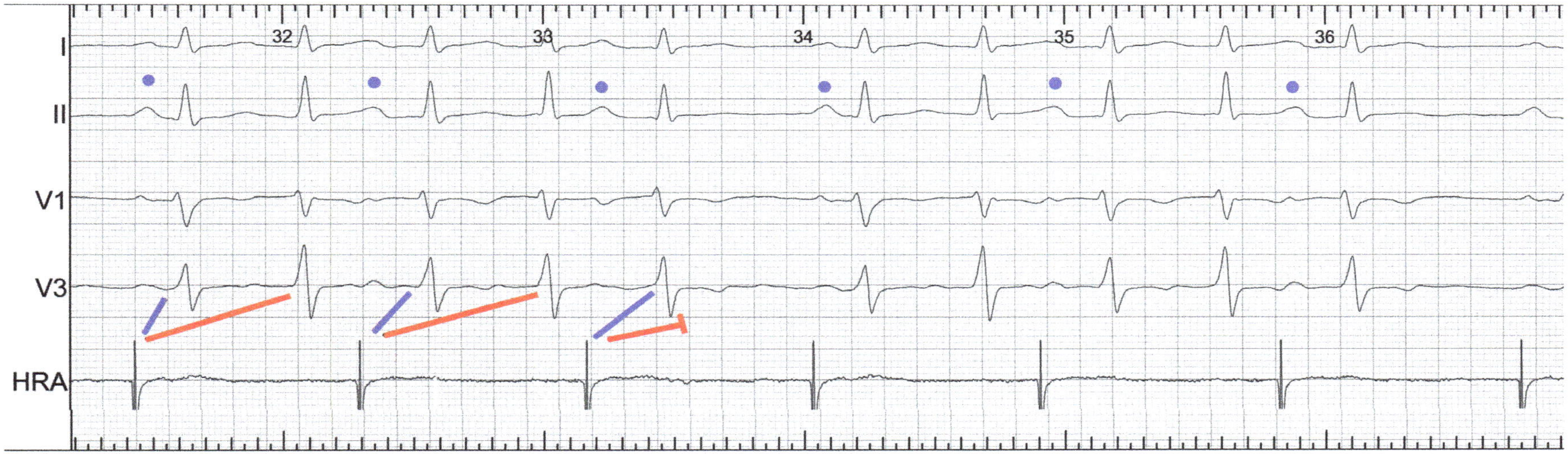

Figure 6-3A

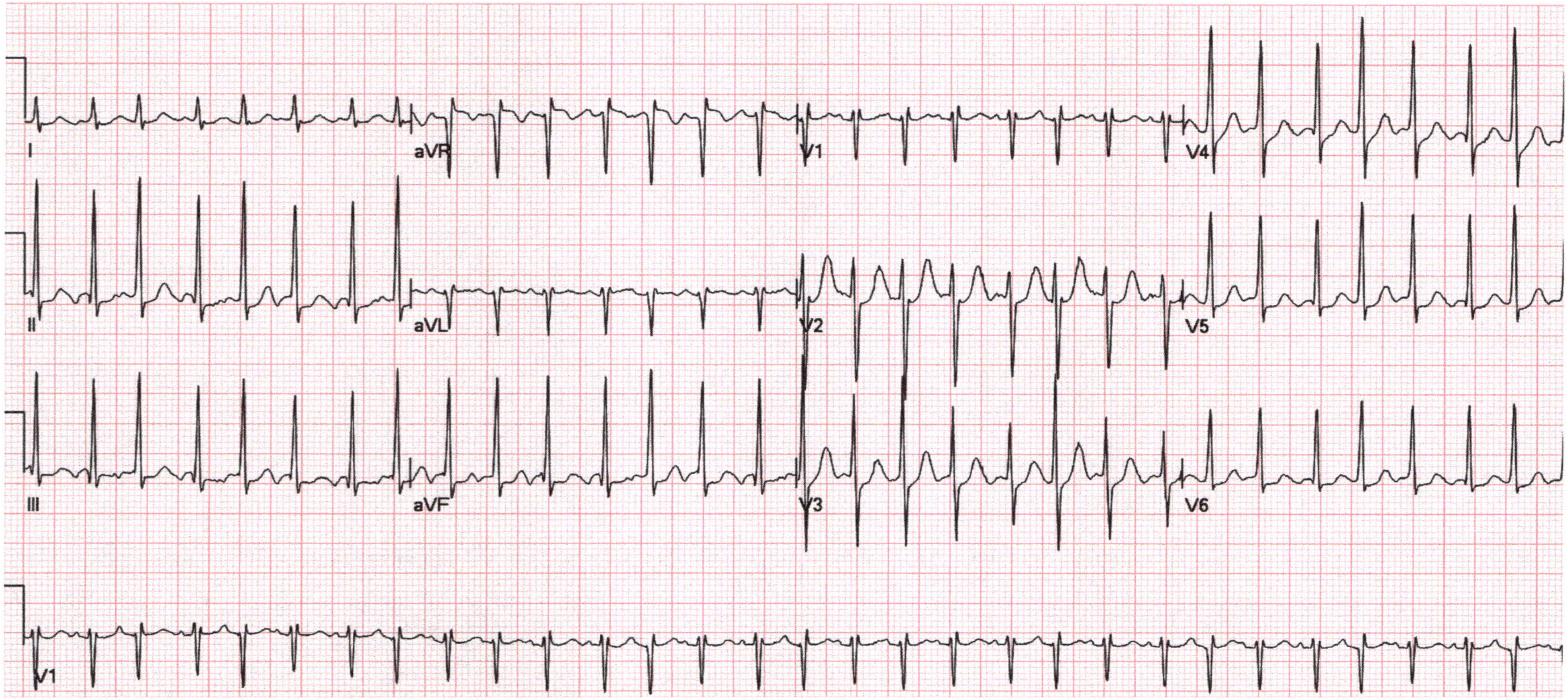

## Question 6-3

Question 6-3

The ECG in **Figure 6-3A** illustrates:

1. AT
2. AVNRT
3. AVRT
4. Sinus with 2:1 AV node conduction

## Answer

The rhythm is irregular and was in fact diagnosed initially as AF by the referring community physician. However, there is clearly a distinct P wave, perhaps best appreciated in lead $V_1$, and the P and QRS have a 1:1 AV relationship. The P wave in the frontal leads has a "low-to-high" activation sequence (negative initial forces in leads 2, 3, and aVF), but this only rules out sinus tachycardia, which should have a "high-to-low" atrial activation sequence.

If we carefully measure successive PR and RP intervals in a magnified portion of the tracing (**Figure 6-3B**), it becomes apparent that both the PR and the RP intervals are oscillating, with a longer RP generally heralding a shorter PR. This would not be expected in AT, where the PR usually stays relatively constant, nor in AVRT, where the RP stays relatively constant.

In my experience, atypical AVNRT is the usual mechanism for this unusual SVT pattern, where both the PR and RP vary. This is intuitively reasonable, since both anterograde and retrograde limbs of the circuit can potentially manifest decremental conduction. This was indeed the diagnosis in this instance. See **Questions 6-7** and **6-14** for variants on this theme.

Figure 6-3B

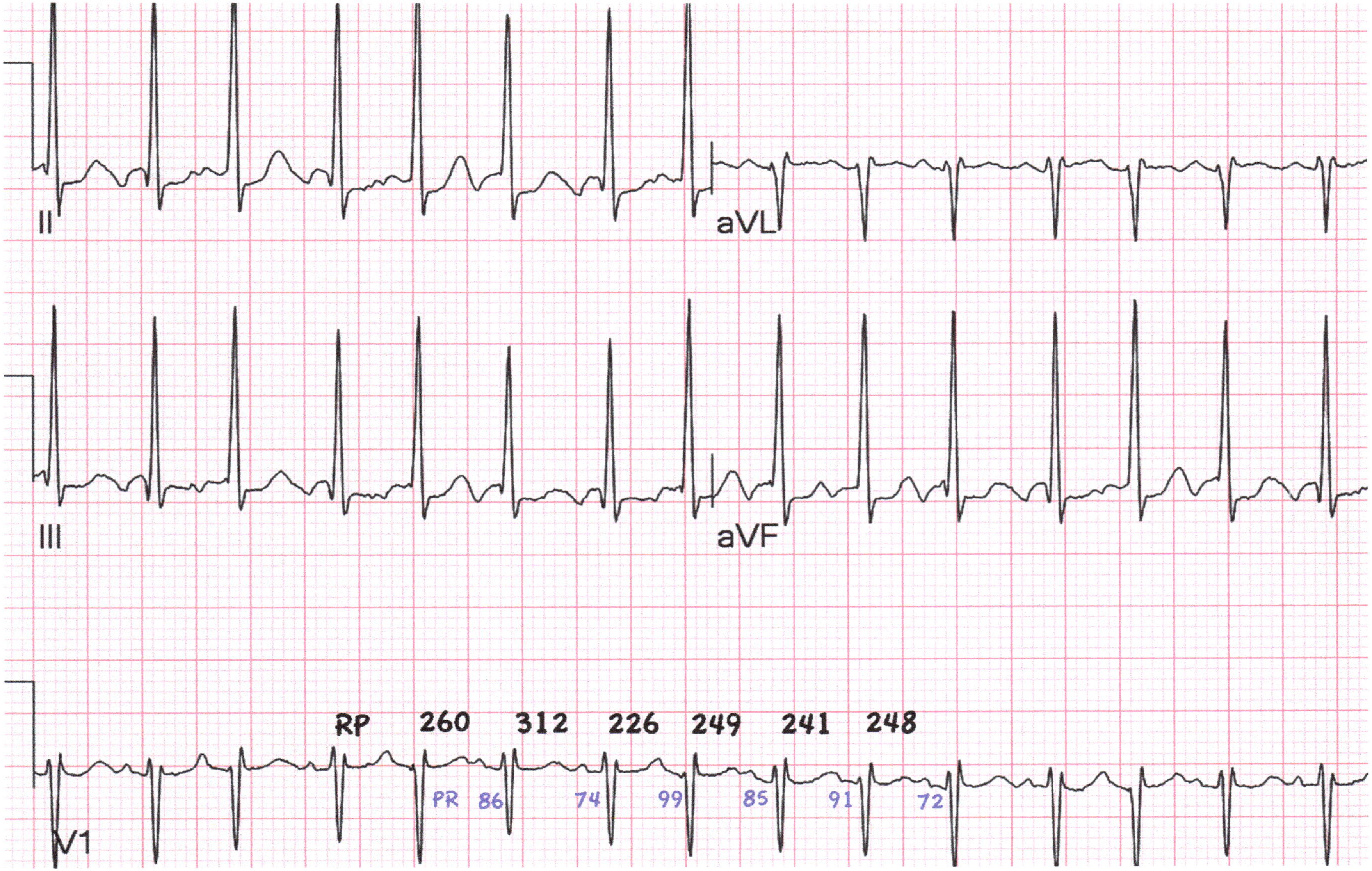
II
aVL
III
aVF
V1
RP
260
312
226
249
241
248
PR
86
74
99
85
91
72

Figure 6-4A

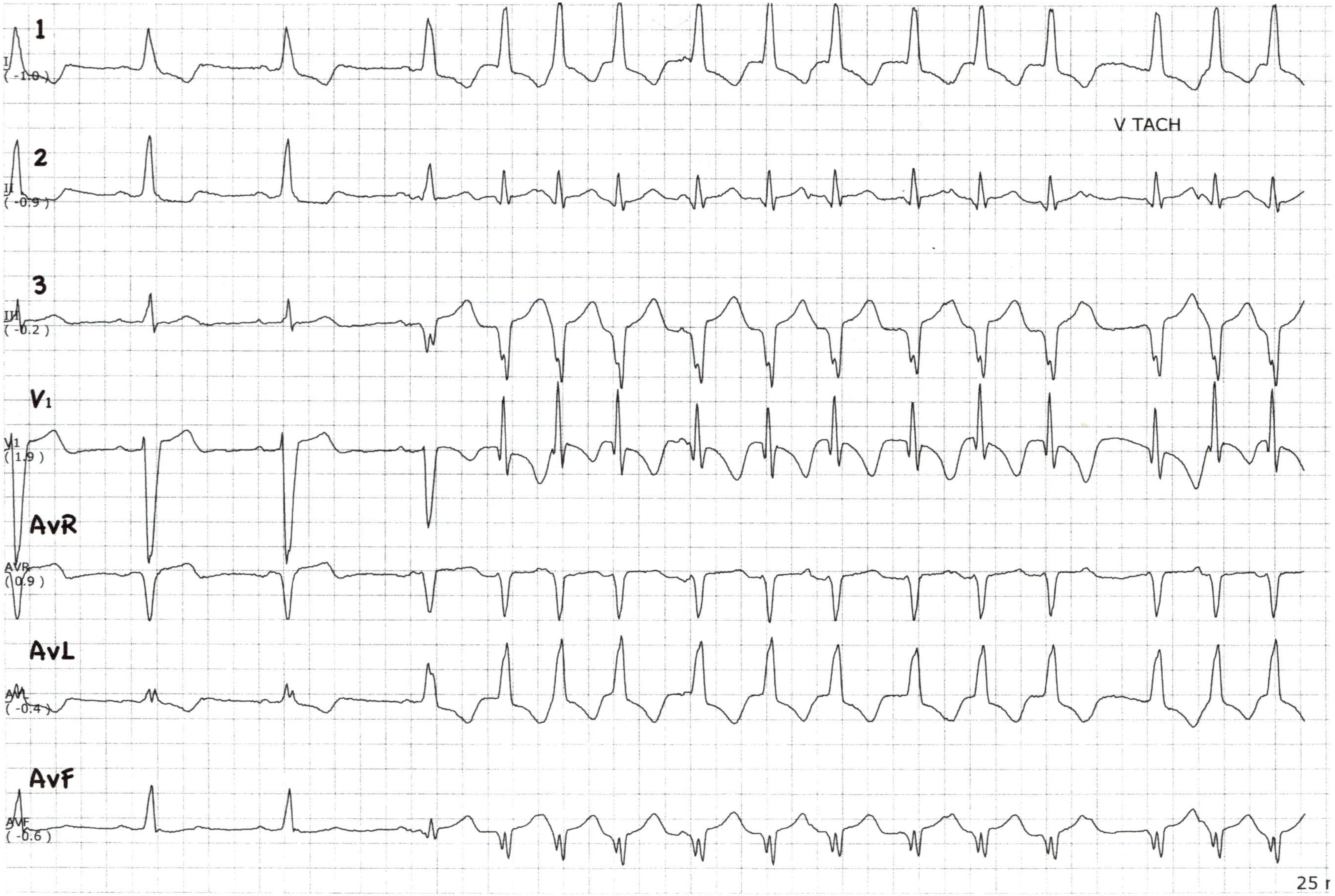
1
I
( -1.0 )
V TACH
2
II
( -0.9 )
3
III
( -0.2 )
V1
V1
( 1.9 )
AvR
AVR
( 0.9 )
AvL
AVL
( -0.4 )
AvF
AVF
( -0.6 )
25

## Question 6-4

The mechanism of wide complex tachycardia (WCT) in the tracing shown in **Figure 6-4A** is:

1. AF with aberrancy
2. VT
3. Preexcited AF
4. Need more data

## Answer

The rhythm is markedly irregular and was diagnosed initially as AF with aberrant conduction. Sinus rhythm is interrupted with a QRS that is a reasonable algebraic summation of the initial sinus QRS and the WCT QRS—a plausible fusion beat (labeled **F** in **Figure 6-4B**). A subtle "shortening" of the PR interval is noted on this beat as the first VT QRS preempts and merges with the sinus QRS. AV dissociation is present and relatively apparent in lead 2 (**blue dots** indicate P timing).

Finally, the QRS morphology during WCT resembles right bundle branch block (RBBB) somewhat in $V_1$ but would be considered most atypical for RBBB in general (for example, development of deep and wide QS in leads 3 and aVF), and thus also confirm a diagnosis of VT.

In spite of the gross irregularity, there is no doubt that the rhythm is ventricular, and irregularity alone should never be a reflex criterion to rule it out. This patient was asymptomatic with no obvious clinical heart disease, and the arrhythmia was considered idiopathic.

Figure 6-4B

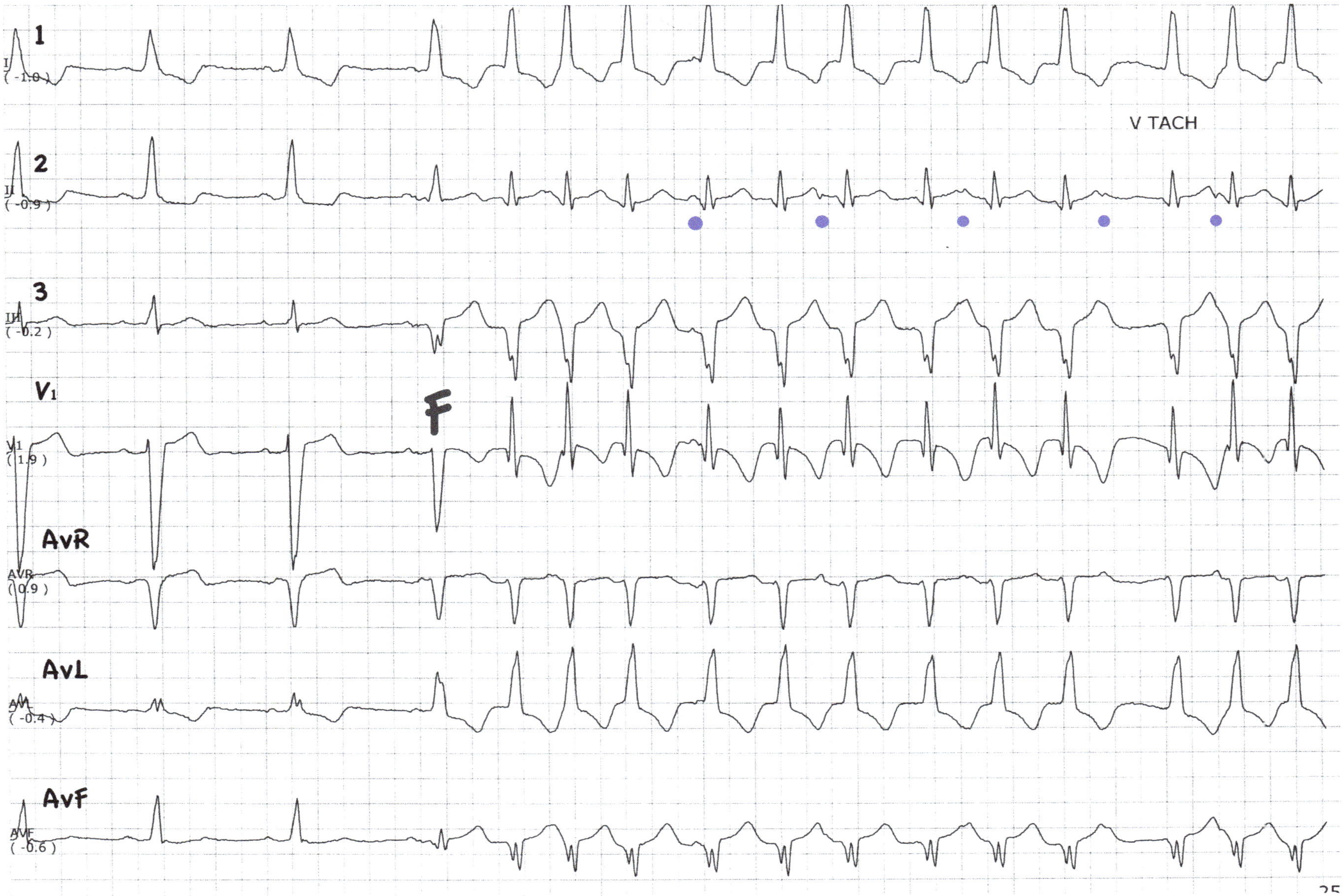
1
I
( -1.0 )
V TACH
2
II
( -0.9 )
3
III
( -0.2 )
V1
F
V1
( 1.9 )
AvR
AVR
( 0.9 )
AvL
AVL
( -0.4 )
AvF
AVF
( -0.6 )

Figure 6-5

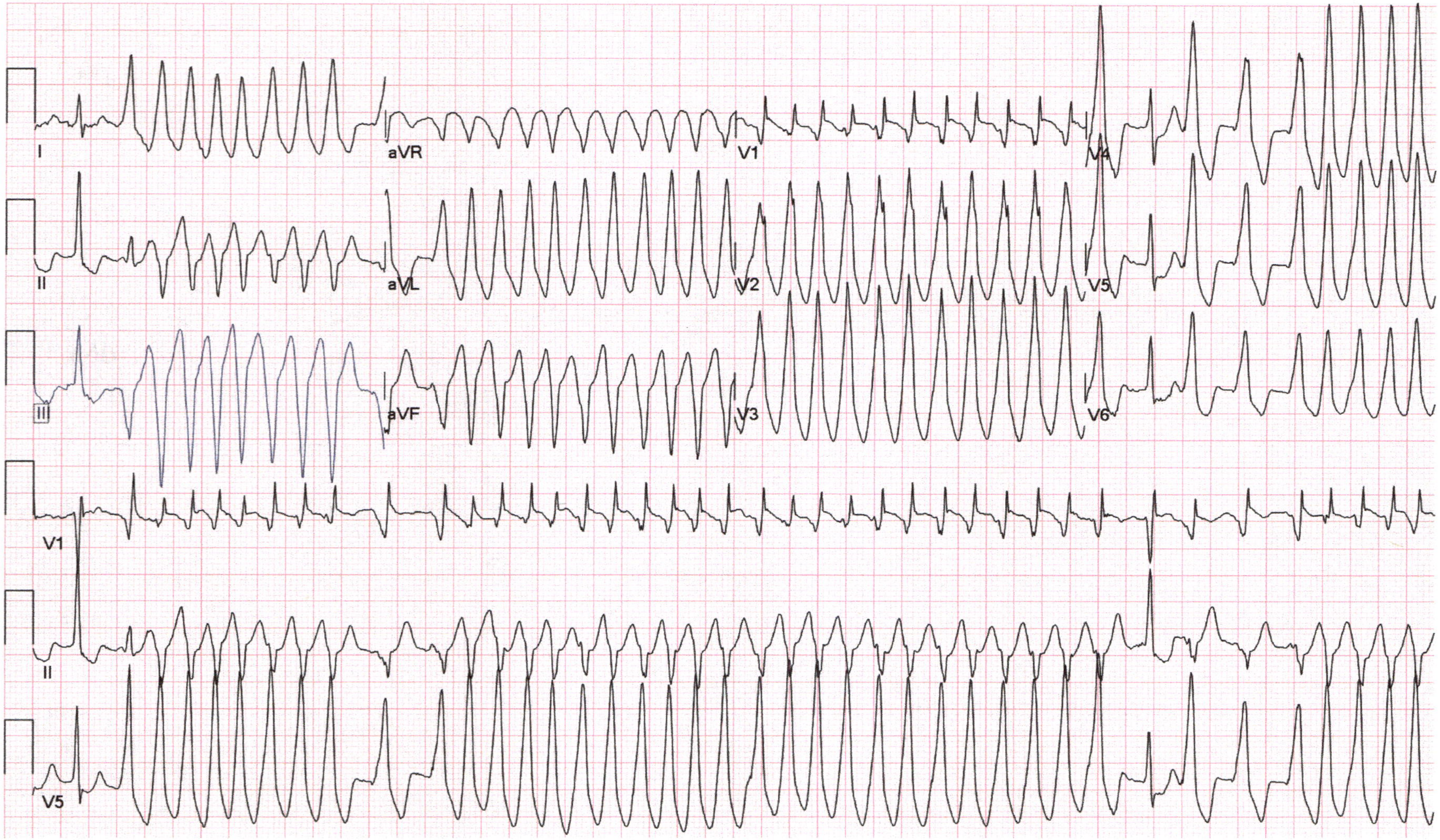


Question 6-5

## Question 6-5

Question 6-5

The patient whose ECG is shown in **Figure 6-5** is a 29-year-old man, previously well. The mechanism of WCT is:

1. AF with aberrancy
2. VT
3. Preexcited AF
4. Need more data

## Answer

The rhythm is "irregularly irregular" and predominately WCT of a single morphology, with 2 cycles (first and sixth from end) probably normal, and 2 (10th, 11th) with a slightly different WC morphology.

The predominate WCT morphology (QS in the inferior leads and QS in $V_1$) is not compatible with a bundle branch block pattern and is clearly "ventricular" or preexcited. With this scenario involving a young man with a totally irregular tachycardia, the rhythm is most probably preexcited AF over a posteroseptal accessory pathway (AP), as this was. The 2 cycles with intermediate WC morphology may be due to fusion of AP and normal QRS or possibly a second AP (not found at electrophysiology study).

From solely a QRS morphology viewpoint, there is nothing that rules out VT breaking out at the ventricular insertion of the AP, in this case the posteroseptal ventricular region.

Figure 6-6A

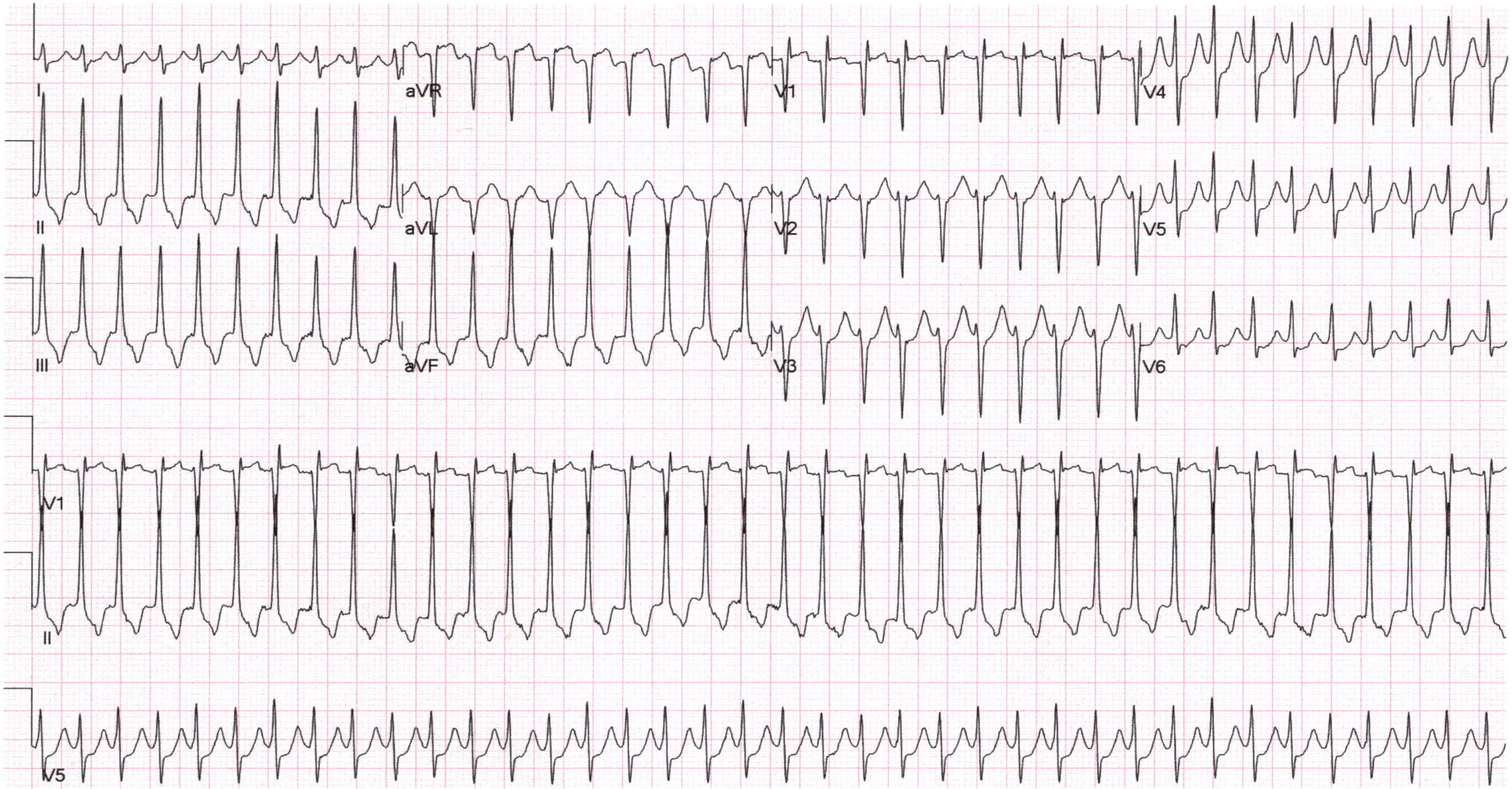

## Question 6-6

The patient is a 32-year-old woman, otherwise well, with paroxysmal tachycardia occurring over the last 2 years, the last being documented and presented in **Figure 6-6A**.

The mechanism of tachycardia is most probably:

1. AT
2. AVNRT
3. AVRT
4. JT

## Answer

The tachycardia (Figure 6-6A) is a relatively regular, normal QRS tachycardia with a suggestion of atrial activity in the middle of the ST segment (leads 2, 3, aVF) with a low-to-high activation sequence. We can thus frame our problem as an SVT with a 1:1 relationship between the QRS and the P waves.

Electrocardiographically, there is no absolute proof of mechanism, and all of our multiple-choice options are theoretically possible. The question is nonetheless worded in such a way ("most probably") that other information can be used to answer the question.

JT would be a very uncommon paroxysmal tachycardia in a in a healthy young adult. The RP interval is too long for typical AVNRT. One also observes an alternation in QRS amplitude (**Figure 6-6B**) that is associated with a slight variability of the R-R interval. This "alternans" has been correlated with AVRT rather than AT or AVNRT, although others have suggested that it is purely a function of high heart rate. In my personal experience, it is has been usually associated with AV reentry, as was the case in this patient.

Figure 6-6B

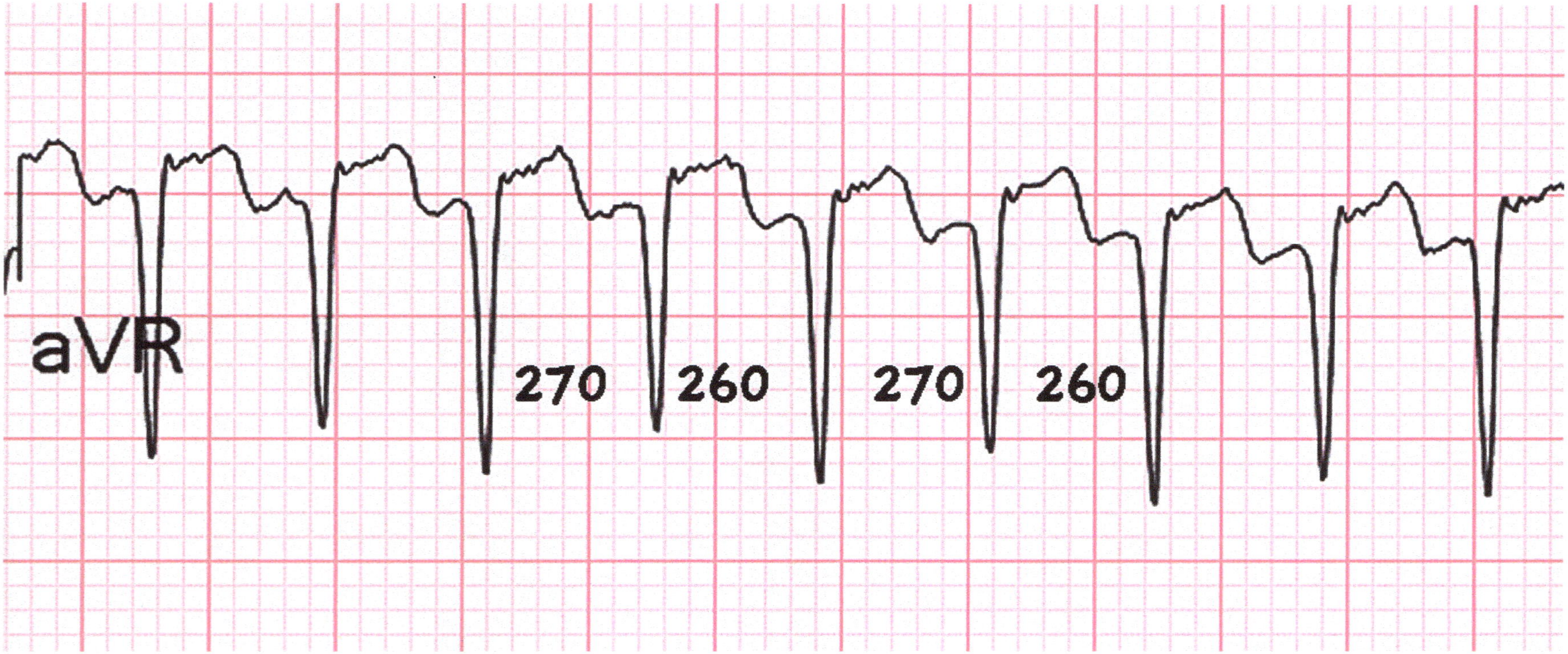

Figure 6-7A

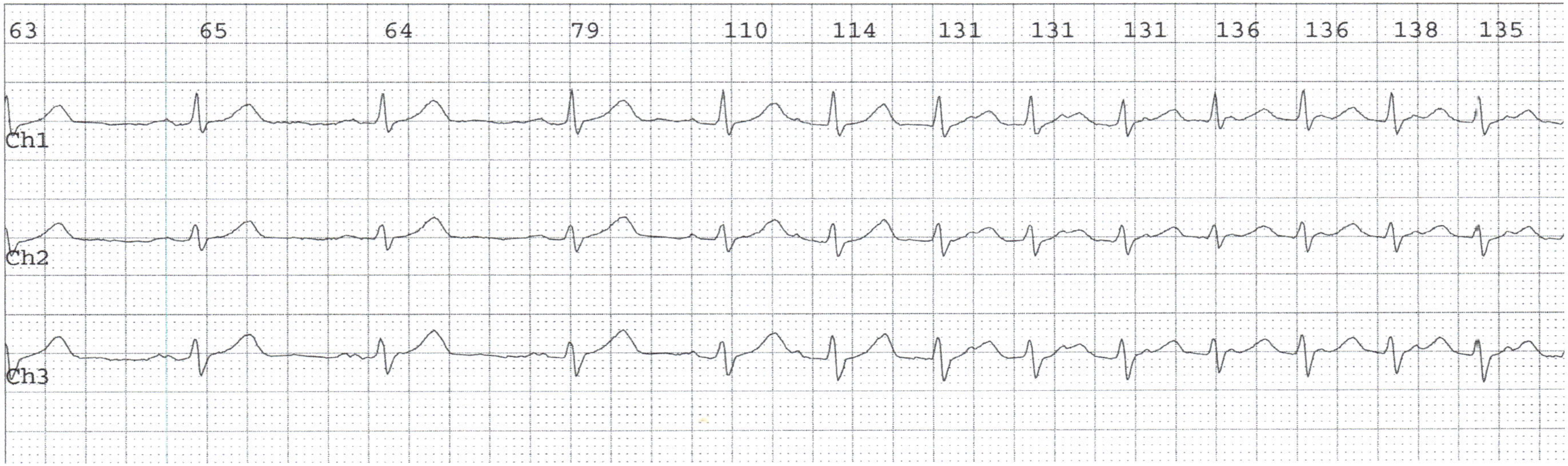




## Question 6-7

The mechanism of tachycardia shown in **Figure 6-7A** is:

1. AT
2. AVNRT
3. AVRT
4. JT

## Answer

The key to this arrhythmia is identifying the P wave right from the onset of tachycardia (**Figure 6-7B, blue dots**). A premature atrial contraction (PAC) with an upright P wave in the 3 monitored frontal leads is similar to sinus rhythm and starts tachycardia with slight prolongation of the PR interval.

Although AVNRT and AVRT each generally require PR prolongation to start tachycardia after a PAC, *prolongation of the PR interval doesn't help narrow the mechanism, since it is the usual physiological response to a sufficiently early PAC regardless of the mechanism of the subsequent arrhythmia.*

The P waves can then be tracked, all with a similar upright P wave, which would not be expected in AVNRT. Subsequent PR intervals are considerable longer, consistent with conduction over a "slow" AV nodal pathway. The wide fluctuation in the apparent RP interval would be most unusual in AVRT.

The correct diagnosis is AT with AV conduction over a slow AV nodal pathway.

One would not expect this patient to have either retrograde conduction over the AV node or AVNRT. The atrial rhythm has blocked in the anterograde fast AV nodal pathway and moved to the slow pathway. This might be expected to result in AV nodal echo cycles or AVNRT if a return AV nodal pathway were available for conduction.

Figure 6-7B

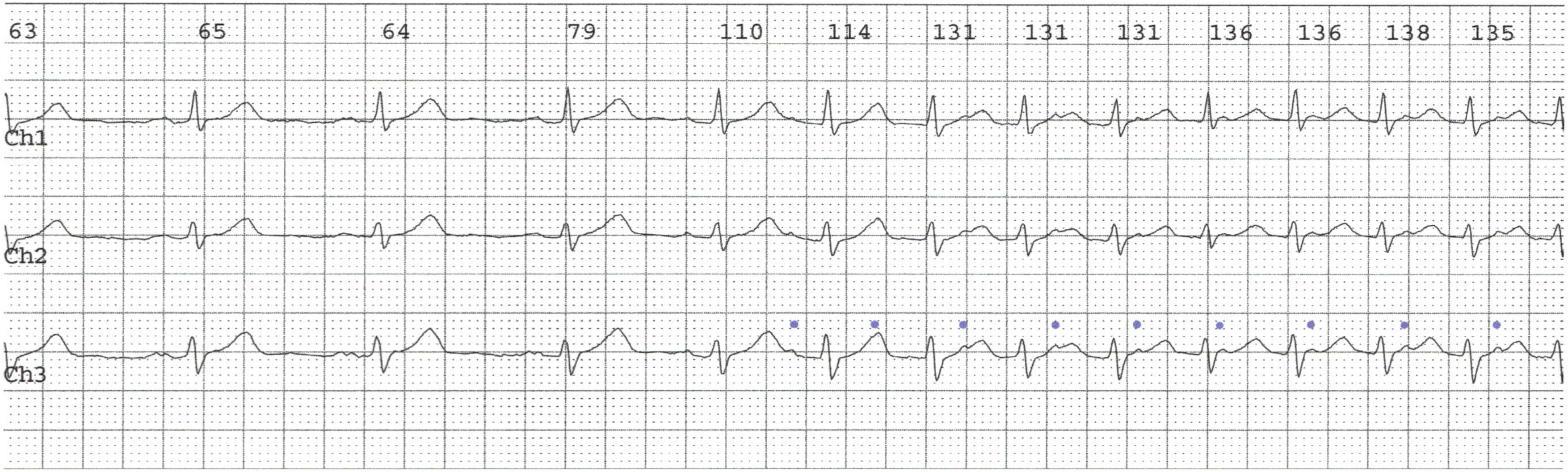

Figure 6-8A

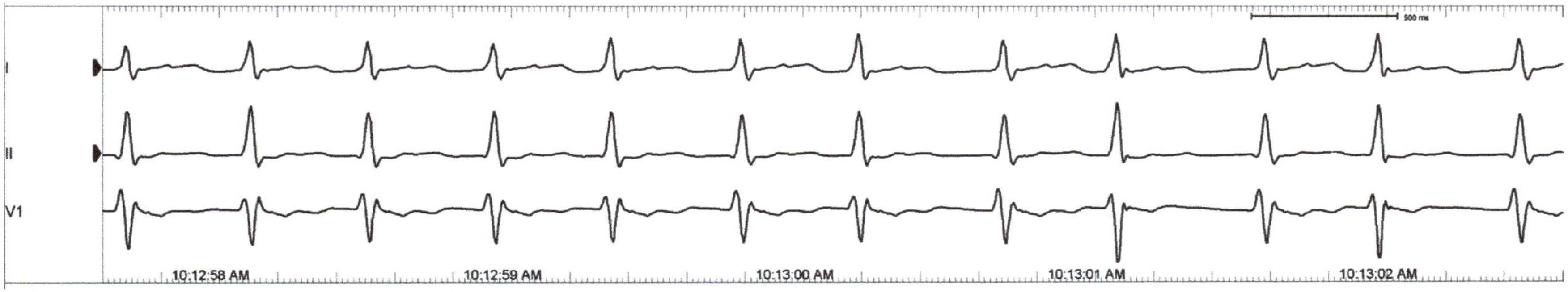




## Question 6-8

The mechanism of tachycardia shown in **Figure 6-8A** is:

1. AT
2. AVNRT
3. AVRT
4. JT

## Answer

The striking observation for this narrow QRS tachycardia is "regular irregularity" from about the middle of the tracing. Long cycles alternate with shorter cycles.

If one identifies the P waves (**blue dots** in magnified **Figure 6-8B**) and measures, the RP interval (**red**) stays constant while the PR alternates between 200 and 320 ms. This *cannot be* AT, since prolongation of the PR interval alters the arrival time of the next P wave, and thus the tachycardia rate is dependent on AV node conduction (i.e., the change in the QRS to QRS interval *precedes* the subsequent change in the P to P interval so that it can't be AT).

This pattern almost invariably occurs with AVRT when retrograde conduction is relatively fixed while anterograde conduction alternates between 2 AV nodal pathways, a fast and a slow. This was indeed the case in this example.

Again, as in **Question 6-7**, one would not expect this patient to have retrograde conduction over the AV node or AVNRT since there are no AV nodal echo cycles after the long PR interval beat. The latter should provide the opportunity for retrograde AV node conduction if it were possible.

This is another example of how dual AV node pathways can influence the manifestation of an arrhythmia without being directly involved in the mechanism. AP ablation should resolve this tachycardia. It seems reasonable to speculate that slow AV node pathway alone in this patient would render clinical tachycardia less symptomatic and generally self-terminating, since spontaneous block in the fast AV nodal pathway would then also stop tachycardia.

Figure 6-8B

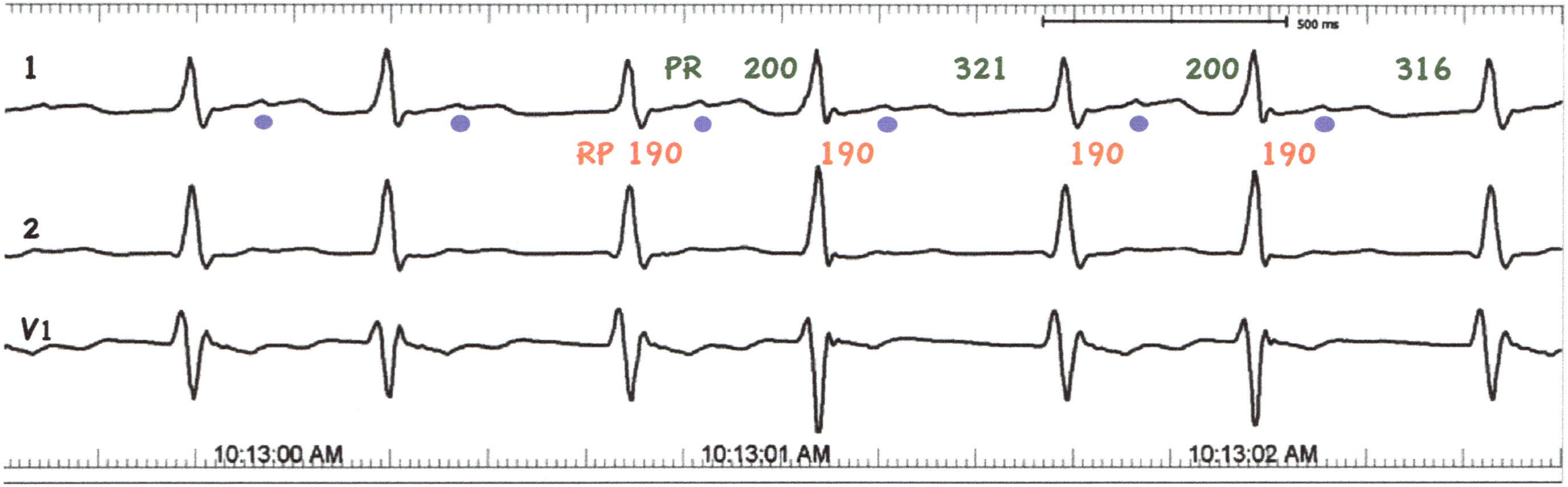

Figure 6-9A

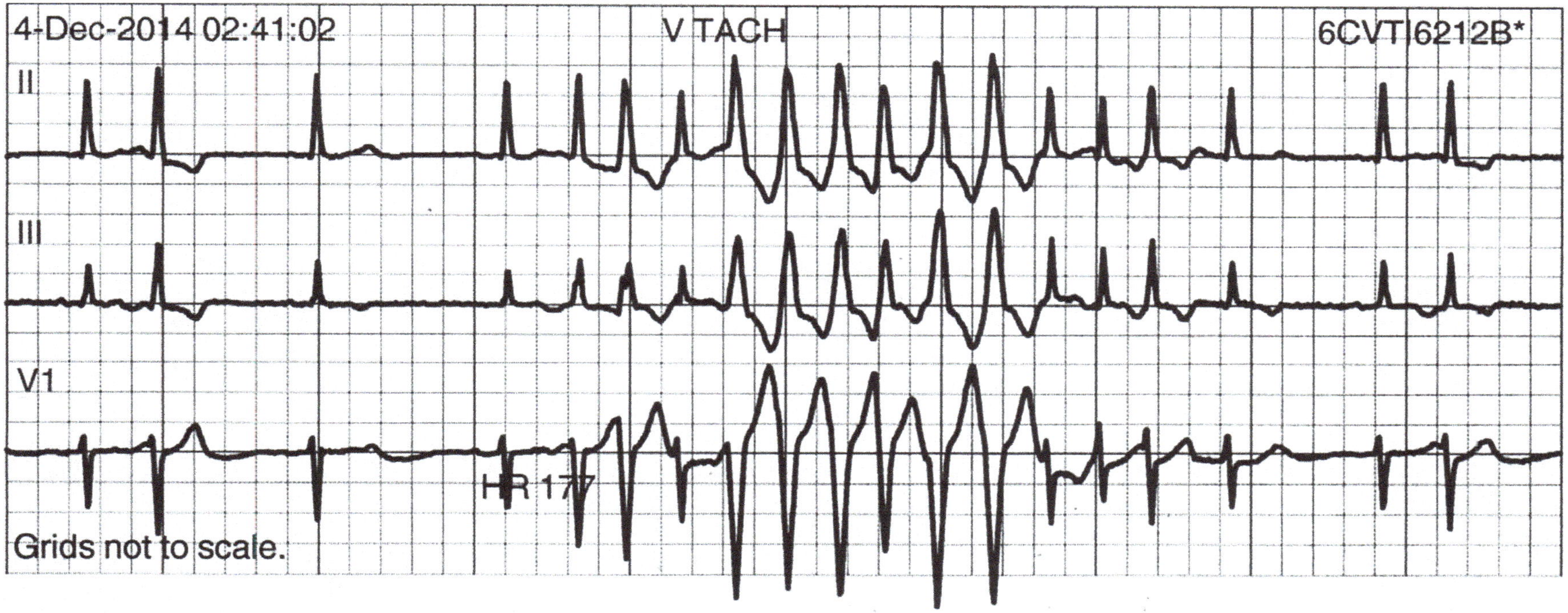


## Question 6-9

The wide QRS cycles in **Figure 6-9A** are attributed to:

1. VT
2. Aberrancy
3. Intermittent preexcitation
4. More data needed

## Answer

The diagnosis of WCT in the context of AF and atrial flutter (AFL) may be clinically important and can be challenging.

The recording of the onset of WCT during a baseline sinus rhythm is very useful and usually diagnostic, since it can be determined if the initial premature event is atrial or ventricular, the latter generally strongly favoring VT. This information is not possible during baseline AF and AFL, and other clues need to be sought. **Questions 6-9** to **6-13** will deal with variations on this theme.

This rhythm strip (Figure 6-9A) shows sinus cycles with PACs both at the beginning and end of the record. The tachycardia in the center is rapid and slightly irregular and most compatible with non-sustained AF. The wide QRS portion is "sandwiched" in by normal QRS complexes of essentially the same cycle length. *VT of similar CL and irregularity to the ambient AF would be most unlikely.*

Additionally,

1. The QRS morphology in $V_1$ has a very rapid downstroke, more compatible with left bundle branch block (LBBB) aberration than VT.
2. The last cycle of the wide QRS run is followed by a *normal* QRS of the same CL as the wide QRS rhythm. This would not be expected with VT, since some degree of retrograde concealed conduction into the AV node would be expected for the first normal cycle after the wide rhythm ("compensatory pause" after ventricular ectopy in AF).
3. The ventricular rate during AF is relatively rapid and rapid ventricular rates in AF and large fluctuations in cycle length generally favor aberrancy.

**Figure 6-9B** is recorded from the same patient at a different time. The AF is now associated with both RBBB and LBBB aberrancy in addition to normal QRS, all at similar CLs during AF. There is no reason why the presence or absence of BBB should influence the CL pattern if it is all AF with aberrancy. The bundle branches are downstream from the AV node, which is generally responsible for the irregularity of response during AF.

Figure 6-9B

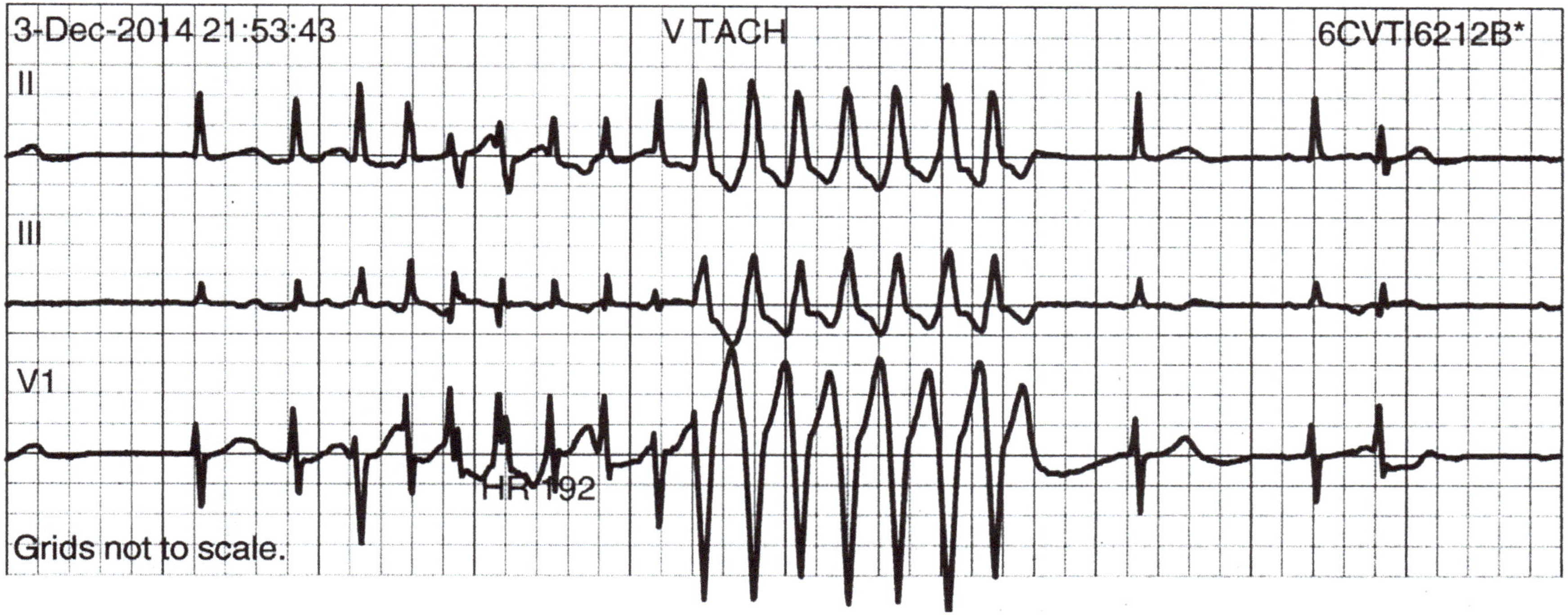
3-Dec-2014 21:53:43
V TACH
6CVTI6212B*
II
III
V1
HR 192
Grids not to scale.

Figure 6-10

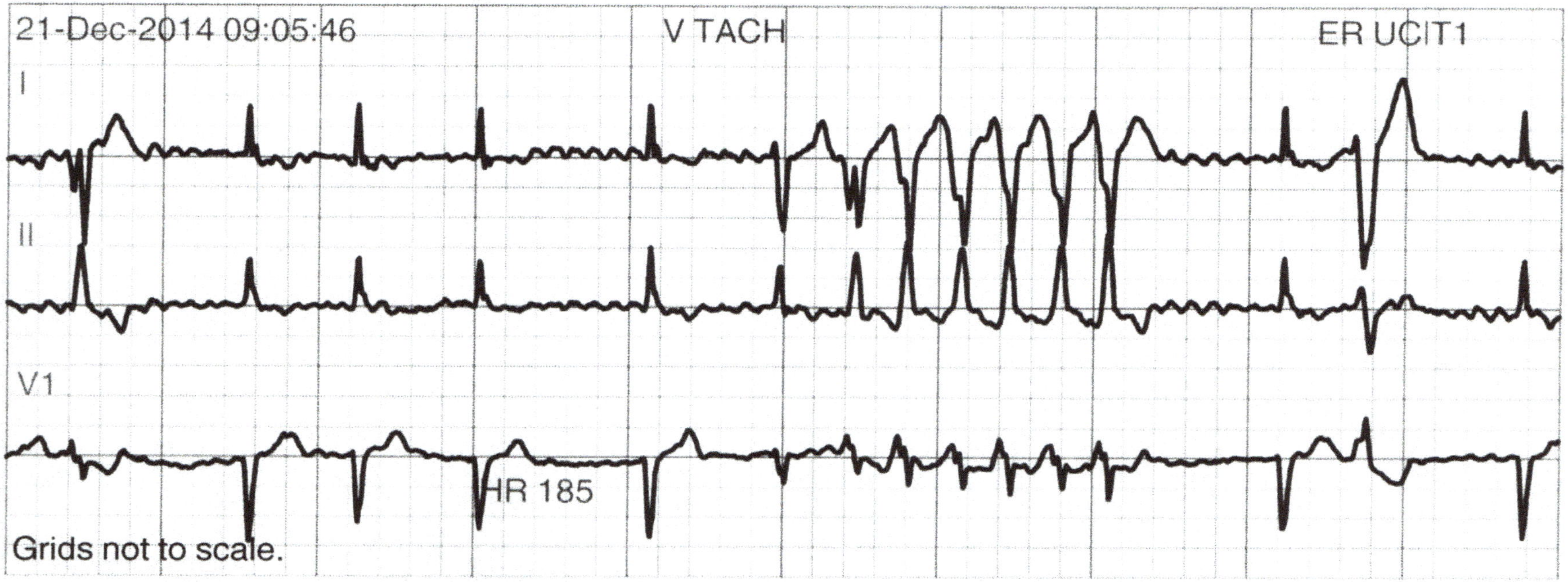


Question 6-10

## Question 6-10

The wide QRS cycles in **Figure 6-10** are attributed to:

1. VT
2. Aberrancy
3. Intermittent preexcitation
4. More information needed

## Answer

There are 2 useful features to help us with this tracing.

First, the ambient rhythm is relatively slow, and this generally favors a diagnosis of ventricular ectopy and VT.

Secondly, we have 3 standardized leads and can use QRS morphology to guide us. Lead 1 is particular useful since it is a wide QS complex; that is, ventricular activation is proceeding from far left to right. The normal leads do not suggest an infarction pattern, so this can only be VT, as this activation sequence is not tenable with a bundle branch block aberration pattern. Of course, it may theoretically be preexcitation, although it would be unusual to see a run of rapid preexcited beats during AF when they don't appear during the relative preceding bradycardia.

One may also note that the first cycle of VT has QRS morphology intermediate between the normal and the WCT QRS and is a very plausible "fusion" cycle.

Figure 6-11A

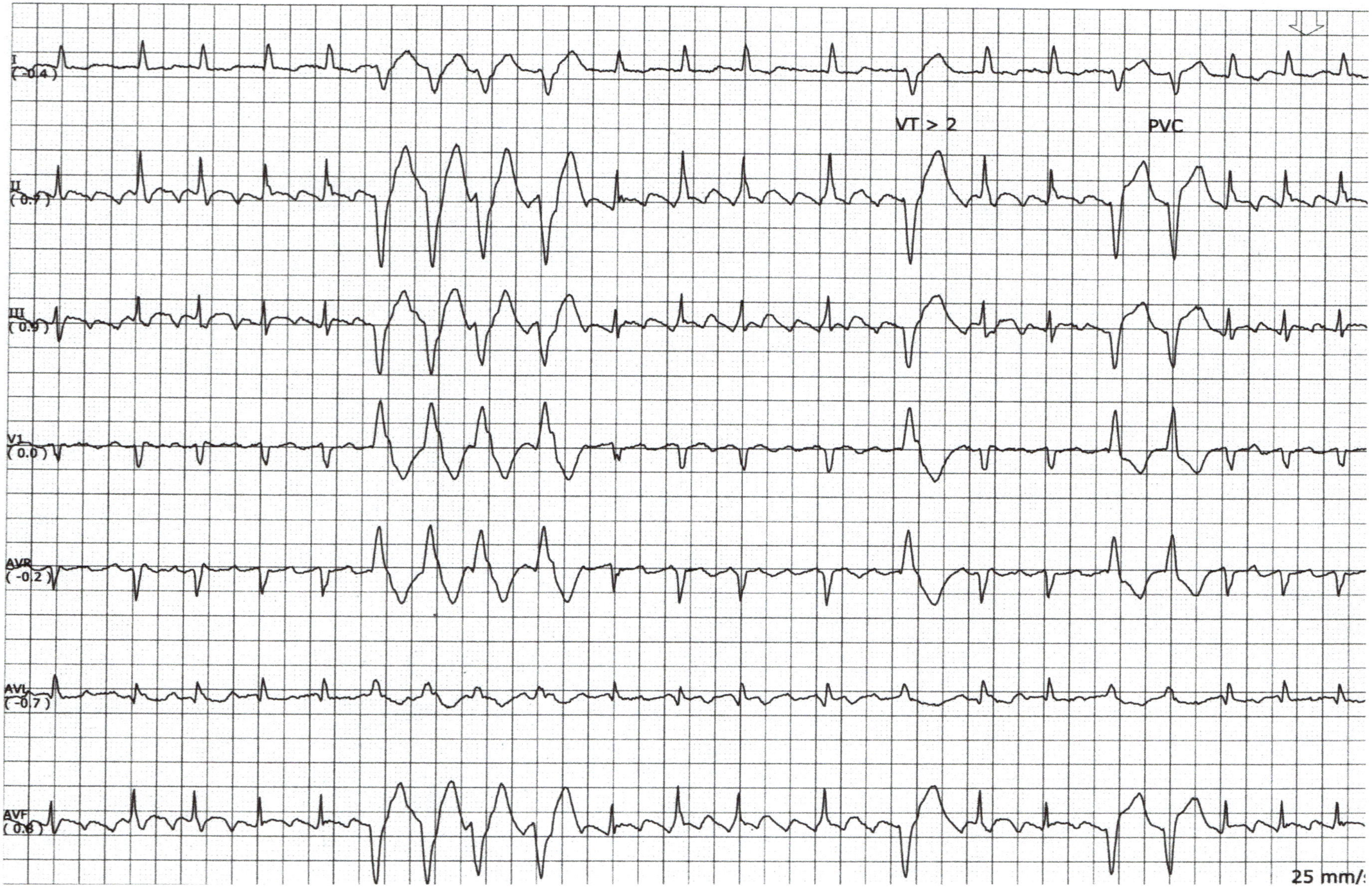


Question 6-11

## Question 6-11

The wide QRS cycles in **Figure 6-11A** are attributed to:

1. VT
2. Aberrancy
3. Intermittent preexcitation
4. More information needed

## Answer

The ambient rhythm is typical AFL, and we are fortunate enough to record the WCT with multiple surface ECG leads. We observe during normal QRS rhythm that the QRS is narrow without infarction pattern or substantive abnormality. We would then expect any bundle branch block aberration to have a relatively "typical" bundle branch block pattern. Such is not the case with QS complexes in lead 1 and inferior leads and a "northwest" axis, which is not compatible with bundle branch block aberration (nor with preexcitation, for that matter) and can only be VT.

We now measure the flutter CL (**Figure 6-11B**) and see that it is 230 ms (2 cycles measured in the figure). One generally expects the CL of the conducted QRS complexes in AFL to be a *multiple of the flutter CL*, and such is not the case with the WCT complexes as noted. This is again consistent with a diagnosis of VT.

Figure 6-11B

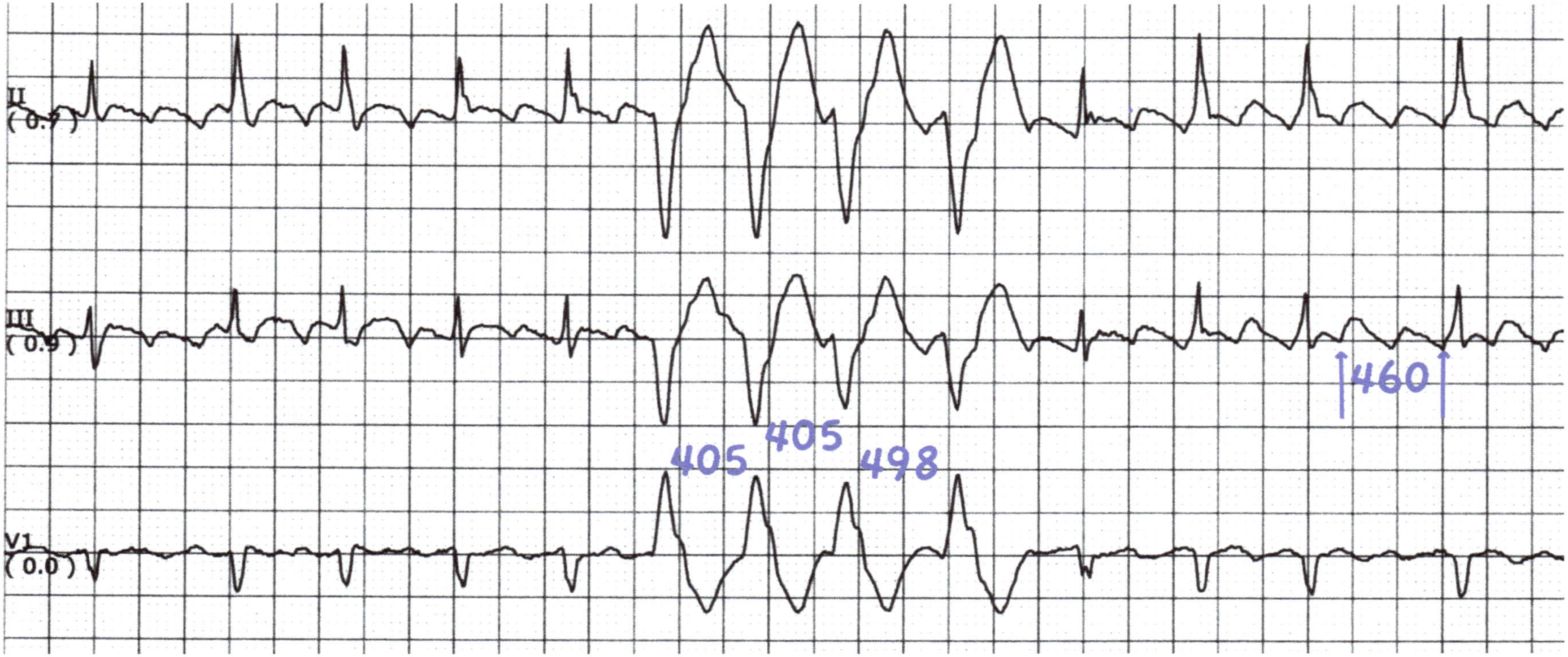

Figure 6-12

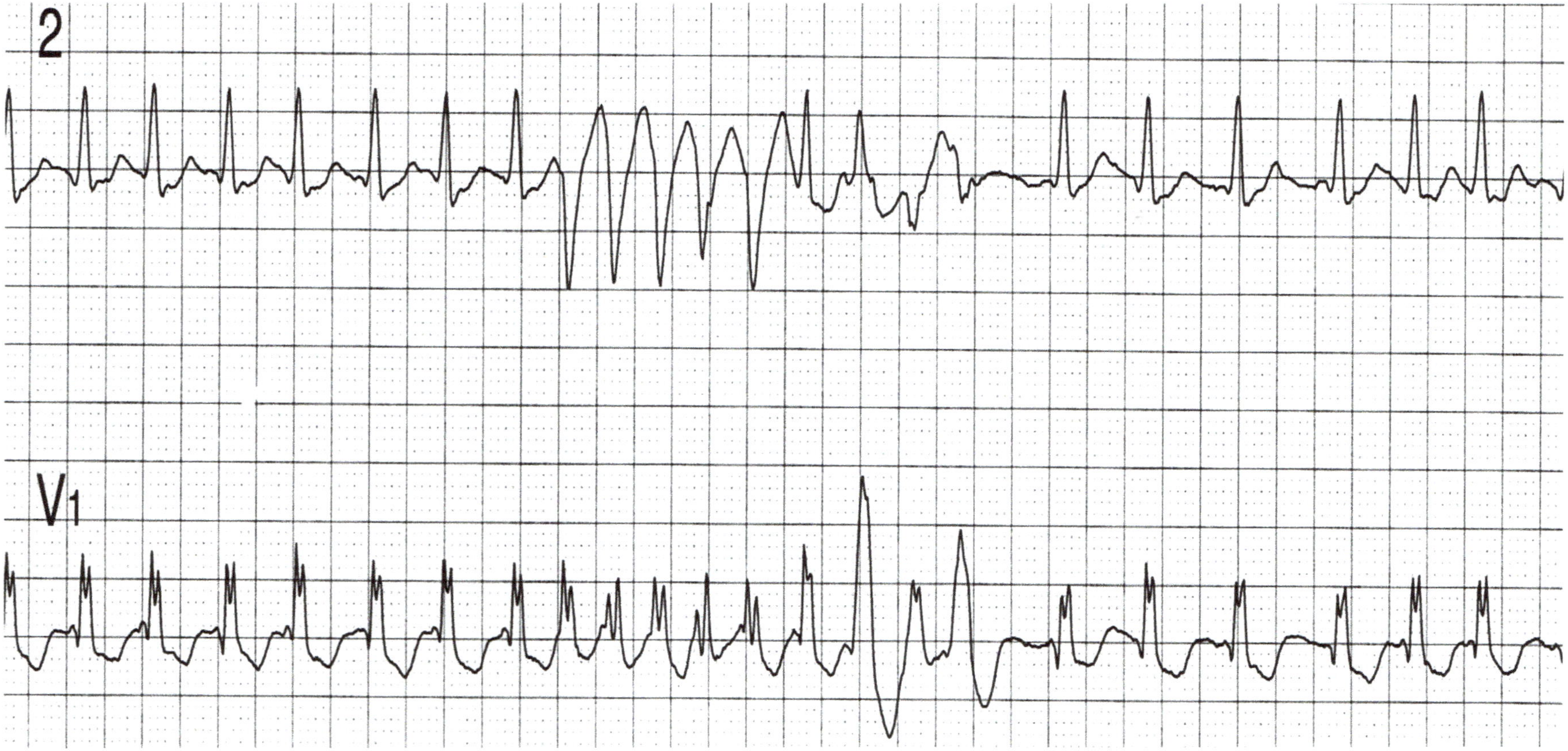

Question 6-12

## Question 6-12

The 2 leads shown in **Figure 6-12** are simultaneous. This individual had long-standing RBBB with known paroxysmal atrial fibrillation.
The wide QRS cycles are attributed to:

1. VT
2. Aberrancy
3. Intermittent preexcitation
4. More data needed

## Answer

The ambient rhythm is AF, and our challenge is to comment on the WCT at the center of the tracing.

Our most important clue here is the presence of baseline right bundle branch block (RBBB). Most of the WCT complexes are *different* than the ambient QRS (deep QS in lead 2), and this, in my experience, is a very useful clue to the diagnosis of VT. This is intuitively rational, as one might imagine LBBB aberration to cause complete AV block in the presence of established RBBB.

One might also note that the last cycle of WCT is followed by a pause relatively longer than the average CL. This suggests the last cycle of WCT at the least is ventricular (concealed retrograde conduction into the AV node would be expected to delay the next supraventricular cycle).

Figure 6-13

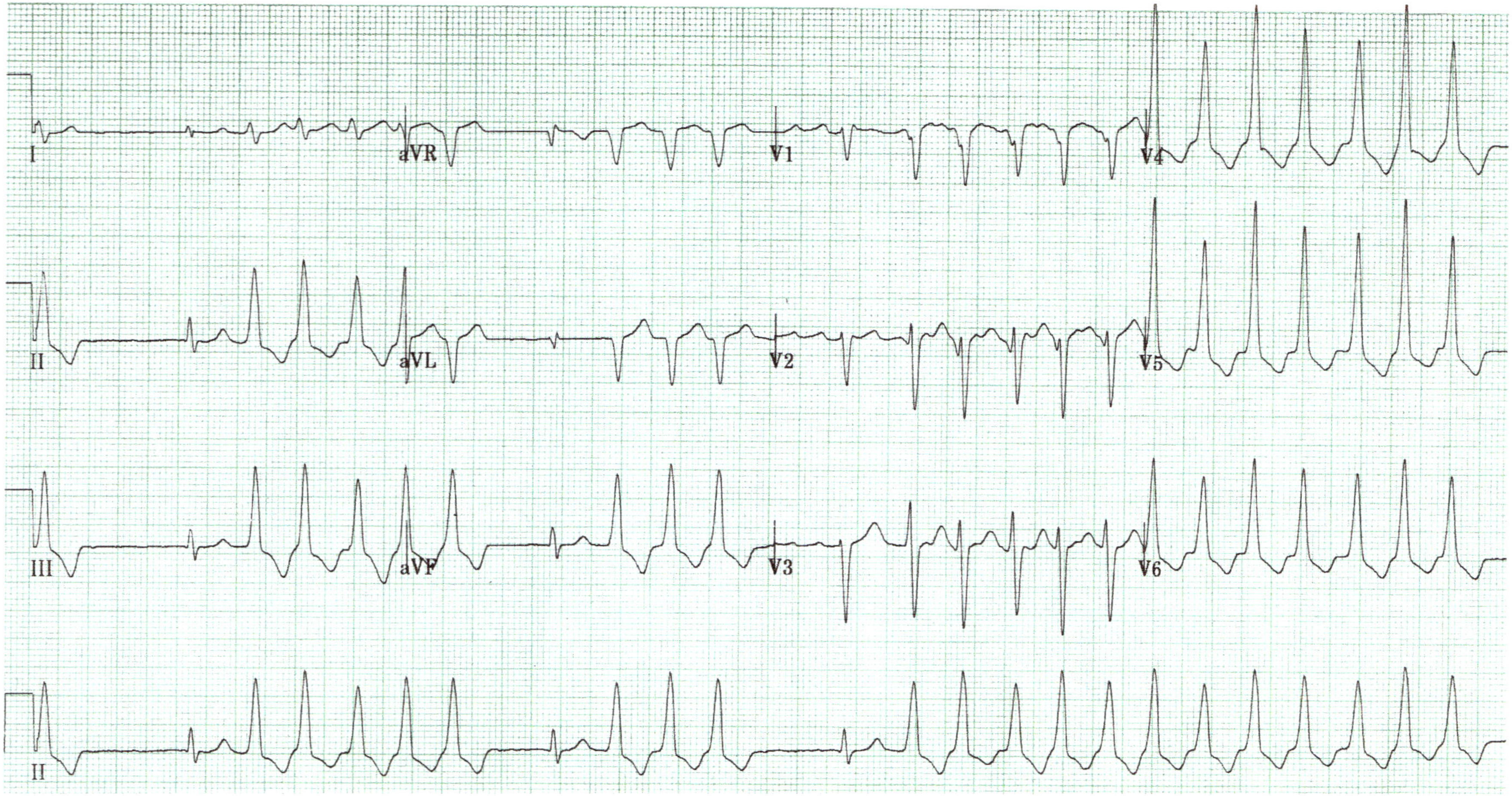


Question 6-13

## Question 6-13

The individual whose ECG is shown in **Figure 6-13** had long-standing AF.
Most probable mechanism of WCT:

1. VT
2. AF with aberrancy
3. Intermittent preexcitation
4. More data needed

## Answer

The baseline is relatively flat, especially in the frontal leads, but fibrillatory activity is more obvious in the precordial leads $V_1$ to $V_3$, and a conclusion of background AF is reasonable. We are hampered by not seeing longer runs with normal QRS, which would give us the opportunity to compare the ventricular pattern (speed, regularity) during AF during normal QRS to the WCT. The former and latter would be similar, all things being equal, if it were all just AF, sometimes with aberrancy. We do, however, observe that the WCT is quite regular, and this favors the diagnosis of VT.

There are 3 separate onsets of WCT, and all have virtually the same coupling interval to the previous normal QRS. This also favors ventricular ectopy, since these intervals should differ somewhat if it were all just AF. PVCs, on the other hand, are frequently coupled mechanistically to a preceding normal beat with this coupling interval often relatively constant. Constant coupling intervals favor VT.

Finally, we are fortunate enough to see the WCT in all 12 leads. The QRS resembles LBBB but $V_1$ and $V_2$ are certainly somewhat "atypical" with a rather slurred onset and qrS pattern rather than the sharp rS pattern seen typically. More compellingly, the frontal axis is strongly downward, suggesting a high ventricular, such as right ventricular (RV) outflow, origin of depolarization. The latter would be most atypical for LBBB and strongly favors a diagnosis of VT.

Putting it all together, the most likely answer is VT, and we have a "double tachycardia," namely, both AF *and* VT.

Figure 6-14A

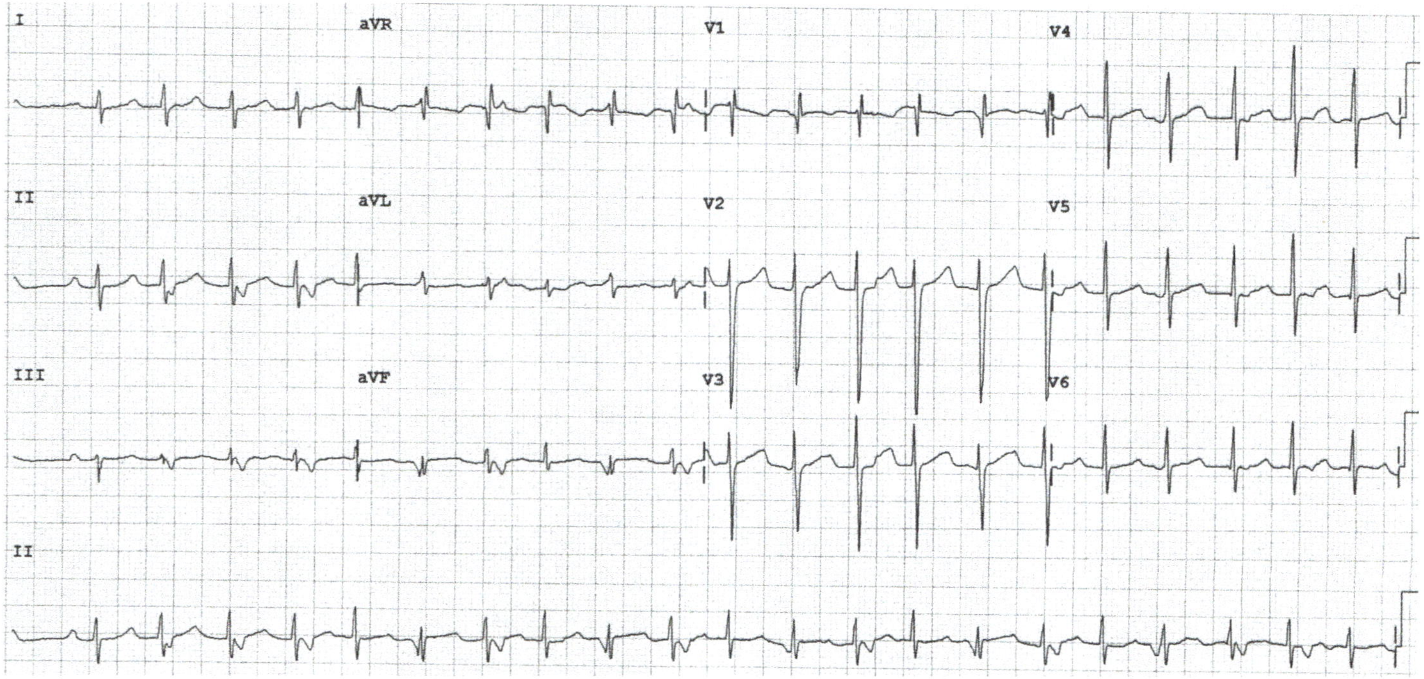


Figure 6-14B

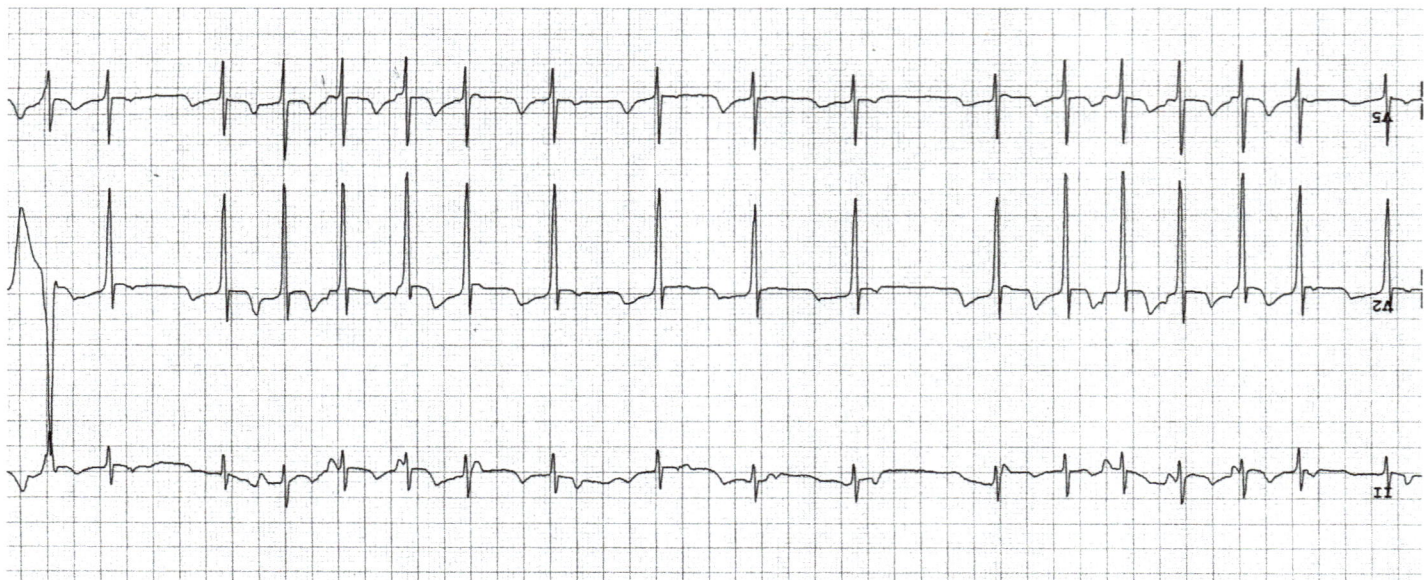

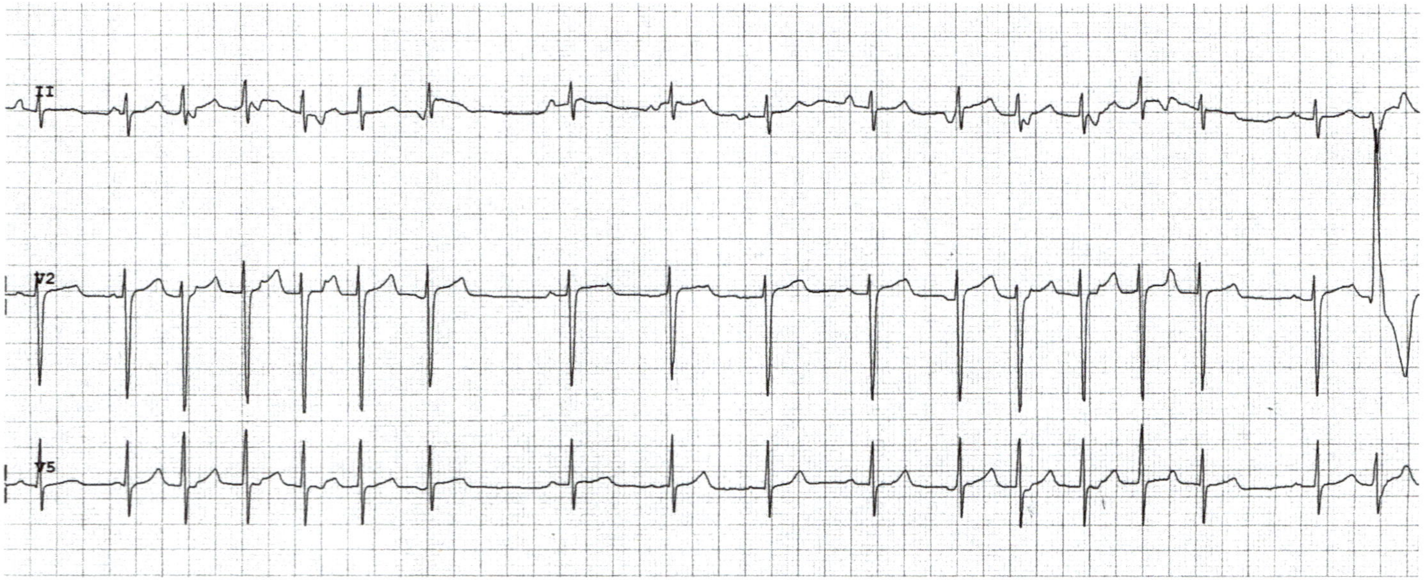

Question 6-14

## Question 6-14

The most probable mechanism for the tachycardia in **Figures 6-14A** and **6-14B** is:

1. AT
2. AVNRT
3. AVRT
4. JT

## Answer

We have 2 ECGs (Figures 6-14A and 6-14B) available from this individual with paroxysmal tachycardia. How does one start to interpret this obviously complex record—what is a useful strategy?

We start by making some global observations: note that the QRS complex is normal with no significant repolarization abnormality. The rhythm is irregular, and there is no obvious consistent relationship between the P waves and QRS complexes. Atrial activity is identifiable, and the P waves are inverted in the in inferior leads, i.e., "low-to-high" atrial activation. There is a suggestion of a recurring pattern although not perfect.

We now need to focus on some details, and I will initially focus on a segment that appears to be less complex. The rhythm strips (Figure 6-14B) show 2 tachycardia stops and starts. The onset is particularly useful, so we will start there. We can divide this strip into several "zones," and I have chosen the latter part of the figure, magnified in **Figure 6-14C**, since it shows a sinus beat followed by SVT, as well as spontaneous termination—also usually informative. This segment resembles the repeating pattern in the complete 12 lead.

When P waves and QRS complexes are identified, it is easy to exclude AVRT, which requires a 1:1 relationship between P and QRS and a minimal RP interval. The latter is too short for some and P waves even precede the QRS at times. AVRT is unequivocally out.

The onset in Figure 6-14C shows an inverted P wave as the first tachycardia event followed within 60 ms or so by the QRS. This apparent PR interval is too short to be physiological in the absence of preexcitation (of which there is no suggestion anywhere). An AT is possible and would, of course, begin with a P wave, but if this were the case in this instance, one would have to postulate a coincidental junctional extrasystole just after the first tachycardia P wave if we don't believe that there is enough time for the P wave to make it to the ventricle.

We move on to measure some intervals to clarify the relationship between P and QRS. On making a few measurements, one immediately notes that *the atrial rate (CL in **blue**) is actually slower than the ventricular rate (CL in **red**)*, a fatal contradiction for a diagnosis of AT—which can thus be reasonably excluded. It is interesting that this relationship is made clearer by simply writing the intervals on the strip!

With a faster junctional rate than atrial rate, we now only have 3 finite possibilities, namely JT, AVNRT, or possibly nodoventricular tachycardia (the latter using a circuit including the normal AV conducting system (AVCS or atrioventricular conducting system) anterogradely and a nodoventricular pathway linking the ventricle back to the AV node).

JT would not be expected to be this irregular, and JT isn't a common paroxysmal arrhythmia (certainly in adults), but it can't be entirely excluded. AVNRT would be the best fit *since neither the atrium nor the ventricle are essential to the AV nodal reentrant circuit*, and it is not untenable that variable conduction from the circuit reaches both atrium and ventricle differently. The same might also be said for the very rare nodoventricular tachycardia (anterogradely over normal AVCS, retrogradely back to the node via a nodoventricular pathway). It is usually a better bet to pick an unusual manifestation of a common problem (namely AVNRT) than a very rare one.

Figure 6-14C

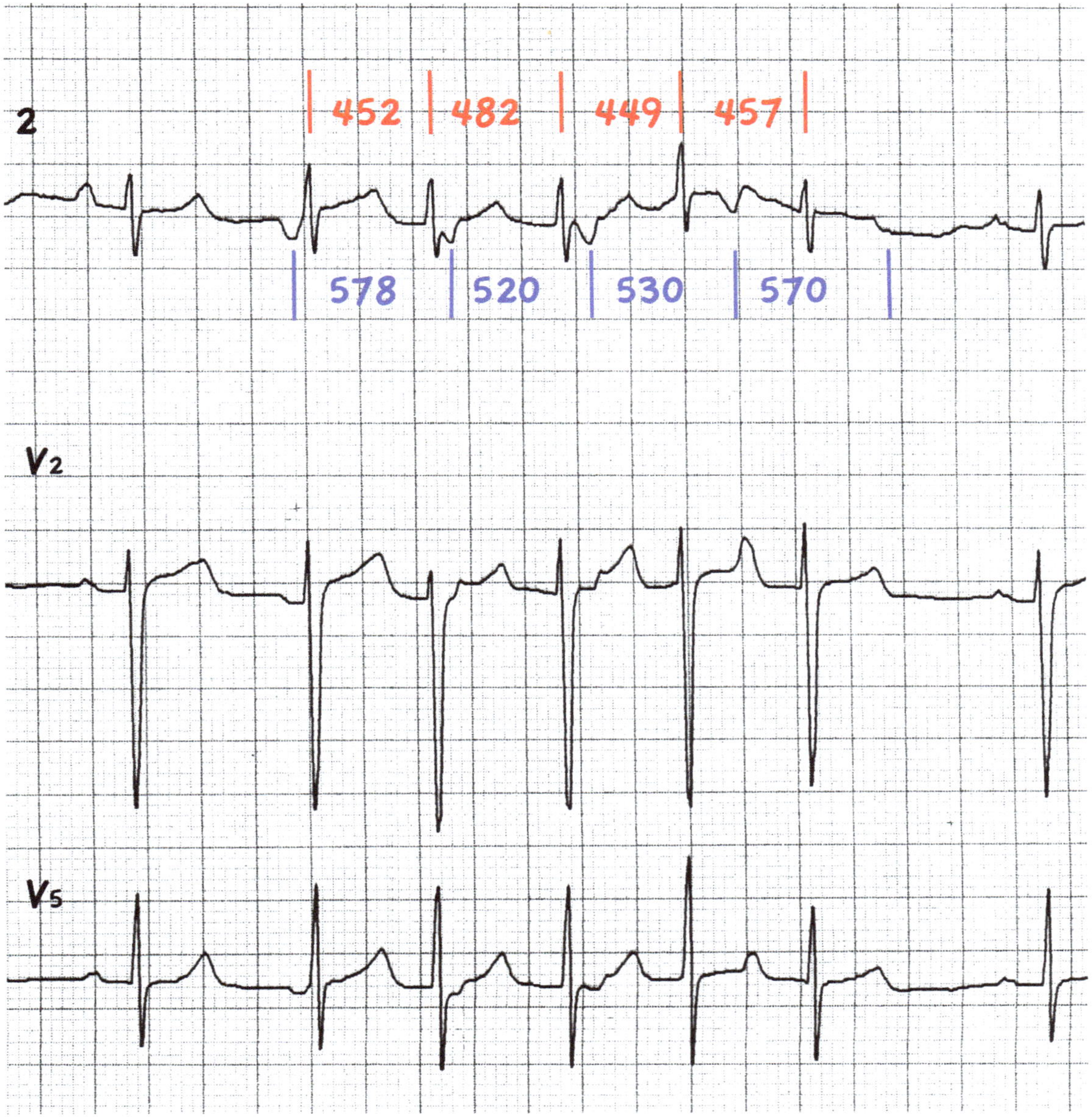

Thus, the most probable diagnosis, after all is said and done, is AVNRT, and this would be the best answer (although not uncontested!) to the multiple-choice question. The final diagnosis by electrophysiology testing was AVNRT. AVNRT can be very cryptic and a great masquerader and is frequently the culprit when one is confused!

It is appreciated that this is a complex ECG, but the case illustrates well the strategic approach—namely, making general observations, focusing on a region initially more readily understandable, magnifying areas of interest, careful measurement and hypothesis testing to come incrementally to a diagnosis or at least a "short list."

*Acknowledgments:* Original tracings were courtesy of Dr. Ray Sy.

Figure 6-15A

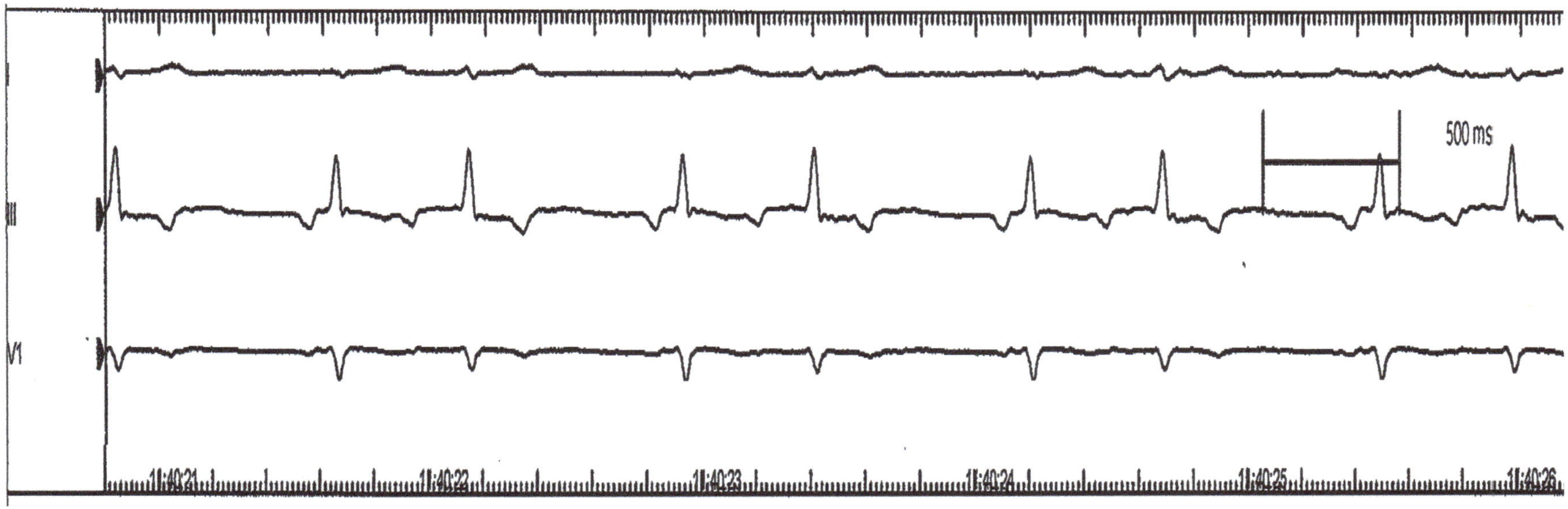




## Question 6-15

The most probable mechanism for the tachycardia shown in **Figure 6-15A** is:

1. AT
2. AVNRT
3. AVRT
4. JT

## Answer

This is a "regularly irregular" rhythm with a recurring pattern. The most glaring observation is that there are more P waves than QRS complexes, informing us that whatever the mechanism, it does not require ventricular participation. There are only 3 possible mechanisms for an SVT that doesn't require ventricular participation, and these are enumerated in the question.

We can now make some measurements and further observations (**Figure 6-15B**). The P wave is negative in lead 2 (low-to-high atrial activation), but this does not rule out any of our possibilities.

There is a recurring pattern or "group beating" (**horizontal arrows**) and the atrial CL is irregular. JT does not require atrial or ventricular participation and can theoretically conduct to the atrium while blocking to the ventricle. However, this is very rarely (if ever?) observed and can be relegated to the very unlikely category.

AT would be expected to be more regular as a rule so this is a less likely possibility. Additionally, one notices that the recurring pattern suggests Wenckebach periodicity with the PR interval prolonging prior to every blocked P wave. Notably, the atrial CL *follows* this pattern and also prolongs, making the atrial CL irregular. Thus, *the atrial CL is variable (prolongs within each recurring segment) and each CL prolongation is preceded by prolongation of the PR interval.* This would essentially rule out AT.

The only plausible diagnosis left is AVNRT (obviously "atypical") where anterograde AV nodal conduction is linked to retrograde conduction, even though one can only guess at the "micro" anatomy that is the substrate for this connectedness in our example.

The above is a clear example where the correct answer is really only arrived out by *excluding* those options that are clearly not compatible with the observations after the universe of options is laid out.

Figure 6-15B

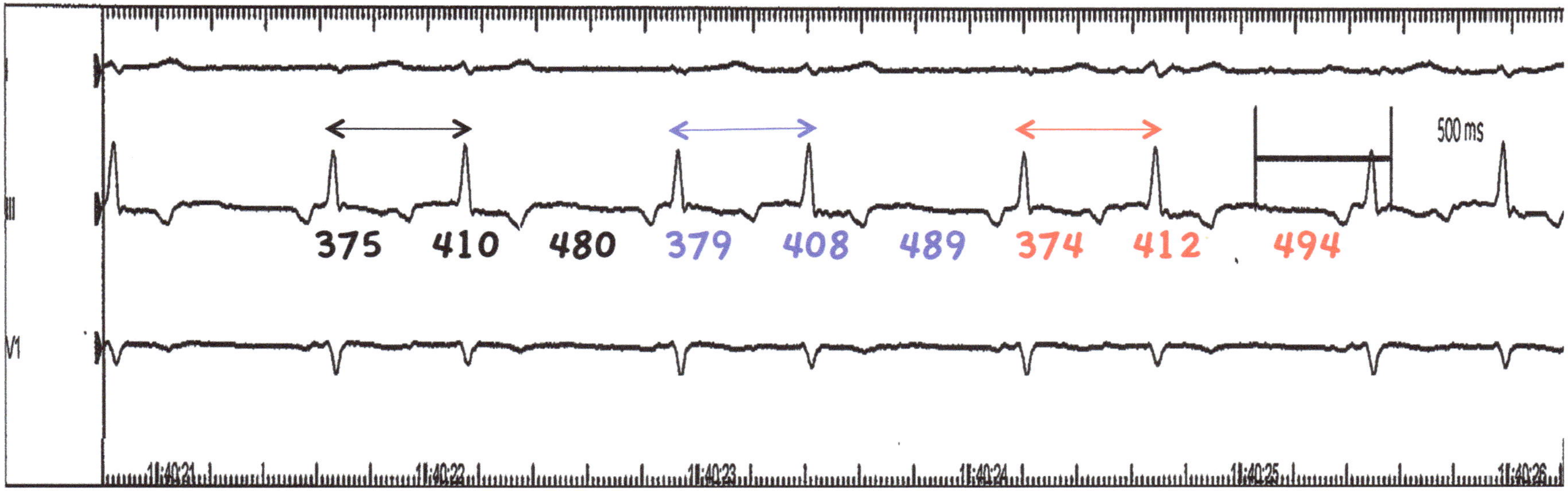
I
III
V1
500 ms
375
410
480
379
408
489
374
412
494
11:40:21
11:40:22
11:40:23
11:40:24
11:40:25
11:40:26

# Chapter 7

## Application of Strategies: Further Practice

Question 7-1

Figure 7-1

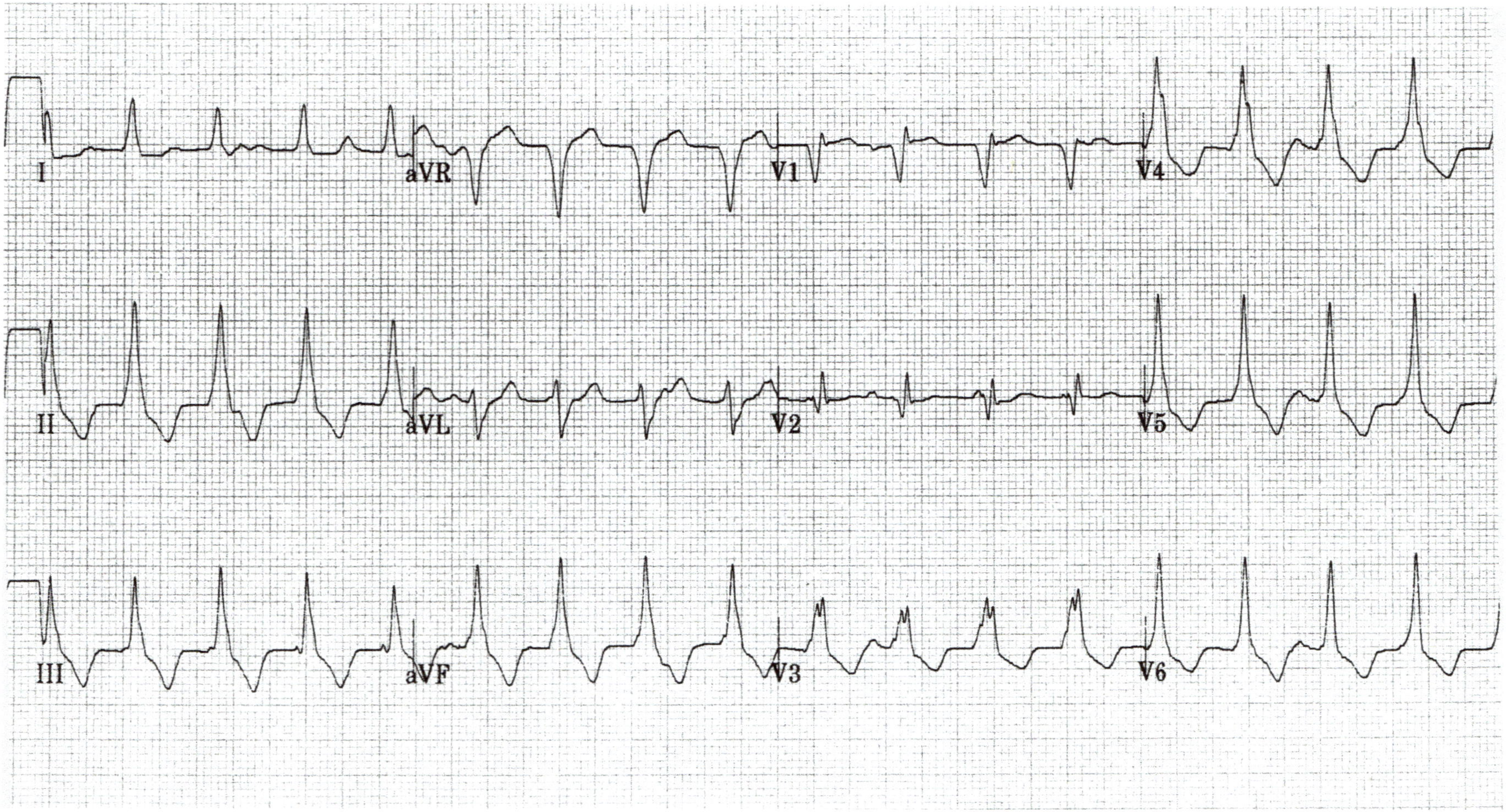

## Question 7-1

The ECG in **Figure 7-1** is from a 45-year-old man, previously well, presenting with palpitations.
The baseline ECG was normal.
The tachycardia mechanism is:

1. Ventricular tachycardia (VT)
2. Supraventricular tachycardia (SVT) with aberrancy
3. Preexcited tachycardia
4. Need more data

## Answer

Figure 7-1 shows a regular tachycardia with QRS duration of at most 120 ms, and less in some leads. Most of the readers of this book should not have great difficulty with this tracing, but it does highlight a few important principles.

P waves are not apparent in the all the leads and probably most obvious in $V_2$, where AV dissociation is evident. *It is useful to remember that atrial activity and AV dissociation are often best appreciated in the leads with the lowest amplitude QRS, as occurs in this example.*

The tracing also shows a relatively narrow "wide QRS" tachycardia often misdiagnosed as SVT by the inexperienced. Further, it highlights the pitfalls of diagnosis from one or a few leads of a rhythm strip, noting here that lead 1 here looks especially "supraventricular" if that were the only one available.

The diagnosis of VT is also evident from the QRS morphology. It is atypical of, if not frankly incompatible with, bundle branch block aberrancy, making SVT with aberrancy untenable.

We remind here, as elsewhere, that essentially all published so-called VT "criteria" are based on the goodness of fit of the putative tachycardia to an acceptable bundle branch block pattern. The more closely it resembles a "typical" bundle branch block pattern, the more likely it is to be bundle branch block aberrancy and vice versa.

In this case, the strikingly inferior axis (high-to-low activation in the frontal plane) would be compatible with VT origin in the ventricular outflow region. Relative narrowness of the QRS in VT may be related in part to a more septal location with cancellation of forces or perhaps good access to the His-Purkinje system.

Figure 7-2A

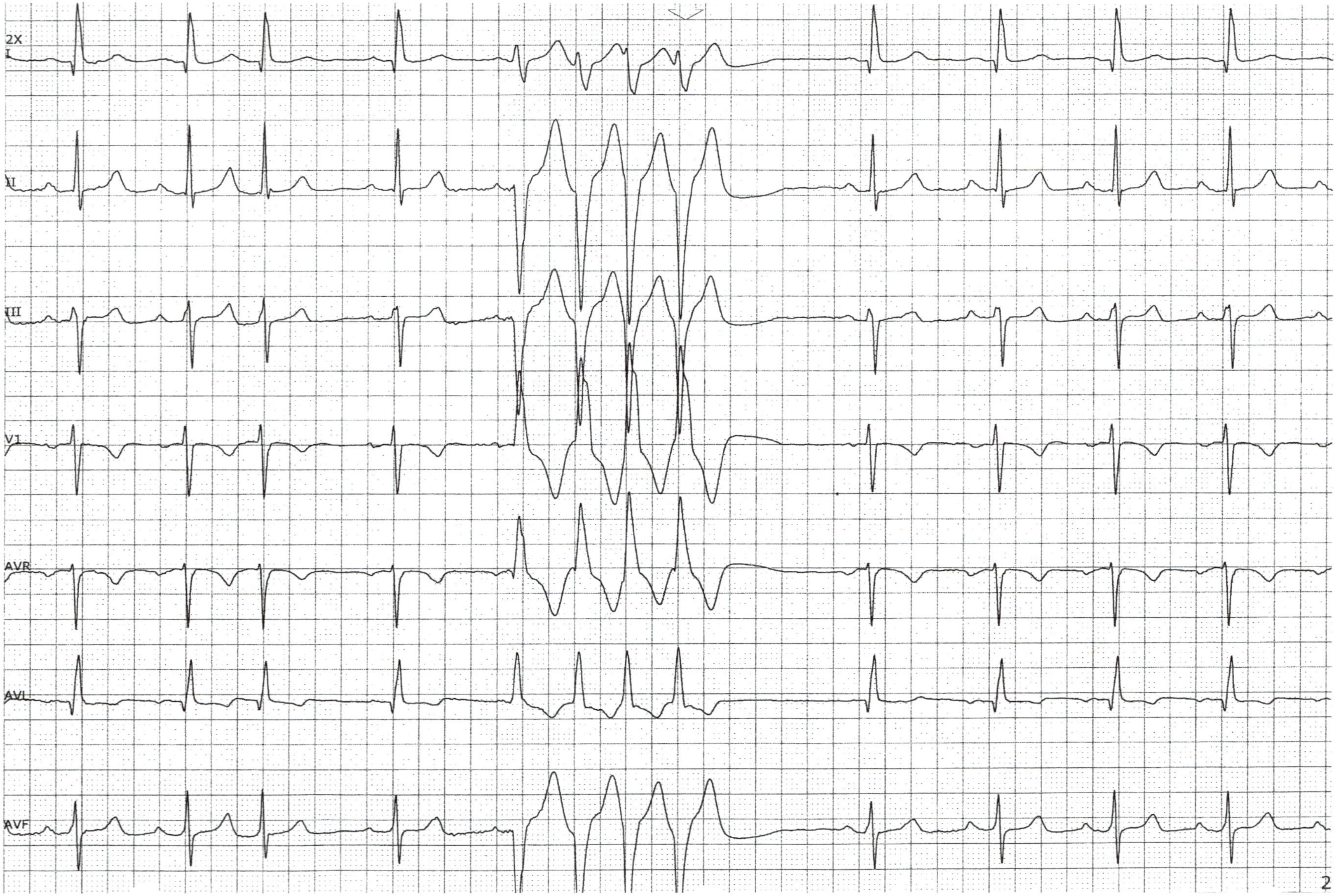

Question 7-2

## Question 7-2

The tachycardia mechanism for the tracing shown in **Figure 7-2A** is:

1. VT
2. SVT with aberrancy
3. Preexcited tachycardia
4. Need more data

## Answer

Although AV dissociation is not evident, the tracing provides multiple leads and is free of artifact. The experienced electrocardiographer should readily identify this tracing unequivocally as VT. For an exercise, however, the reader is invited to pause and enumerate the number of supportive criteria before reading the explanatory section that follows.

Firstly, the QRS morphology resembles right bundle branch block (RBBB) but is very atypical of, if not frankly incompatible with, bundle branch block aberrancy. $V_1$ shows a wide, monophasic complex, the axis is closer to "northwest," and there are wide QS complexes in the inferior leads. *The QRS in sinus rhythm is relatively normal, so that one would expect a relatively "typical" bundle branch block pattern in the case of aberrancy.*

Second, the initial forces between normal and wide QRS are discordant (**Figure 7-2B**, **arrows**), and one would usually expect them to be the same in RBBB since the initial forces in normal ventricular activation are usually related to septal activation by the septal branch of the left bundle branch (LBB) and not affected by RBBB.

Third, the tachycardia begins with a plausible fusion beat (**blue asterisk**), that is a credible summation of the preceding normal and subsequent wide QRS (**red asterisks**).

Finally, the first cycle of the WCT (i.e., the fusion beat) is preceded by a sinus P wave with a shorter PR than the preceding sinus beat (**vertical lines**). This can only happen if the first beat of VT starts to depolarize before the sinus beat makes it through the AV conduction system and is essentially a late-coupled premature ventricular contraction (PVC). It can potentially represent preexcitation but the QRS doesn't fit with the usual accessory pathway (AP) patterns.

Figure 7-2B

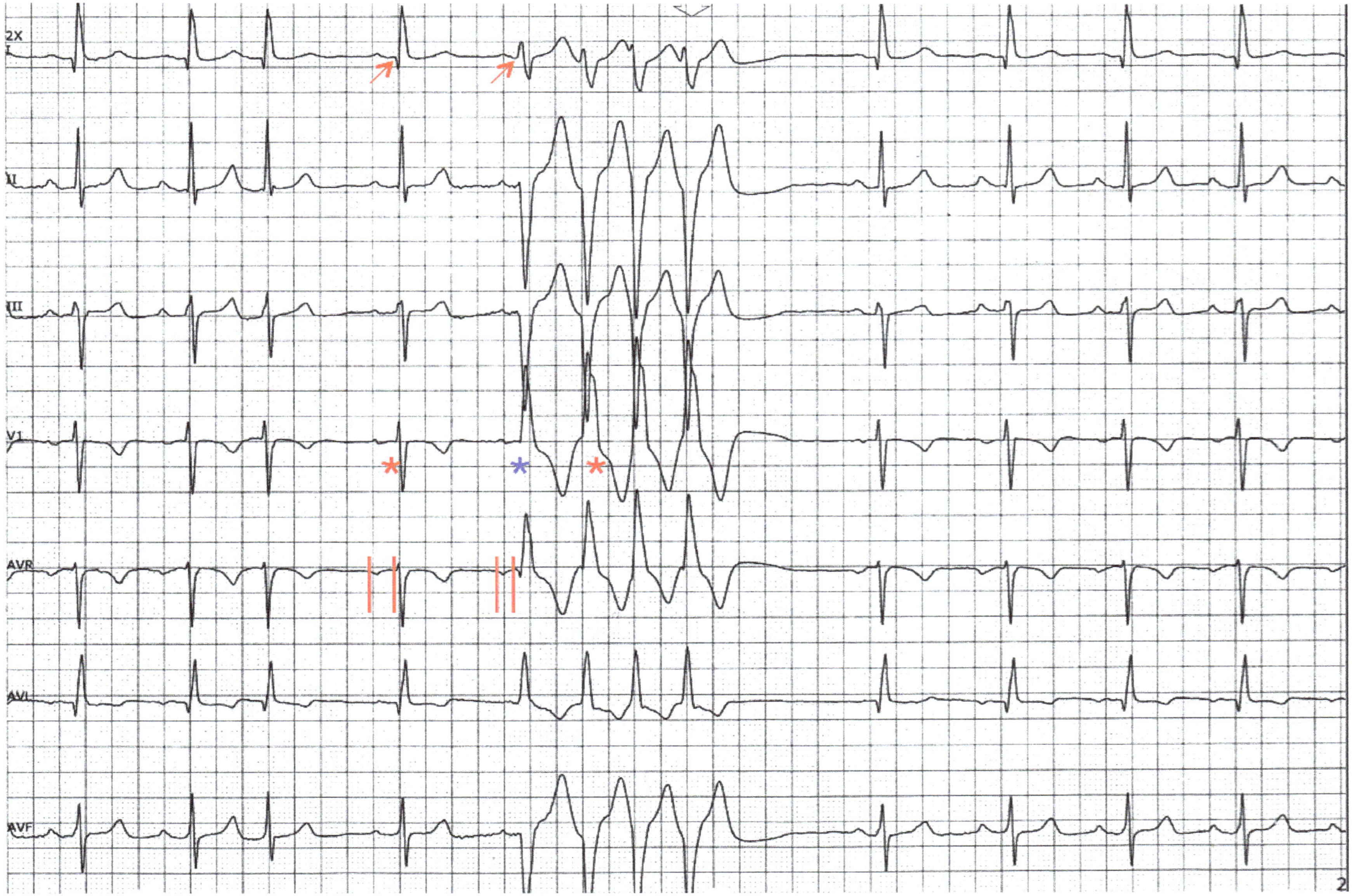

Figure 7-3A

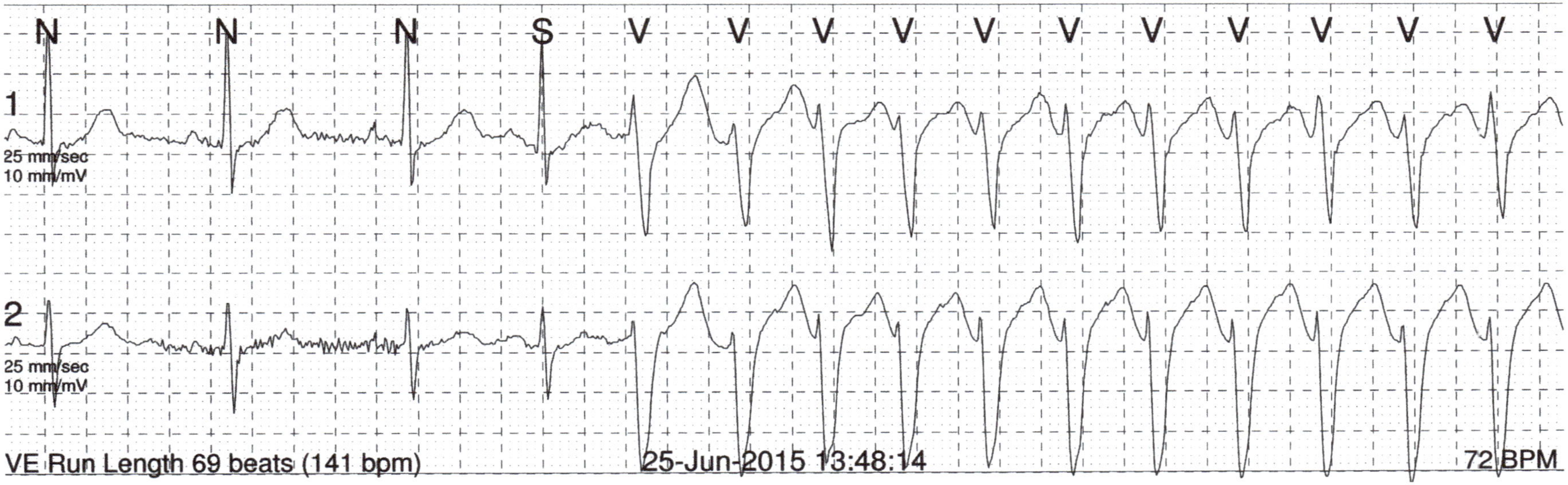


## Question 7-3

The tachycardia mechanism in **Figure 7-3A** is:

1. VT
2. SVT with aberrancy
3. Preexcited tachycardia
4. Need more data

## Answer

This strip only provides 2 leads of unknown location, and furthermore has artifact complicating the situation, but this is often reality. However, the initial forces in the WCT are very "rapid" with very steep downslope, suggestive of activation by the His-Purkinje system (**Figure 7-3B**).

There is a consistent deflection on the upstroke of the ST segment (**blue dots**) most suggestive of a P wave, so that this appears to be wide complex tachycardia (WCT) with a 1:1 AV relationship (although it is unclear whether the P drives the QRS or vice versa).

The best clue comes from the fourth QRS on the left (**blue arrow**), which is clearly a premature atrial contraction (PAC) immediately preceding the WCT. *It would be a large coincidence if this PAC happened to be there at the onset of VT,* and this favors SVT considerably. Contrast this with Figure 7-2 where the first beat of the WCT is *preceded by a sinus P wave on time*, not a premature one.

In addition, channel 1 is relatively free of artifact. The first WCT

Figure 7-3B

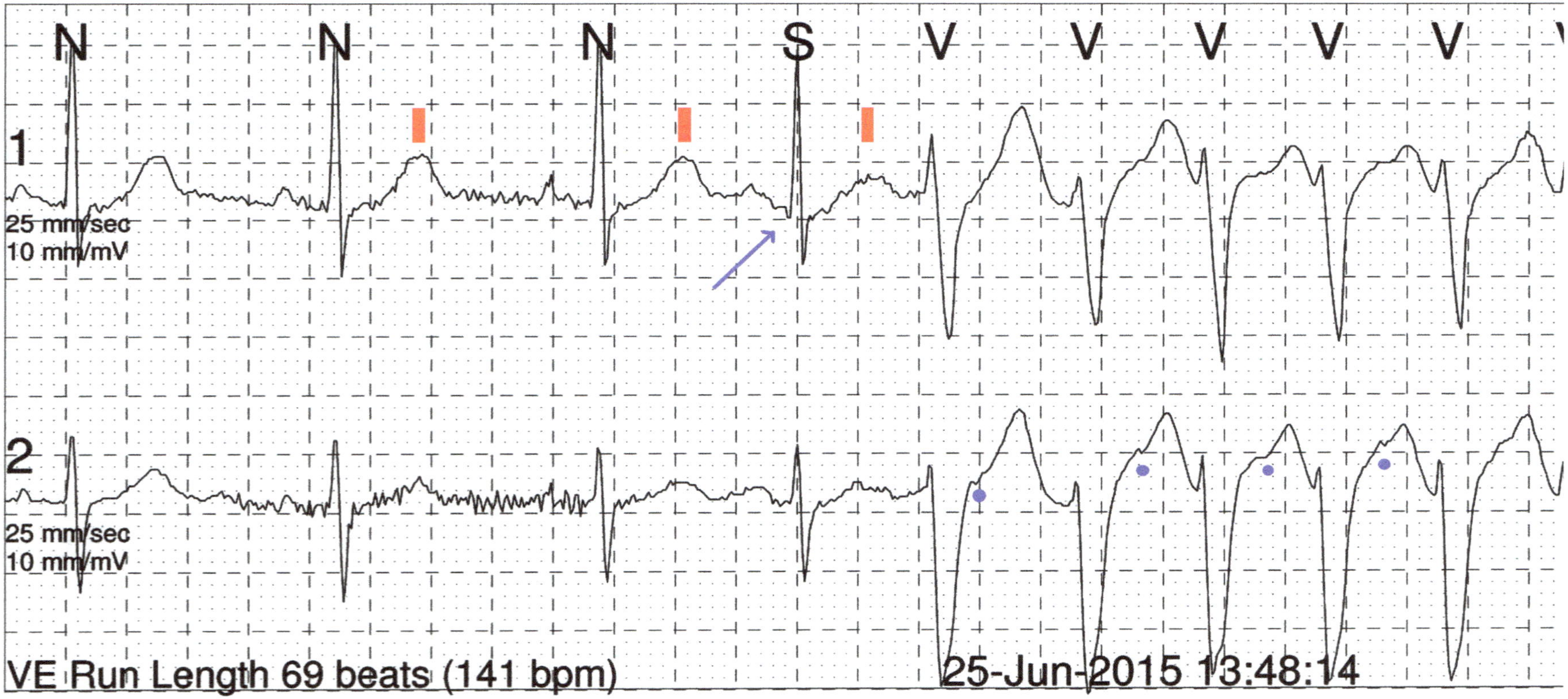

beat is preceded by a T wave that is dissimilar to its predecessors (**red rectangles**) and most probably represents a P wave merging with the T wave and initiating SVT.

This analysis is supported elsewhere in this patient's Holter record (**Figure 7-3C**), where atrial tachycardia (AT) of virtually identical cycle length (CL) is initiated similarly to the WCT.

Figure 7-3C

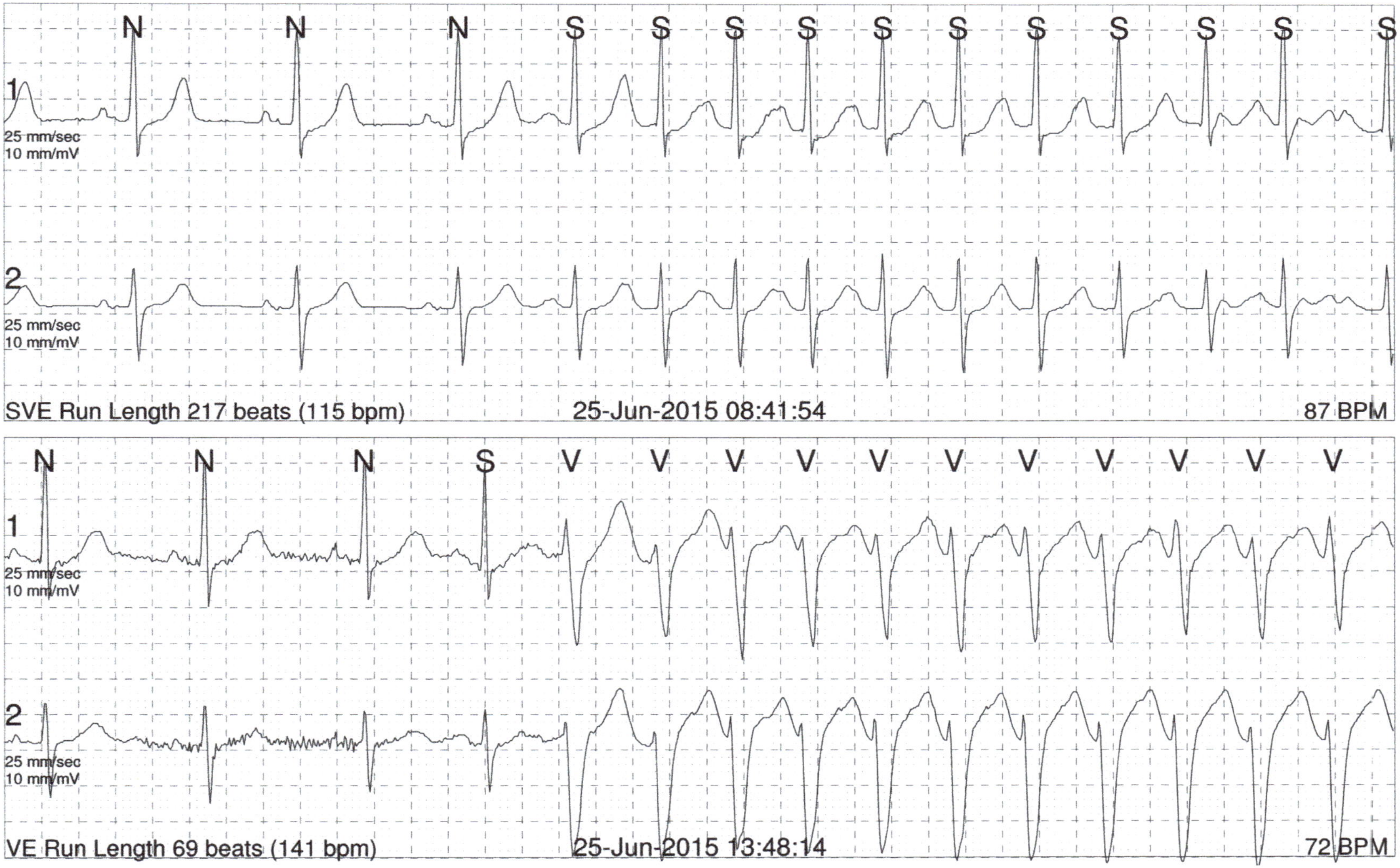

Figure 7-4A

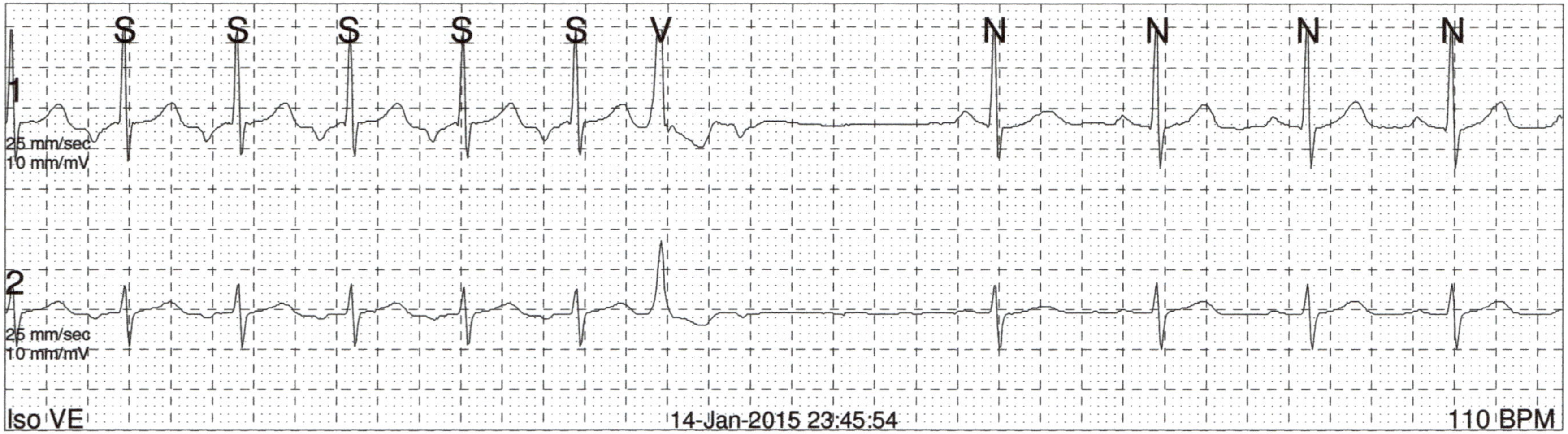
S S S S S V N N N N
1
25 mm/sec
10 mm/mV
2
25 mm/sec
10 mm/mV
Iso VE
14-Jan-2015 23:45:54
110 BPM

## Question 7-4

The tachycardia mechanism in the tracing shown in **Figure 7-4A** is:

1. AT
2. Atrioventricular nodal reentrant tachycardia (AVNRT)
3. Atrioventricular reentrant tachycardia (AVRT)
4. Need more data

## Answer

This tracing is taken from the same individual as illustrated in **Question 3-11** and demonstrates a variant of the same theme. The SVT at the beginning of the trace is a "long-RP" tachycardia with the differential diagnosis including the first 3 options of the question. The tachycardia is regular and terminates after a PVC that is coupled relatively early.

The essential observations are evident on the annotated close-up (**Figure 7-4B**). First, termination of AT with a PVC would be most unusual. The tachycardia ends with a P wave, further making AT unlikely.

The PVC timing results in disappearance of the P wave in the PVC and the timing of the expected P wave is indicated by a **blue dot**. The next P wave is advanced (reset), again mitigating against AT, which should not be reset by a PVC .

We can't really assess if the His was refractory at the point the PVC occurred. Nonetheless, the VA interval of the PVC was within the range considered to be "within the circuit" (difference of VA less than 85 ms), clinching the diagnosis of AVRT (see **Question 3-11**).

Figure 7-4B

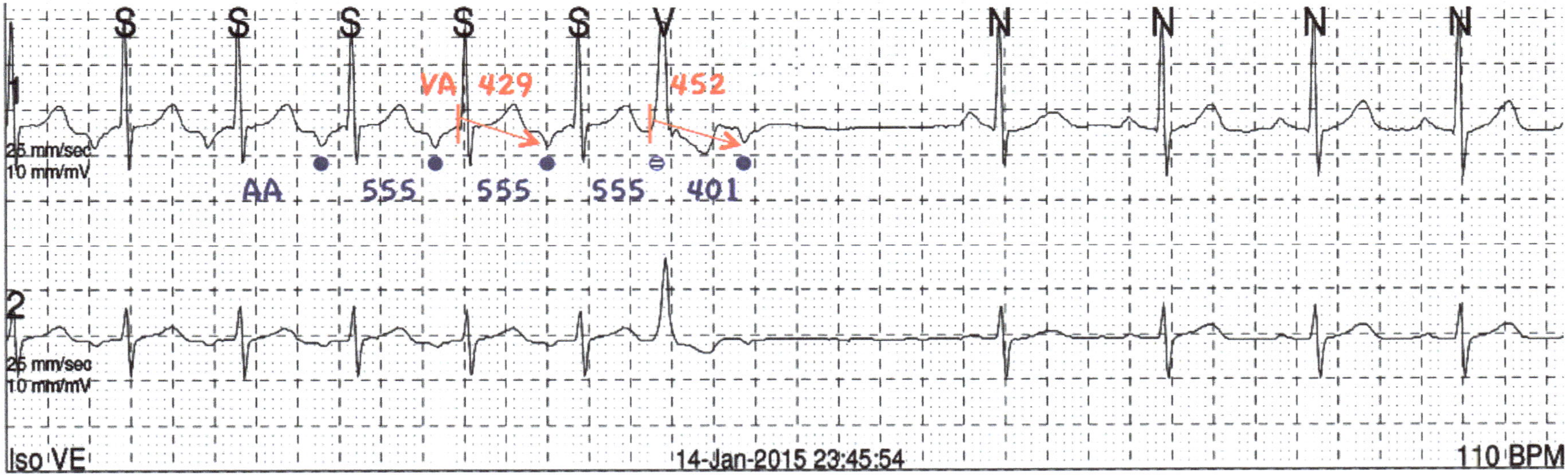
S S S S S V N N N N
1
VA 429
452
25 mm/sec
10 mm/mV
AA
555
555
555
401
2
25 mm/sec
10 mm/mV
Iso VE
14-Jan-2015 23:45:54
110 BPM

Figure 7-5A

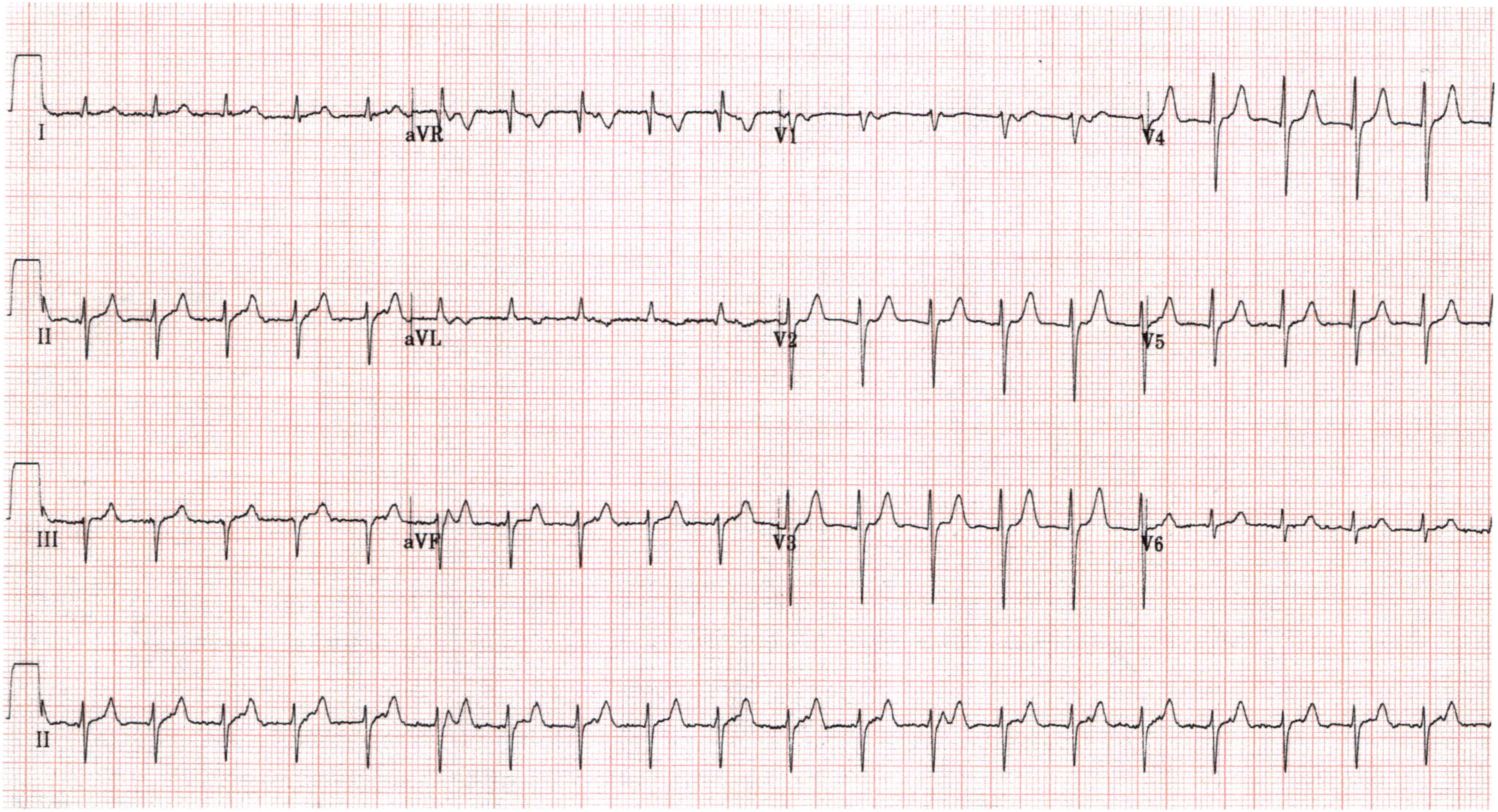


Question 7-5

## Question 7-5

The tachycardia mechanism seen in **Figure 7-5A**, a tracing from an asymptomatic 73-year-old man, is:

1. AT
2. AVNRT
3. AVRT
4. Need more data

## Answer

Figure 7-5A shows a regular tachycardia with CL 440. The QRS is compatible with a supraventricular origin. The search for atrial activity is challenging, but there are 2 "candidate" P waves.

The rhythm strip shows intermittent "sharp" activity in the ST segment (**blue dots** in **Figure 7-5B**) that is distinct, and these could well be P waves. The tracing is otherwise free of noise, making artifact a less likely possibility for this deflection, but certainly still a real possibility.

If this is a P wave, the tachycardia doesn't have a 1:1 AV relationship and the differential diagnosis is confined to AV nodal reentry (most frequent in this circumstance), junctional tachycardia (JT), nodoventricular reentry, or nodofascicular reentry, the latter group not requiring the atrium for tachycardia maintenance.

The other "candidate" P wave is best seen in $V_1$ and indicated by the **blue arrow**. A relatively sharp downward deflection such as this immediately after the QRS would not be expected to result from ventricular repolarization. It is relatively consistent, although not entirely clear in the cycle immediately before the **blue arrow**. If consistent P waves are identified in this region, the diagnosis widens to AVNRT, JT, AVRT, and AT (the latter 2 utilizing a slow AV nodal pathway for anterograde conduction).

In truth, regardless of which candidate P wave is chosen, the honest answer for most of us on this tracing would be "more data are needed." These needed data are found after the maneuver done in the subsequent **Question 7-6**.

Figure 7-5B

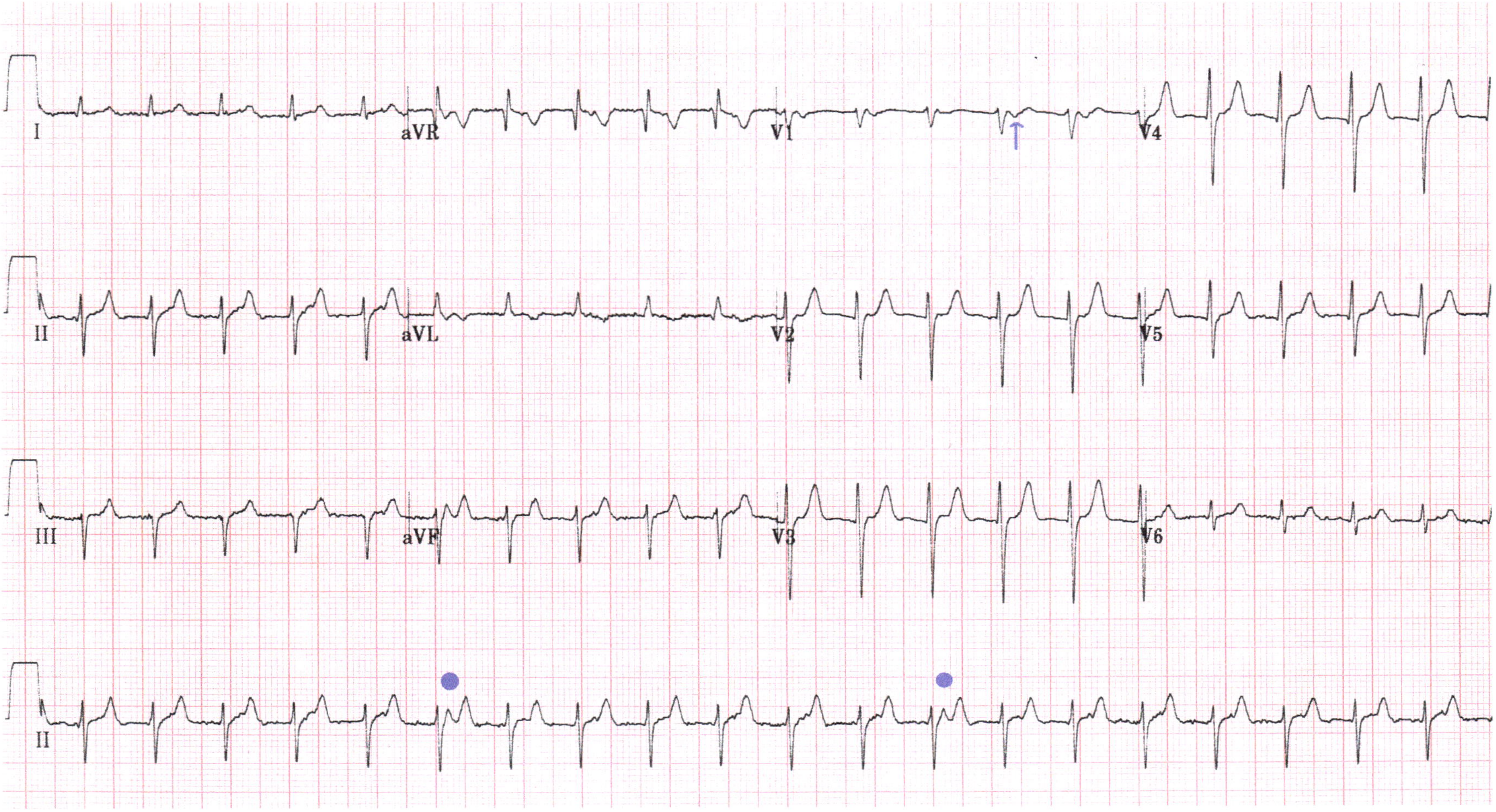

Figure 7-6A

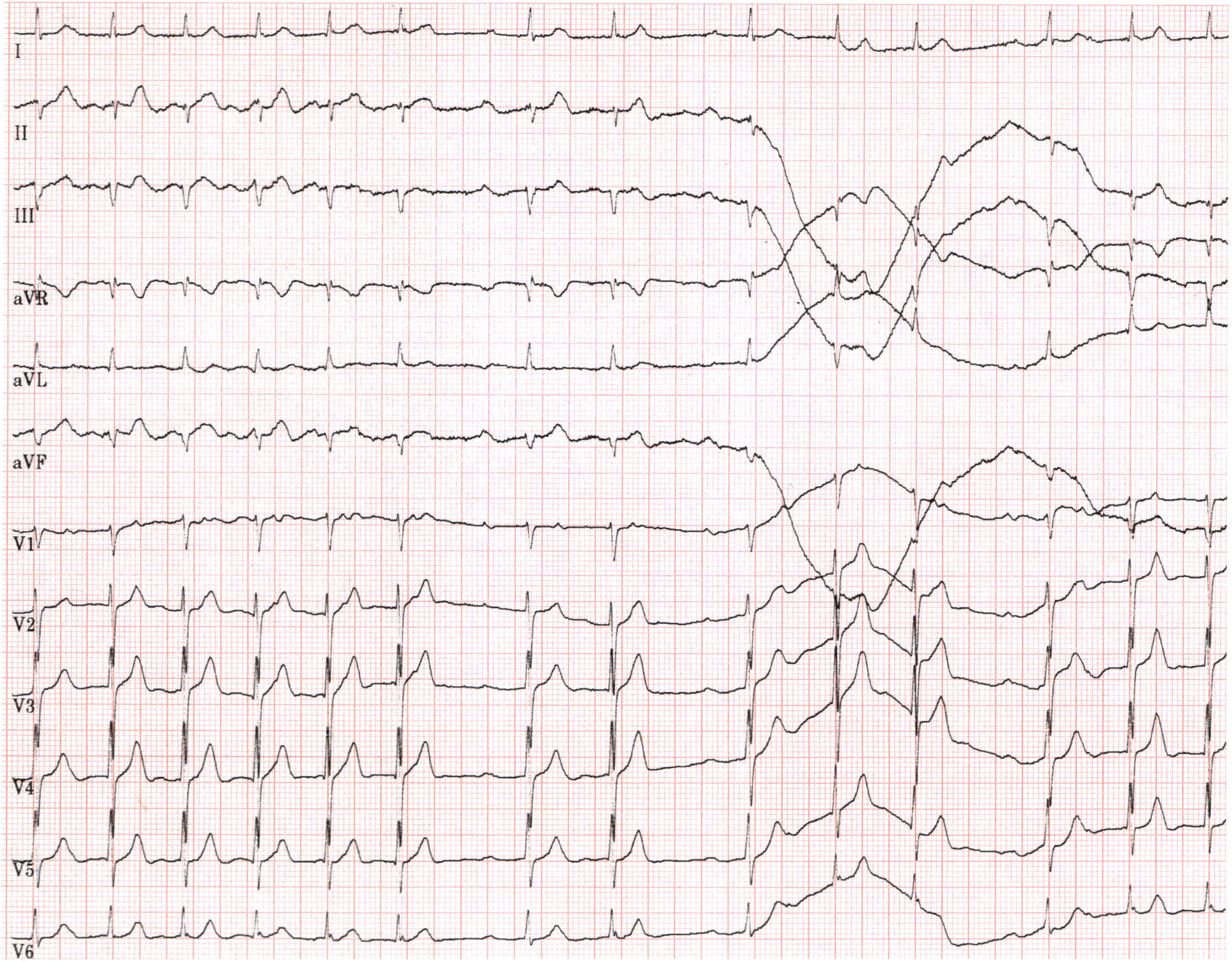


Question 7-6

Question 7-6

## Question 7-6

Carotid sinus massage (CSM) was done during the rhythm recorded in the previous **Question 7-5**. The tachycardia mechanism in **Figure 7-6A** is:

1. AT
2. AVNRT
3. AVRT
4. Sinus tachycardia (ST)

## Answer

Figure 7-6A shows transient AV block without termination of tachycardia, which of course clarifies the diagnosis.

Referring to the annotated version (**Figure 7-6B**), where the P waves are indicated by **blue dots**, facilitates the explanation. It is observed that CSM initially prolongs the PR interval, resulting in a long Wenckebach cycle ending in a dropped QRS. This is followed by graduated prolongation of the PP interval and more Wenckebach block. Thus, the diagnosis is either AT or ST.

The P-wave morphology (positive in leads 1, 2, and 3) unmasked by AV block is certainly compatible with sinus origin or AT originating near the sinus node. The gradual slowing of the sinus rate with CSM makes ST more likely. The time course of CSM effect on the sinus node and AV node need not be exactly the same, and the preponderance of sinus node effect versus AV node effect may also be influenced by whether the right or left carotid sinus is massaged. In retrospect, which is the true P wave in Figure 7-6B? Is there a clue to the diagnosis of AT (see $V_1$).

Figure 7-6B

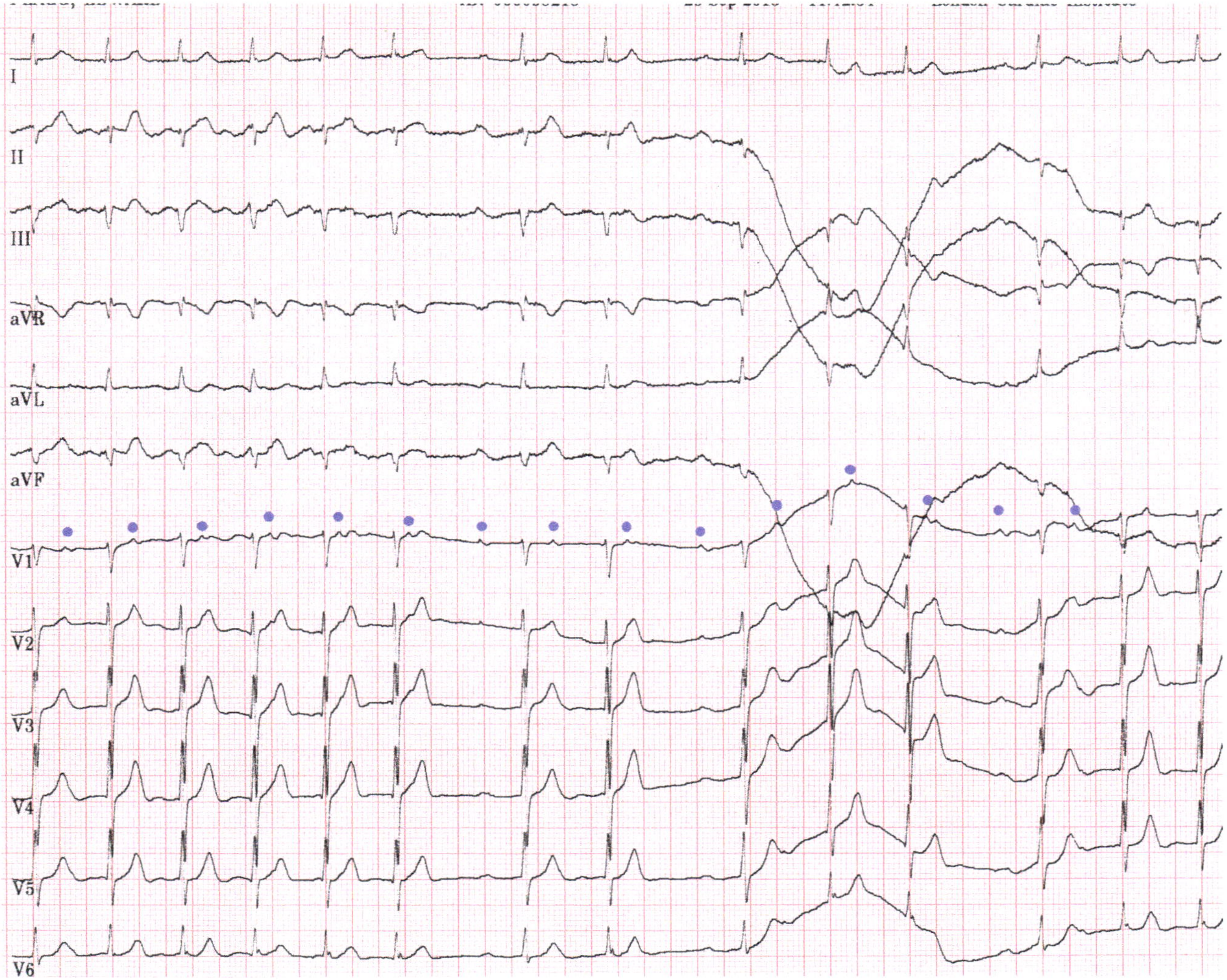

Figure 7-7A

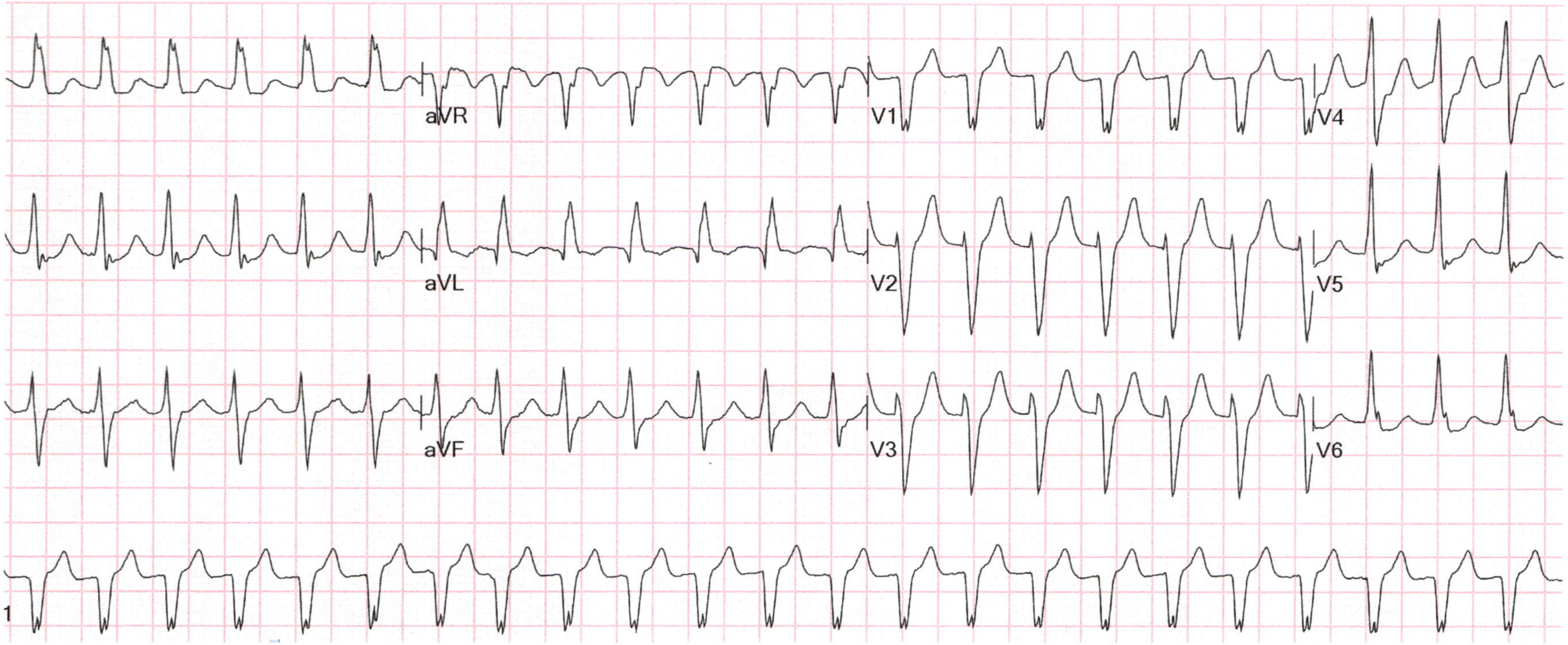

## Question 7-7

The tracing in **Figure 7-7A** is taken from a 71-year-old man presenting with palpitations.
The tachycardia mechanism is:

1. VT
2. AVNRT
3. AVRT
4. Need more data

## Answer

Figure 7-7A shows a regular tachycardia with left bundle branch block (LBBB) pattern. The LBBB pattern is very "typical" for LBBB with a small R wave in $V_2$ and a very rapid downslope, suggesting initial conduction over the His-Purkinje system—less likely to be VT. We are in a little trouble after that.

The rest of the tracing is more cryptic, with no apparent P wave. One might guess that the terminal part of the QRS is slightly notched at the beginning of the ST segment (as in lead 3), but this is tenuous.

A good possibility would be AVNRT, since the P wave in typical AVNRT is usually very close to or actually within the QRS boundaries, that is, subtle or imperceptible. Orthodromic AVRT remains possible, although one would expect to see the retrograde P wave in diastole with this relatively slow tachycardia and noise free tracing. Preexcited tachycardia conducting anterogradely over an atriofascicular AP could resemble typical LBBB, although one would again expect to see a P wave in diastole for AVRT, whether preexcited or not.

Although AVNRT is a leading candidate, there is no unequivocal diagnosis so that the answer to our question must remain Option 4.

The tracing shown in **Figure 7-7B** was recorded on the same day. We note that P waves are readily apparent (**blue dots**) and AT with 2:1 conduction is suggested. The QRS morphology remains

Figure 7-7B

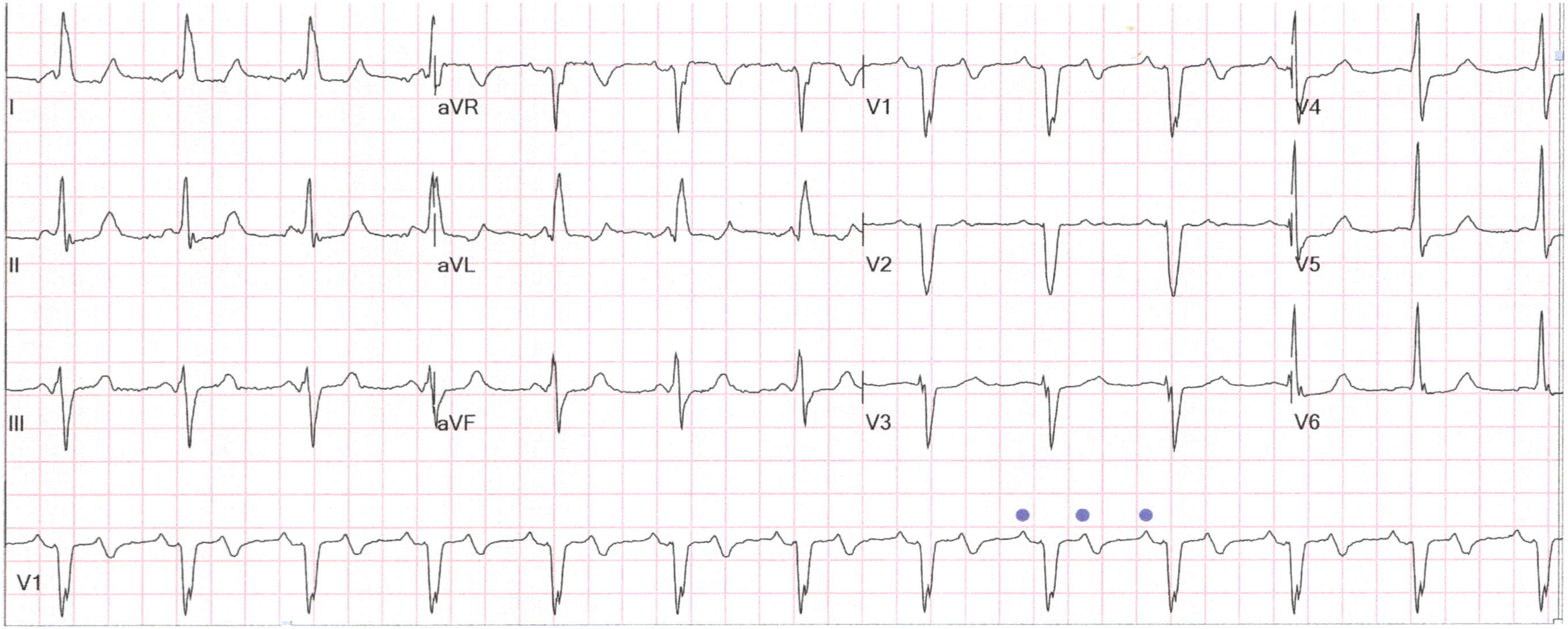

very similar to that above. AVNRT may exhibit 2:1 AV block, but the P wave in this tracing has a high-to-low frontal plane axis (positive in leads 1, 2, and 3), supporting a diagnosis of AT and essentially ruling out AVNRT for this tachycardia.

Is this AT the same tachycardia as in Figure 7-7A, now with 2:1 AV block? The CL of the tachycardia in Figure 7-7A is close to but not exactly twice the CL of the tachycardia in Figure 7-7B. Further, it is difficult to imagine the prominent P wave in Figure 7-7B disappearing entirely during 1:1 AV conduction. This makes it unlikely that the 2 tachycardias have the same mechanism, and we are still short of a diagnosis for Figure 7-7A.

Figure 7-7B, however, is still helpful *in that it provides a QRS template that we know is free of a terminal P wave*, and we can reexamine Figure 7-7A in that light. **Figure 7-7C** compares the lateral precordial leads side by side to facilitate this. We now note subtle differences in the terminal QRS of Figure 7-7A (**blue arrows**). *This supports the presence of a P wave in the terminal QRS of tachycardia of Figure 7-7A and hence a diagnosis of AVNRT.*

This patient reverted to sinus rhythm, and further studies were not pursued, so the final truth in these tracings is unknown. Not knowing does not detract from the thought process and careful observation that underlies the interpretation of such a tracing.

Figure 7-7C

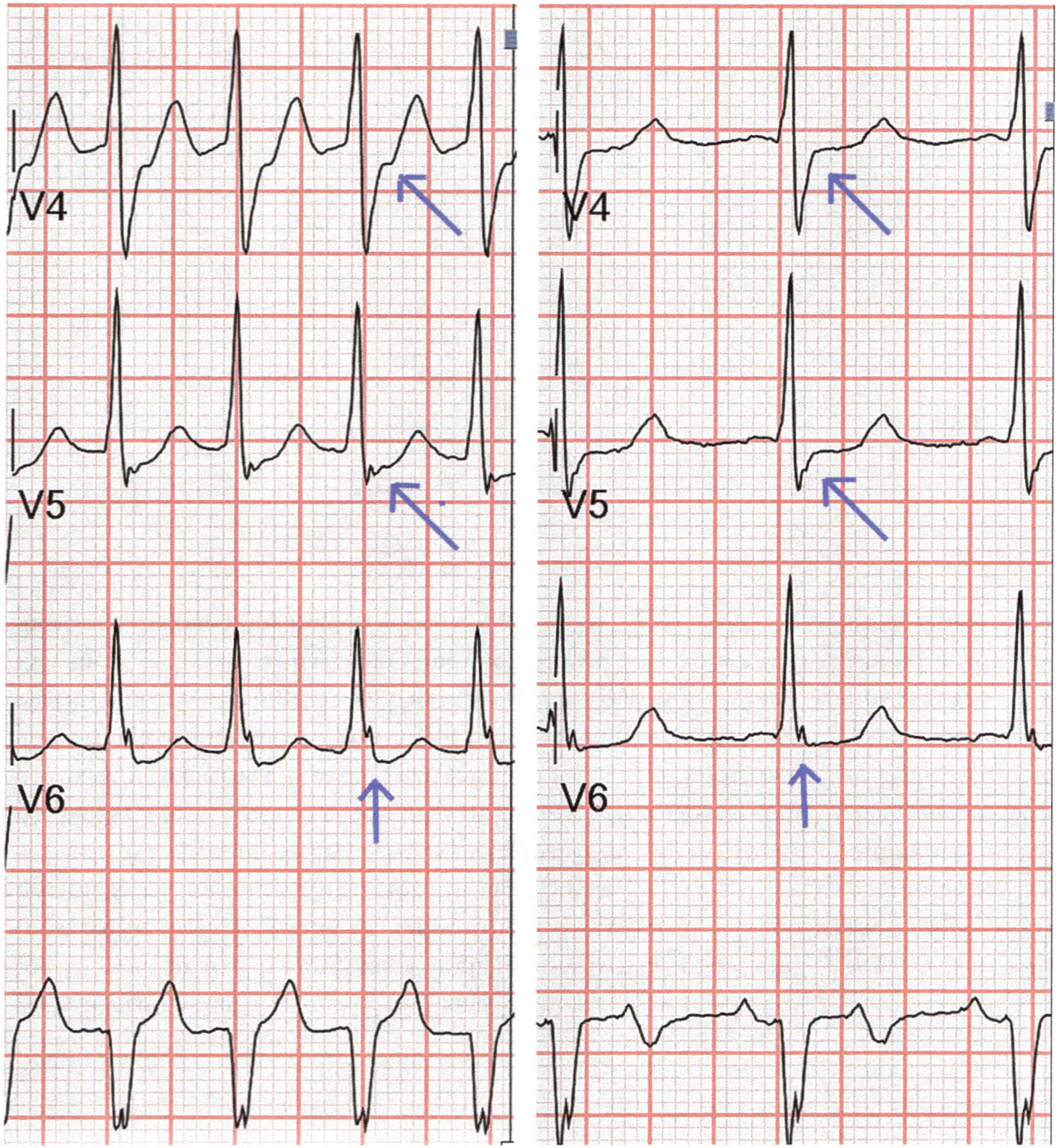

Figure 7-8A

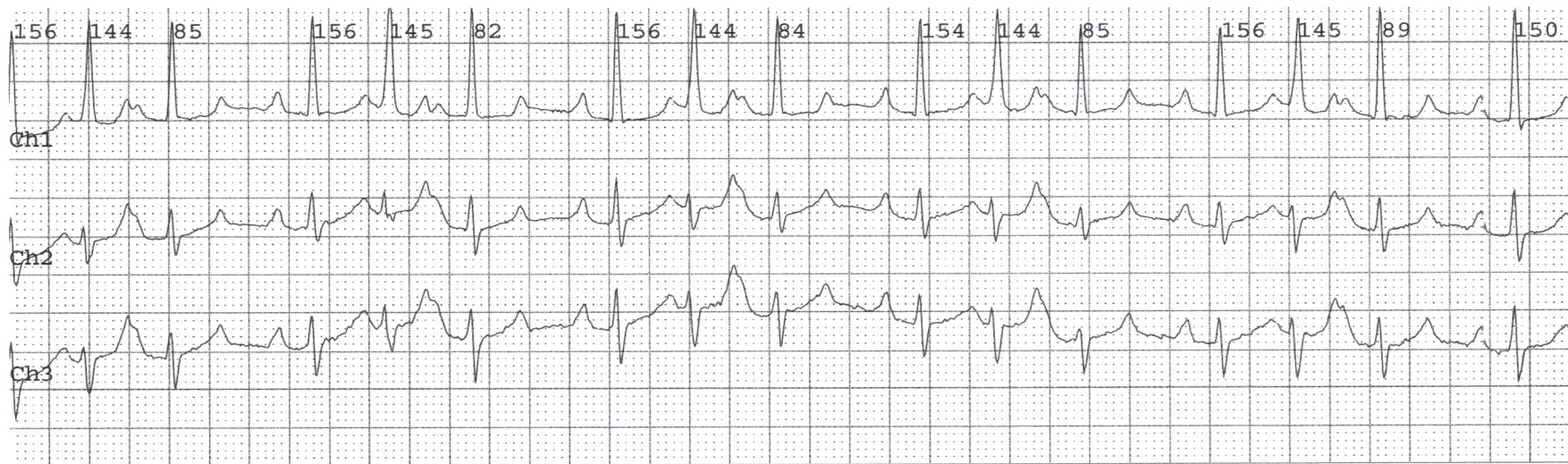

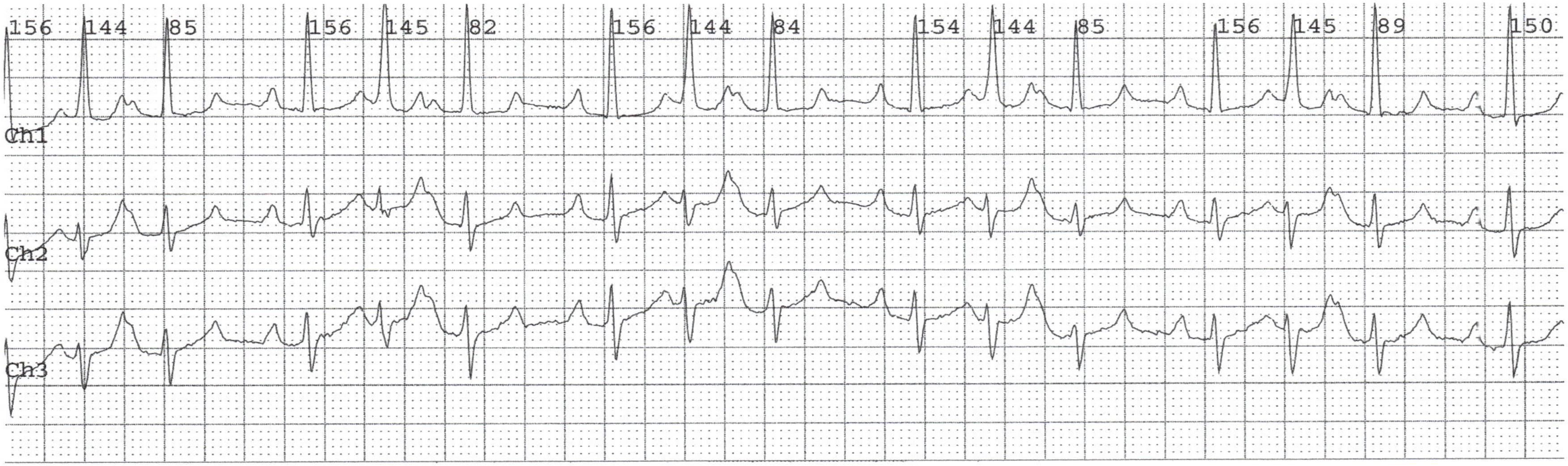


## Question 7-8

The rhythm phenomenon observed in **Figure 7-8A** is primarily a manifestation of:

1. Ectopy
2. Dual AV nodal pathways
3. Concealed conduction
4. Need more data

## Answer

Our question may be a little cryptic but should become clearer after some sense is made of the tracing.

Figure 7-8A shows a recurring pattern of 3 beats separated by a relative pause. Such a pattern of recurrent cycles has been described as "group beating" and may have multiple explanations.

I prefer to begin a complicated tracing with a part of the tracing that I can understand so that I can build upon what is known, rather than just start from left to right. The annotated **Figure 7-8B** identifies 3 repeating beats labeled 1, 2, and 3. Beat 1 is without much doubt a sinus beat.

The key to interpreting this tracing (as with many others, of course!) is identification of P waves. A little "trick," if you will, is to *join 2 consecutive P waves that are identifiable*, as indicated by the ends of the **red arrow**. One then identifies the center point, in this case indicated by the **vertical blue arrow**.

Many electronic calipers provide a centerline between 2 measured points, a feature extremely useful in interpreting such ECG and electrophysiology (EP) data. The **blue arrow** points to a deflection in the ST segment of beat 2 that is a likely P wave candidate. The rest of the pattern now falls simply into place. *This is merely a bigeminal rhythm with beat 2 interpolated between 2 sinus beats.*

The question of where beat 2 comes from is the crux of the multiple-choice question. It could simply be a junctional extrasystole or possibly ventricular, with an origin that provides good access to the specialized conduction system so that it appears to be "supraventricular." One notes that the PR interval of beat 3 is slightly longer than that of beat 1, potentially due to concealed retrograde conduction into the AV node from beat 2.

Alternatively, one might consider that junctional extrasystoles are relatively uncommon. It is also possible that the patient has dual AV nodal pathways, and we are seeing a "2-for-1" phenomenon with a single P wave over the fast pathway causing beat 1 and the same P wave conducting over the slow AV nodal pathway causing beat 2.

Thus, the "correct" answer to our question is Option 4, i.e., we need more data. Our patient was asymptomatic with normal ventricular function so that further studies were not pursued. The true answer here is, again, not as important as the thought process to sort out the tracing.

Figure 7-8B

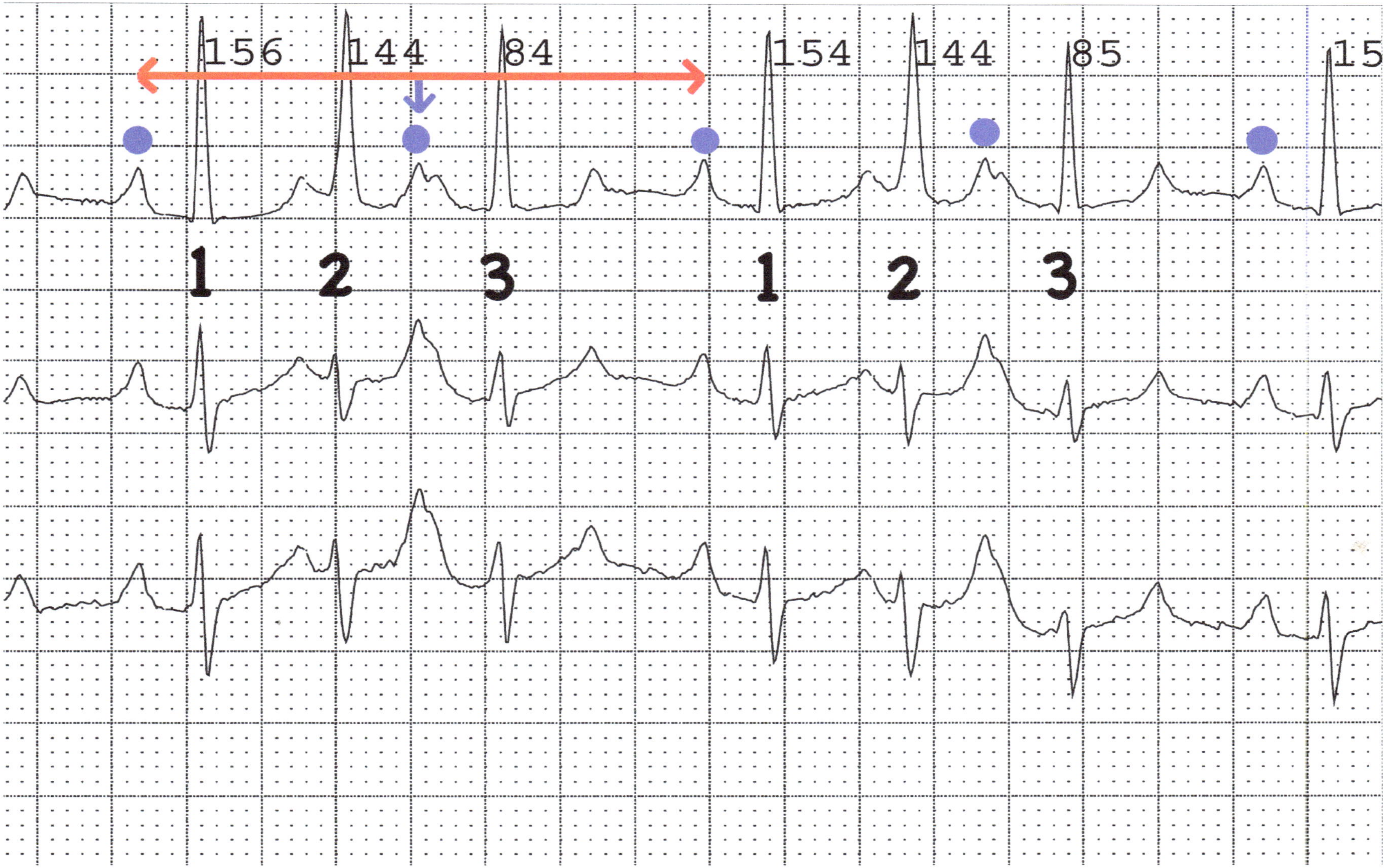

Figure 7-9

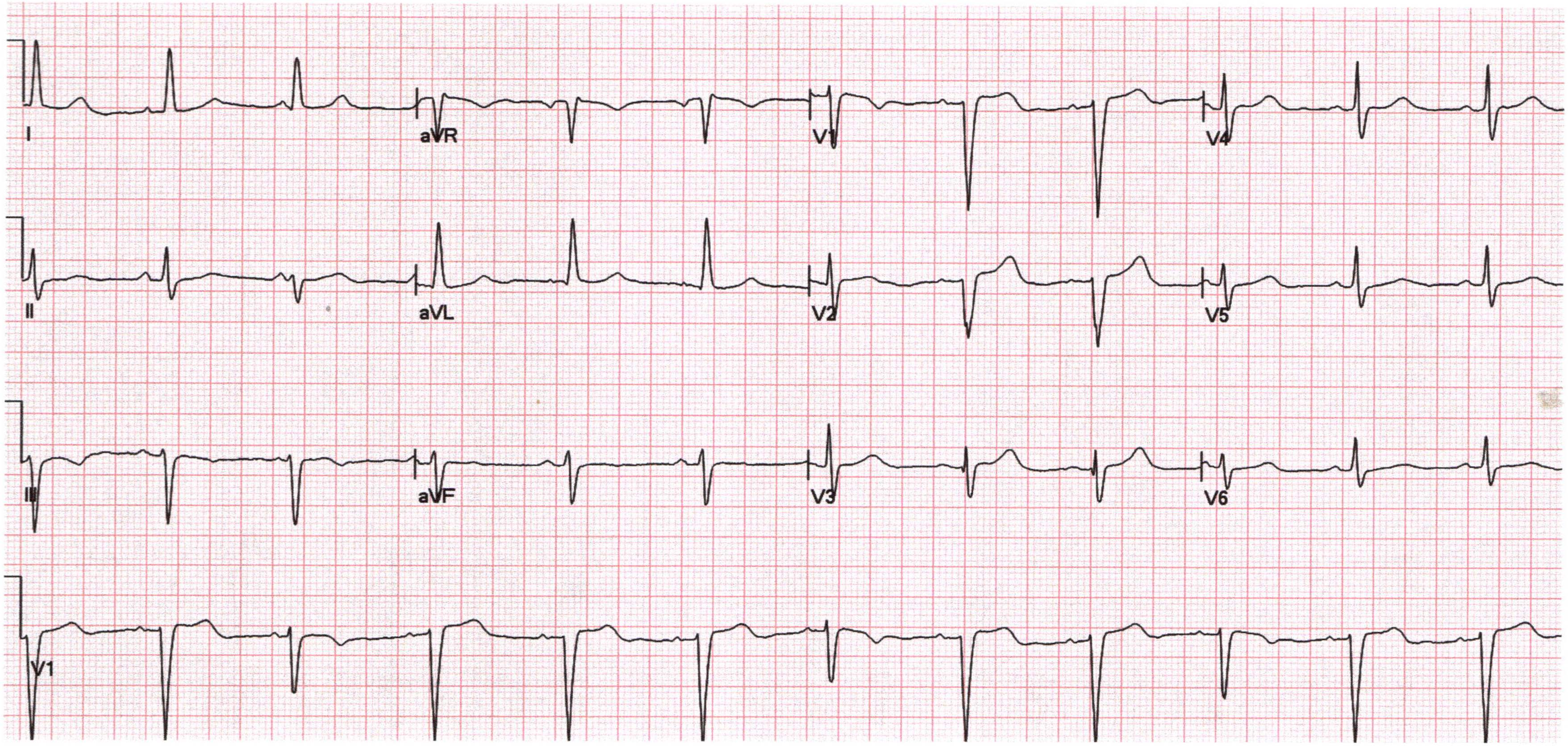


Question 7-9

## Question 7-9

The ECG shown in **Figure 7-9** illustrates:

1. PACs
2. PVCs
3. Intermittent preexcitation
4. "Two-for-one" AV node conduction

## Answer

The ECG is relatively normal except for 3 beats that are different, and this is best appreciated on the rhythm strip. The 3 beats are relatively "narrow," but this is not helpful and does not exclude any of the responses.

There are 2 important observations. The first is that the 3 beats each have a *different* PR interval, with the first in particular shorter than the ambient PR interval. This provides the basis for "framing" our problem—namely, what are the causes of sudden PR shortening?

The list would include all of the above options and additionally would include:

1. Junctional extrasystoles
2. Shortening of the PR interval by resolution of delay in the AV node or His-Purkinje system, perhaps related to a pause or rate slowing
3. Shift to a fast AV nodal pathway in a patient with dual pathways

Of all these possibilities, the most common would be late-coupled PVCs, which interrupt the PR interval, and this should be the presumptive diagnosis, all things being equal.

In our example, one notes that the variability of the PR interval also results in a slight change in the QRS morphology due to variable fusion of the PVC with the normal QRS. This would not be the case with intermittent conduction over an AP, which generally is associated with a constant shorter PR interval at a constant CL.

A PAC might give a shorter PR interval if closer to the AV node, but in our example, the P waves are not premature or different than the ambient P waves.

There would be no reason for a junctional extrasystole to look different than the rest, especially with such late coupling. There is nothing to *absolutely* exclude 2-for-1 AV nodal conduction or shift to a fast AV nodal pathway, but these would be much less common, and there would be no ready explanation for the *variable* change in the QRS complex or the PR interval.

Thus, the "best" answer is Option 2, PVCs.

Question 7-10

Figure 7-10A

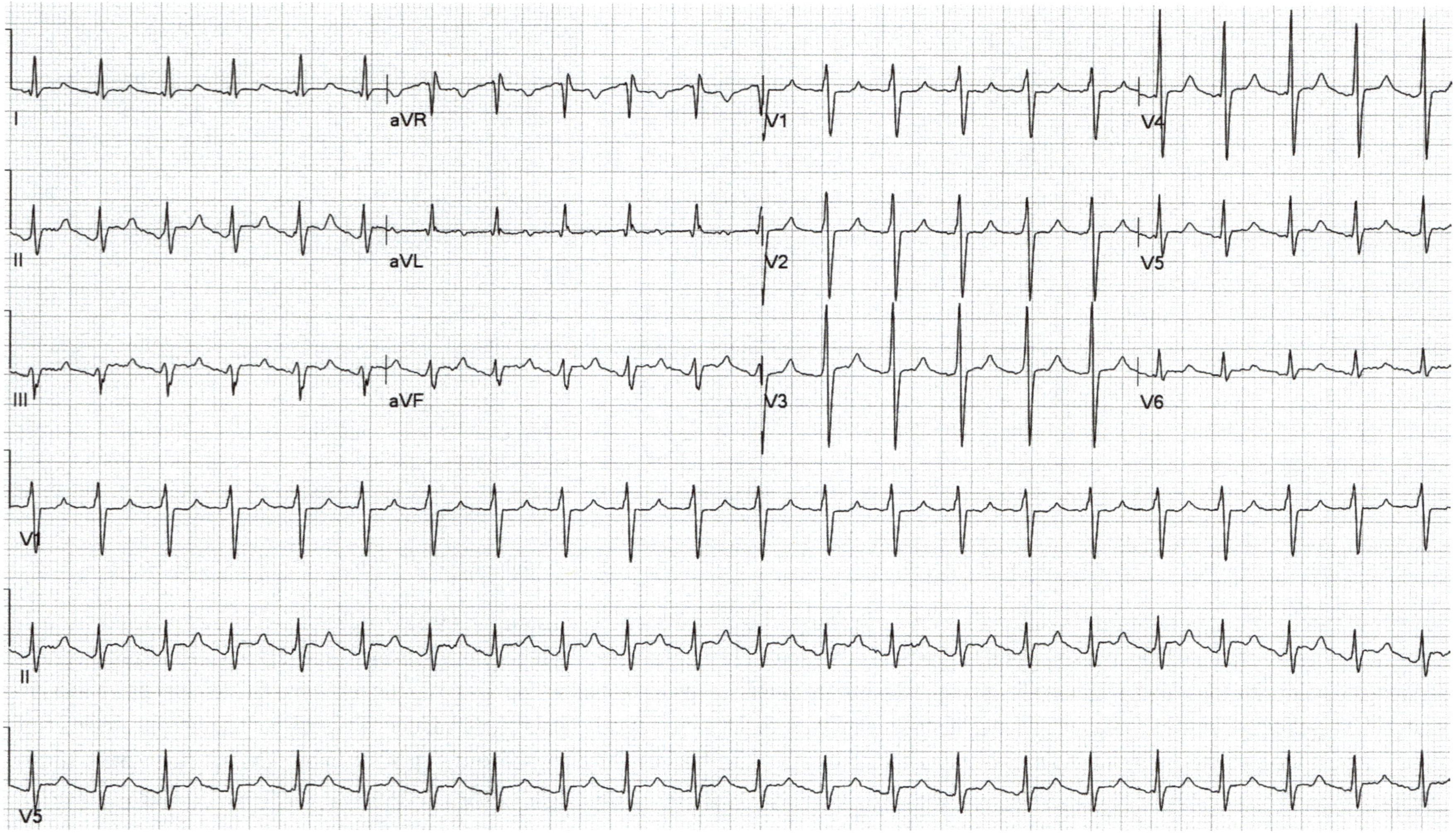

Question 7-10

## Question 7-10

The tachycardia mechanism in **Figure 7-10A** is:

1. AT
2. AVNRT
3. AVRT
4. Atrial flutter (AFL)

## Answer

This ECG is an exercise in attention to detail and looking at all leads available. Atrial activity is not apparent after a superficial look. If we magnify an area of interest (**Figure 7-10B**), atrial activity becomes more apparent.

As we have done before (for example, **Question 7-8**), we identify 2 P waves that are more obvious and draw a line between them (**red arrow**). The *midpoint is identified* (**blue arrow**), and this reveals a notch at the T wave onset that is in all probability a P wave (**blue dots**). The rhythm is now clear: AFL with 2:1 AV conduction.

It may seem obvious, but magnification of the area of interest often facilitates the observation of more subtle features.

Figure 7-10B

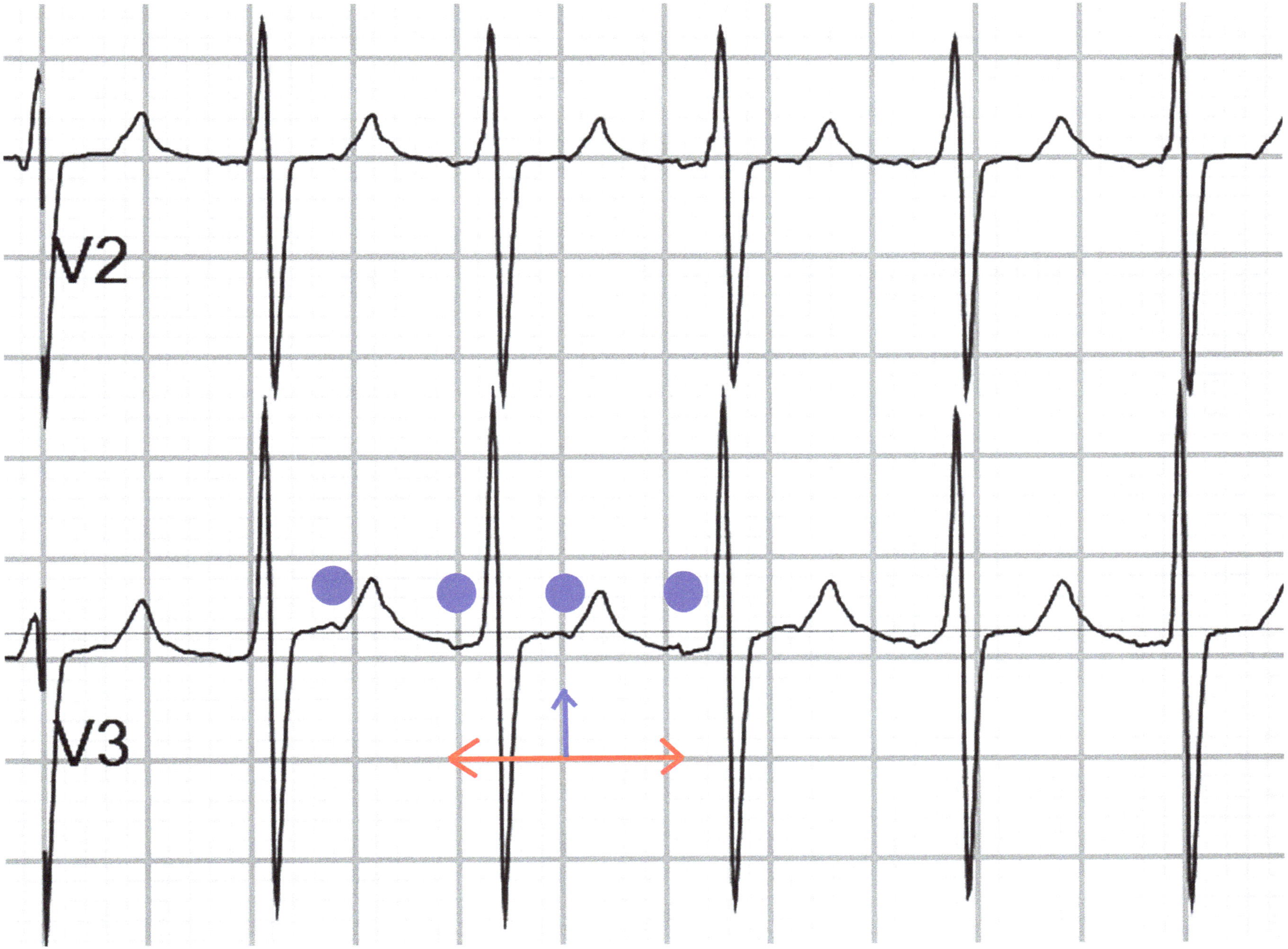

Figure 7-11A

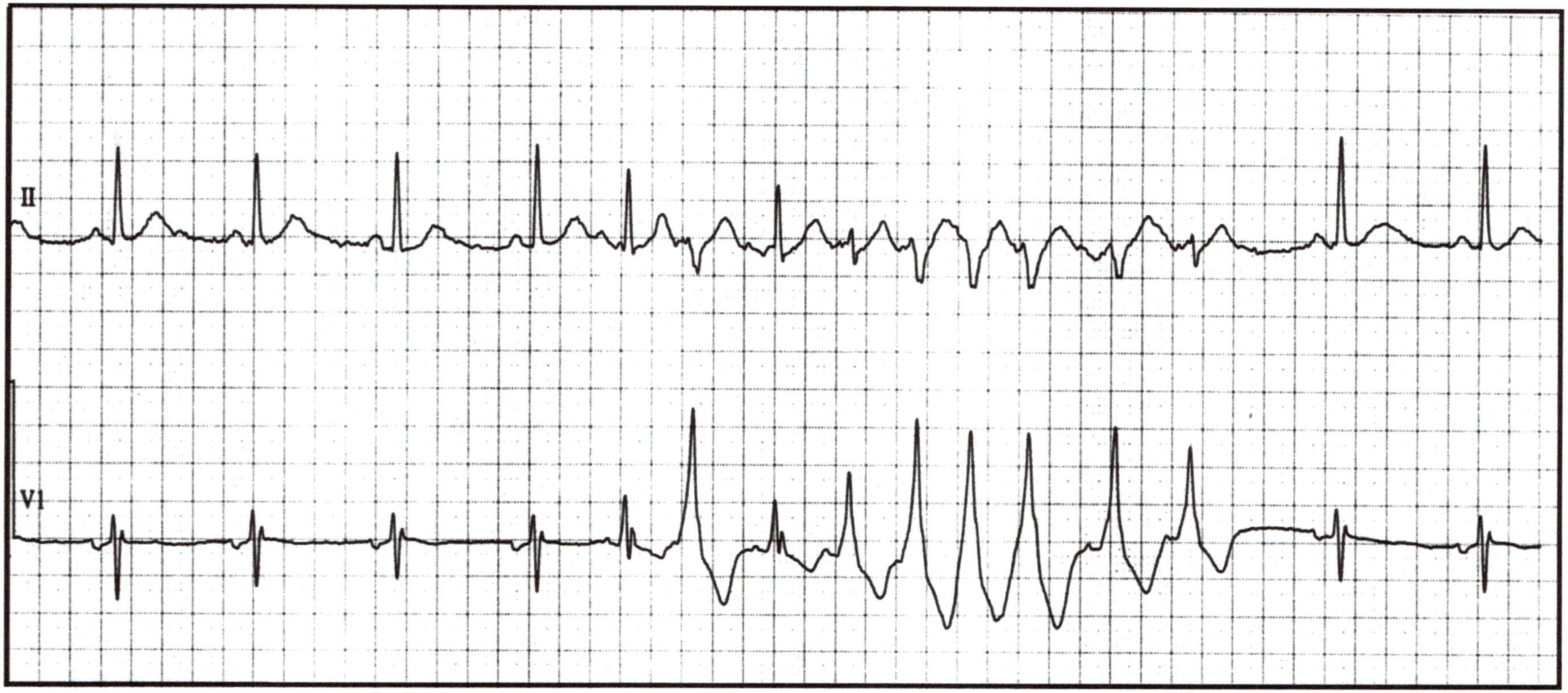

Question 7-11

## Question 7-11

The tachycardia mechanism in the tracing shown in **Figure 7-11A** is:

1. Polymorphous VT
2. Torsades de pointes
3. AT
4. Artifact

## Answer

The tracing begins with sinus rhythm and a normal QRS that is interrupted by an irregular rhythm with multiple QRS morphologies, which immediately suggests polymorphic VT. Artifact should always be considered for such a rhythm, but the tracing is sufficiently "clean" that we can dismiss this.

We are fortunate enough to see the onset of this rhythm and note that the rhythm begins with a PAC **(Figure 7-11B, red arrow)**. *This is a major strike against VT!* It is difficult to see clear atrial activity during this rhythm, but we see some similar to the initiating one reasonably clearly (**blue dots**). It would be very coincidental indeed to have precedent P waves prior to even some VT QRS complexes.

We are thus guided to a diagnosis of AT (albeit irregular), but the QRS morphology in $V_1$ would be very atypical for RBBB aberration. It would not be unusual for a preexcited QRS, and this in fact was a patient with a left lateral AP. The left lateral AP is frequently associated with subtle preexcitation (fusion favoring the normal AV conduction system in sinus rhythm by proximity to the sinus node). PACs and AT from the left atrium, as we may well have here, as suggested by the change in P wave from sinus, would favor the AP and bring out the preexcitation. The changing QRS complexes are compatible with variable fusion over the AV node and AP.

The correct answer is thus AT. The importance of attention to detail without jumping to what seems "obvious" goes without saying.

Figure 7-11B

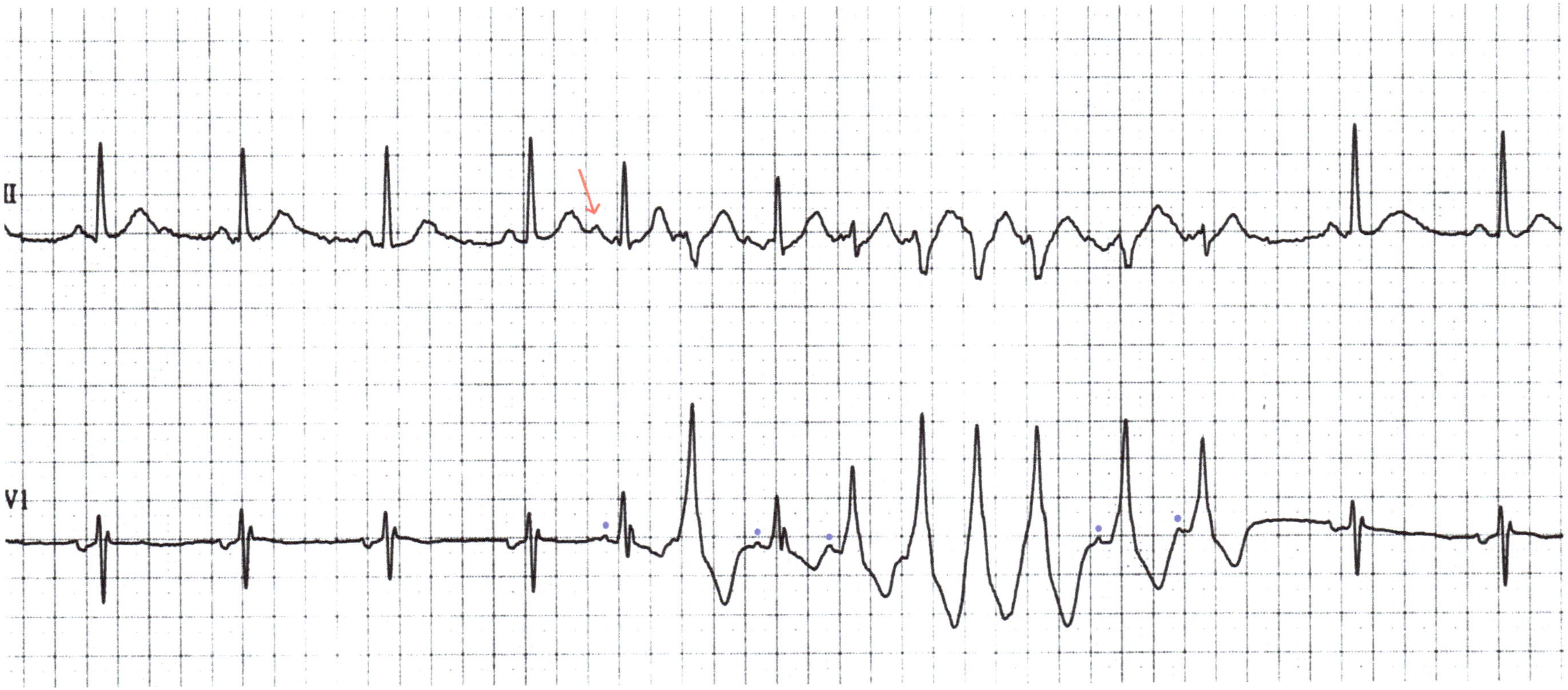

Figure 7-12A

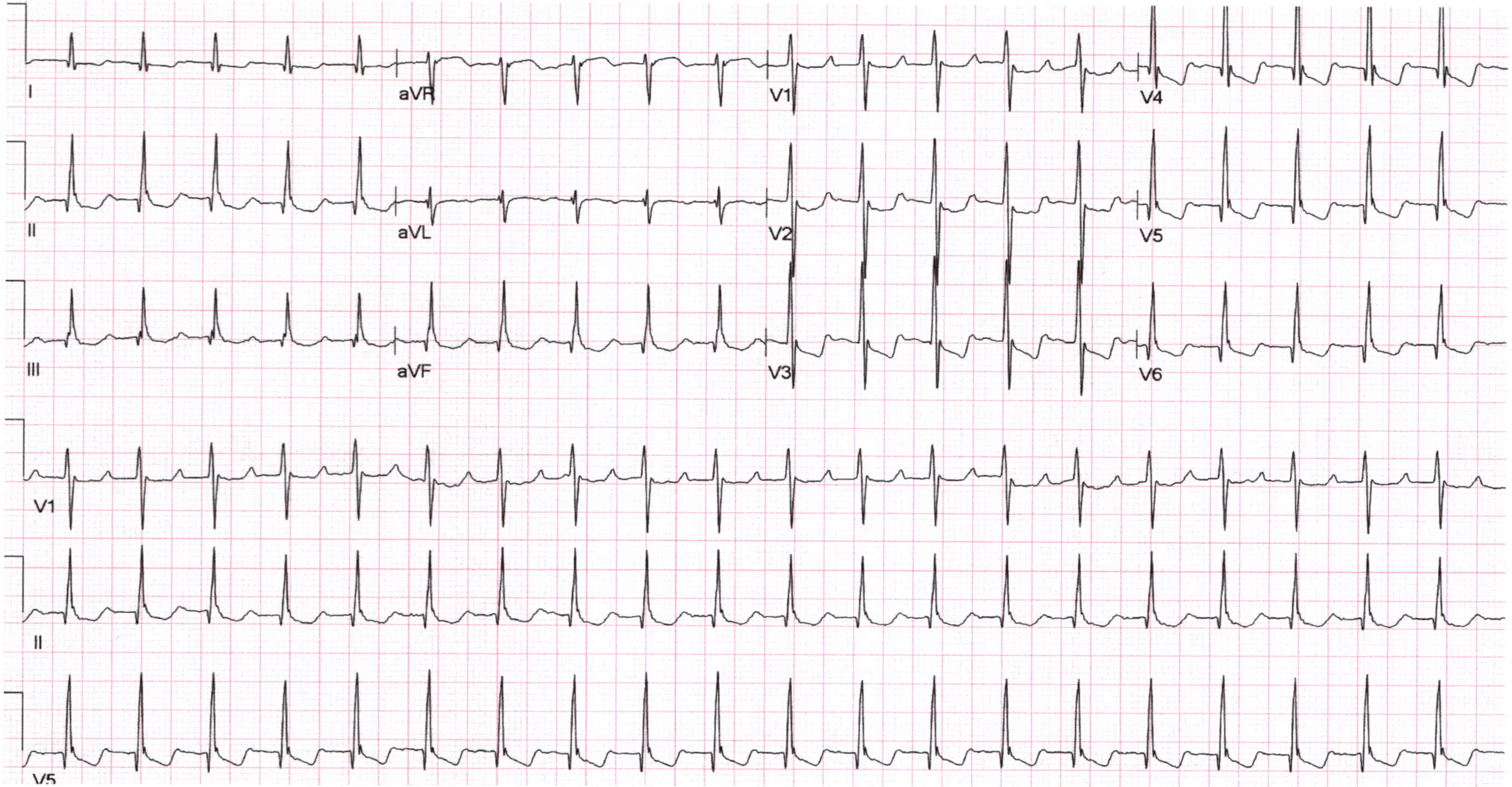


Question 7-12

## Question 7-12

The tachycardia mechanism shown in **Figure 7-12A** is:

1. AT
2. AVNRT
3. AVRT
4. Need more data

## Answer

This tracing falls into the broad category of regular SVT. A good P wave candidate is really only reasonably seen at the end of the T wave in $V_1$, $V_2$, and $V_3$ as a positive deflection in approximately mid diastole. Atrial activity is not clearly apparent elsewhere, and the "obvious" diagnosis here is AT or possibly ST, although the other options are not clearly ruled out.

The key observation here is that the *observed P wave is approximately mid-diastolic.* One should always then ask where a second P wave would be hidden if it were present.

My approach is simply to mark the interval between 2 successive P waves (**solid blue lines** in **Figure 7-12B**) and then establish the midpoint between these (dashed blue line; See also **Question 3-2** to expand this discussion). It immediately becomes obvious that a second P wave, if present, would be largely buried in the middle of the QRS, although a partial P wave may also be suspected from the subtle terminal deflection of the QRS. The

Figure 7-12B

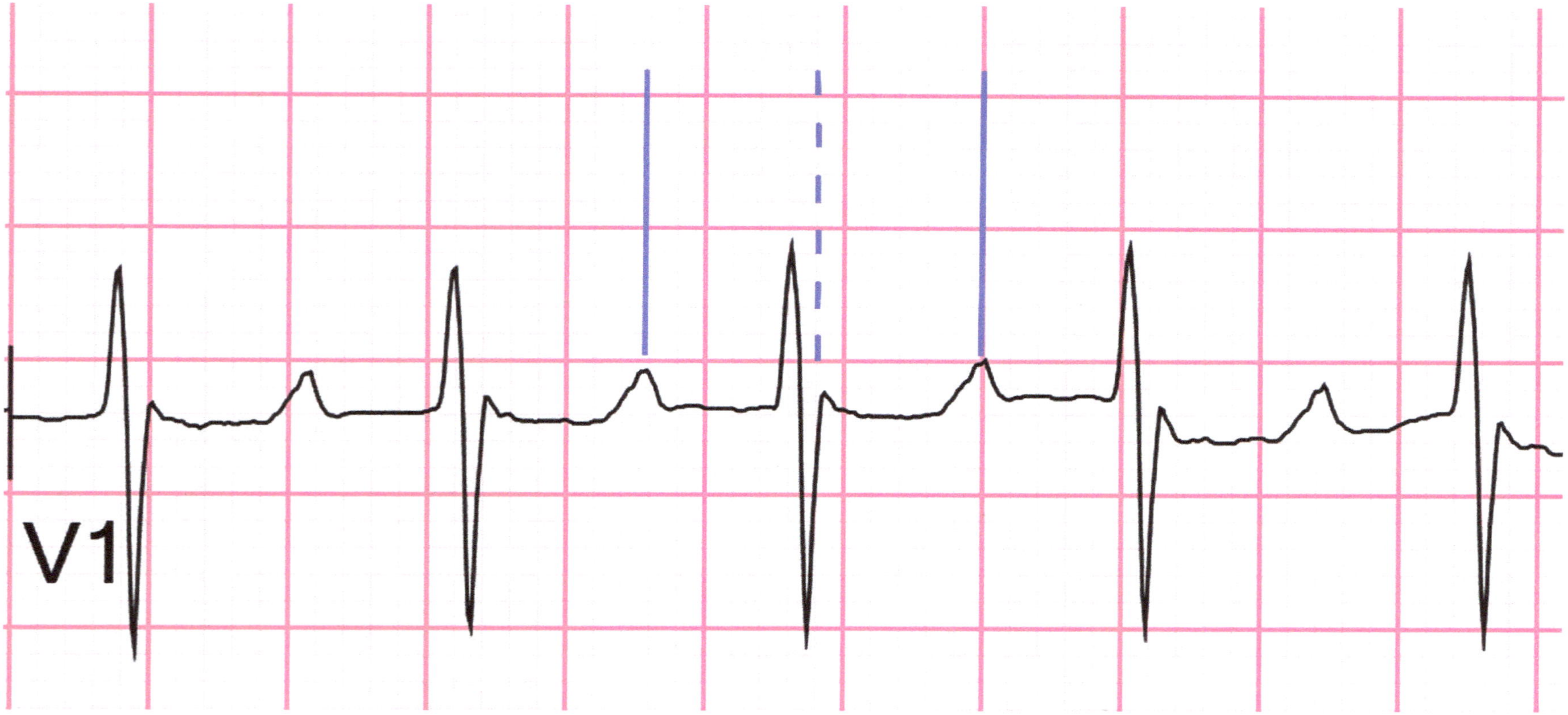

correct answer to our question must be Option 4, in that none of the options are unequivocally ruled out.

Clarification of the issue comes with the subsequent tracing in **Figure 7-12C**, where AFL with variable AV conduction is evident. It then also becomes evident that atrial activity is of very low amplitude with the exception of the anterior precordial leads, adding to our diagnostic difficulty.

*Always* beware of the mid-diastolic P wave!

Figure 7-12C

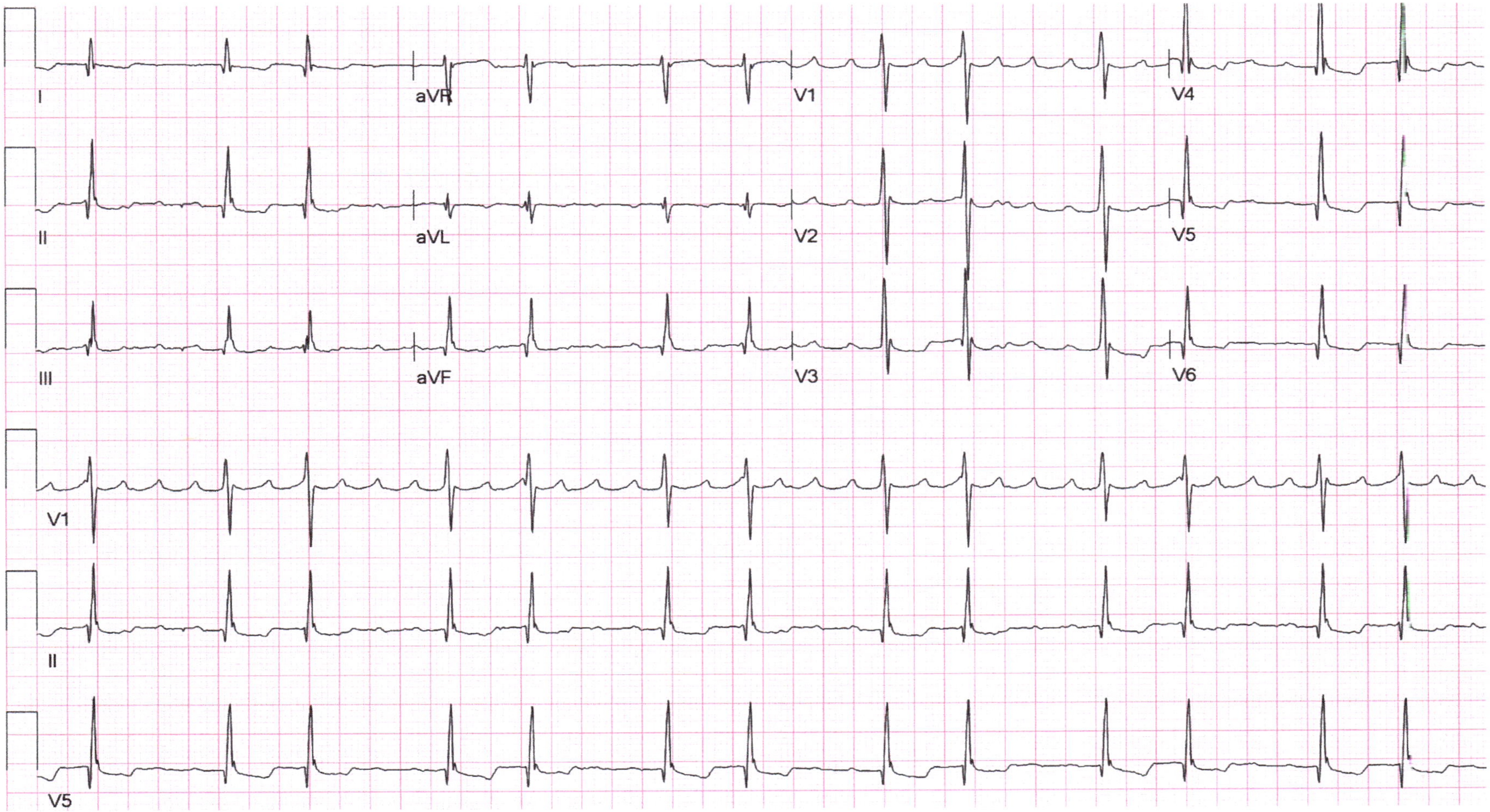

Figure 7-13A

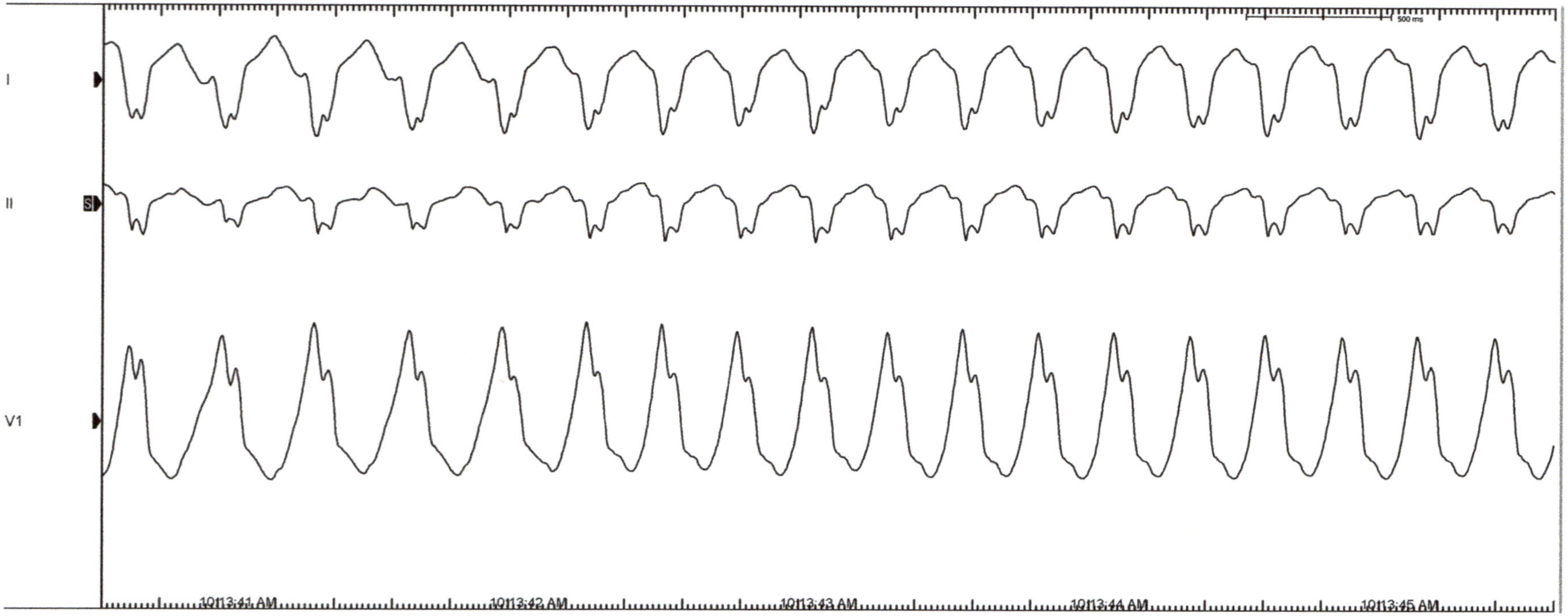
I
II
S
V1
500 ms
10h13:41 AM
10h13:42 AM
10h13:43 AM
10h13:44 AM
10h13:45 AM

## Question 7-13

The ECG in **Figure 7-13A** was obtained during catheter insertion at the onset of an EP study in a 24-year-old man with no known heart disease undergoing study for paroxysmal palpitations. The tachycardia mechanism is:

1. VT
2. SVT with aberrancy
3. Preexcited tachycardia
4. Need more data

## Answer

This is a difficult ECG to interpret, but interpretable using a few basic observations.

Figure 7-13A shows a WCT with leads 1, 2, and $V_1$. The frontal plane axis is strongly "left to right" with a wide QS pattern. $V_1$ indicates a RBBB type of QRS. *This morphology is virtually incompatible with RBBB aberration.* We can thus reasonably narrow our choices to VT or a preexcited tachycardia.

Further elucidation depends on focusing on the transition area (where the tachycardia speeds up rather abruptly at the sixth QRS) and identifying P waves. The annotated **Figure 7-13B** shows us a

Figure 7-13B

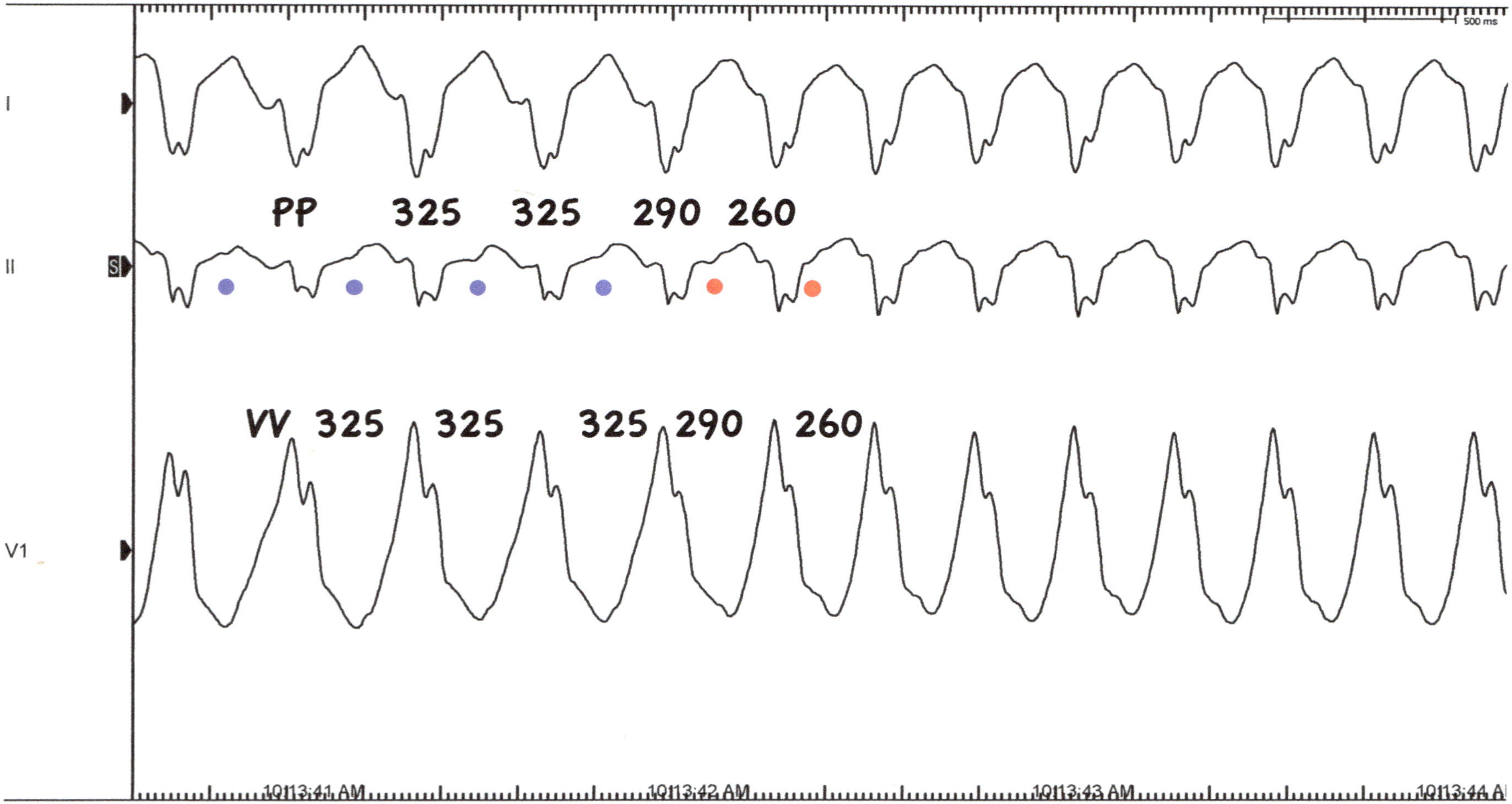

sudden change in CL of the tachycardia, with the sixth QRS being a little premature. The P waves are subtle, indicated by the **dots**, and are easiest to appreciate at the change of CL. Note that the **first red dot** moves earlier into the ST segment and the **second red dot** is earlier still.

One also notes that *the first premature P precedes the first QRS advanced, i.e., the change in the ventricular rate is preceded by the change in the atrial rate. This **cannot be** ventricular tachycardia.* (See the discussion on the value of CL variation with **Question 6-1**.) The cause ("site") of sudden CL change can't be "downstream" from the initially observed site of change. An AT is ruled out if the QRS moves before the P wave and vice versa.

In this example, the tachycardia was antidromic, with the antegrade limb being a left lateral AP (as you would expect from the QRS morphology) and the retrograde limb being the normal atrioventricular conduction system (AVCS or AV conduction system) (**Figure 7-13C**).

The longer CL was related to *retrograde* LBBB, which prolonged the circuit by forcing retrograde conduction over to the RBBB (**Figure 7-13C, panel A**). This resulted in a longer time to get through the ventricle to the atrium, i.e., a longer QRS to P (or "ventriculo-atrial" ) interval. Resolution of retrograde LBBB (**Figure 7-13C, panel B**) shortened the circuit by allowing conduction directly from the left lateral accessory pathway to the AVCS via the LBB. Hence the QRS to P time (ventriculo-atrial time) shortened.

Figure 7-13C

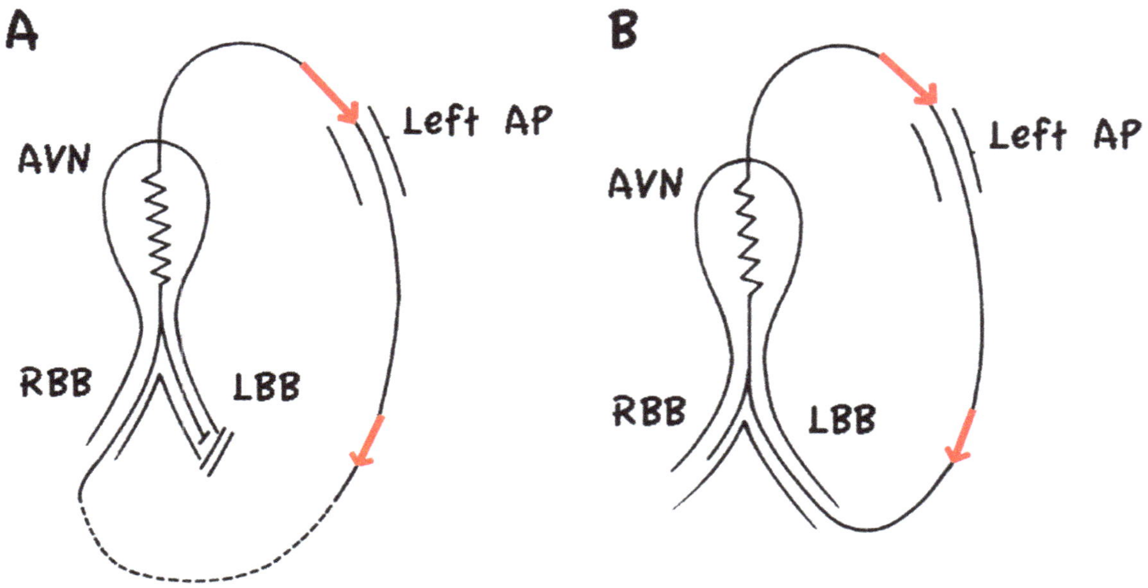

Question 7-14

Figure 7-14A

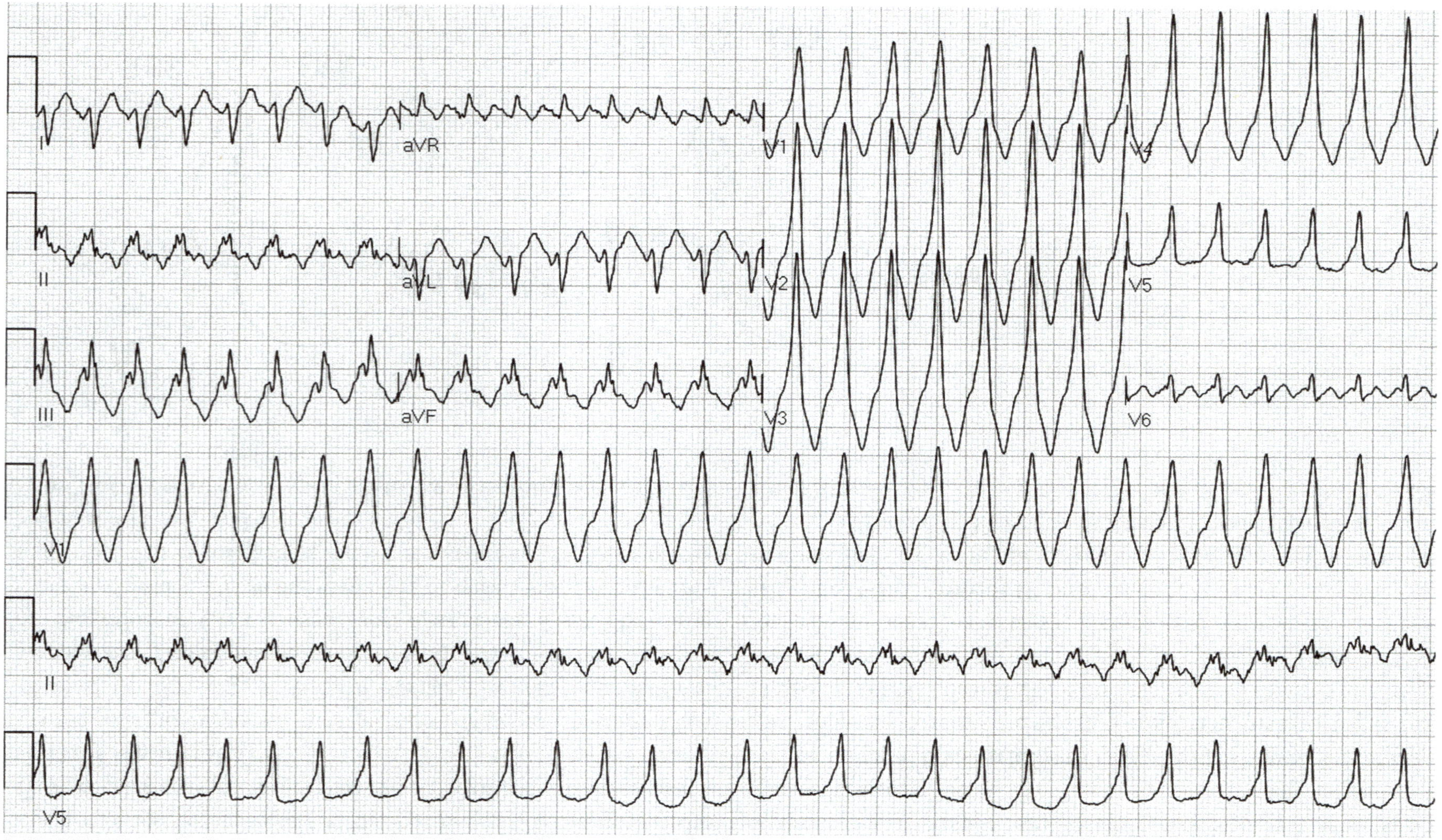

## Question 7-14

The tachycardia mechanism in **Figure 7-14A**, from a previously well 16-year-old woman, is:

1. VT
2. SVT with aberrancy
3. Preexcited tachycardia
4. Need more data

## Answer

As we have done previously, we approach this 12-lead WCT (Figure 7-14A) by initially asking ourselves if this QRS reasonably resembles a bundle branch block pattern or not. The answer to this question is *no, not at all.*

Although $V_1$ is positive and would be classified as a RBBB type pattern, the QRS is monophasic and peaked. Further, most of the V leads ($V_1$ to $V_5$) have upright QRS and could be said to be "positively concordant," which would not be seen in RBBB. The frontal axis is a little difficult to calculate due to all the notching in the QRS but is certainly strongly rightward—again, not expected in usual RBBB.

This tachycardia has an activation pattern more typical of a ventricular origin. The positive concordance in the precordial leads suggests a basal (near the AV ring) origin of activation compatible with VT or a left AP that inserts into the ventricle in that region.

Even after a diligent search magnifying regions of interest, it is very difficult to be confident about identifying atrial activity. The QRS morphology alone tells us that this is very unlikely to be SVT with aberrancy but doesn't categorically distinguish VT vs. preexcited tachycardia. The correct answer to our question would thus be Option 4, need more data.

A spontaneous termination was fortuitously observed (**Figure 7-14B**), and we might now ask our question again. There are 2 significant observations. One is made after the resumption of sinus rhythm where the QRS is unequivocally preexcited after an initial PVC. This, of course, enhances the probability of preexcited tachycardia as a diagnosis, although strictly speaking doesn't prove it.

The more compelling observation is the gradual slowing of the tachycardia before termination. The QRS to P interval prolongs with slight slowing of the atrial rate, and the P waves become clearly visible over the last 5 cycles or so before the break. *Notably, the last event is a QRS without a following P wave.*

This makes VT untenable. It would be most unlikely if a spontaneous termination of VT were associated coincidentally with retrograde block to the atrium at the instant of VT termination.

One might perform a little additional exercise by magnifying the last 4 or 5 cycles in $V_5$ several-fold to facilitate finer measurement (**Figure 7-14C**). It would then be observed that a CL change in the PP interval preceded the change in the QRS-QRS interval, an occurrence incompatible with VT.

This was a preexcited tachycardia, specifically antidromic tachycardia using the AP as the anterograde limb of the circuit and the normal AV conduction system as the retrograde limb. The latter is often the "weak limb" of this circuit, as it was in this case.

Figure 7-14B

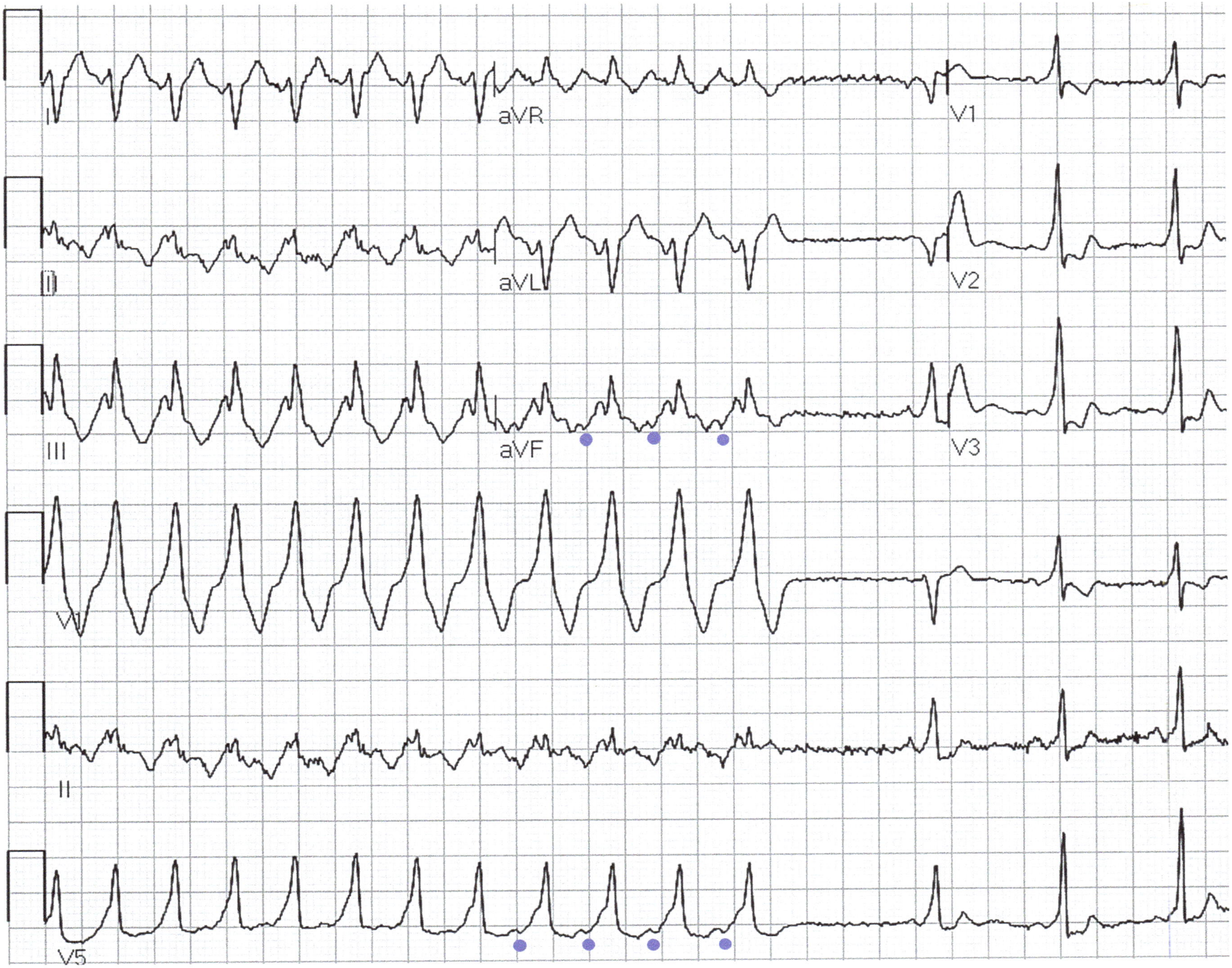

Figure 7-14C

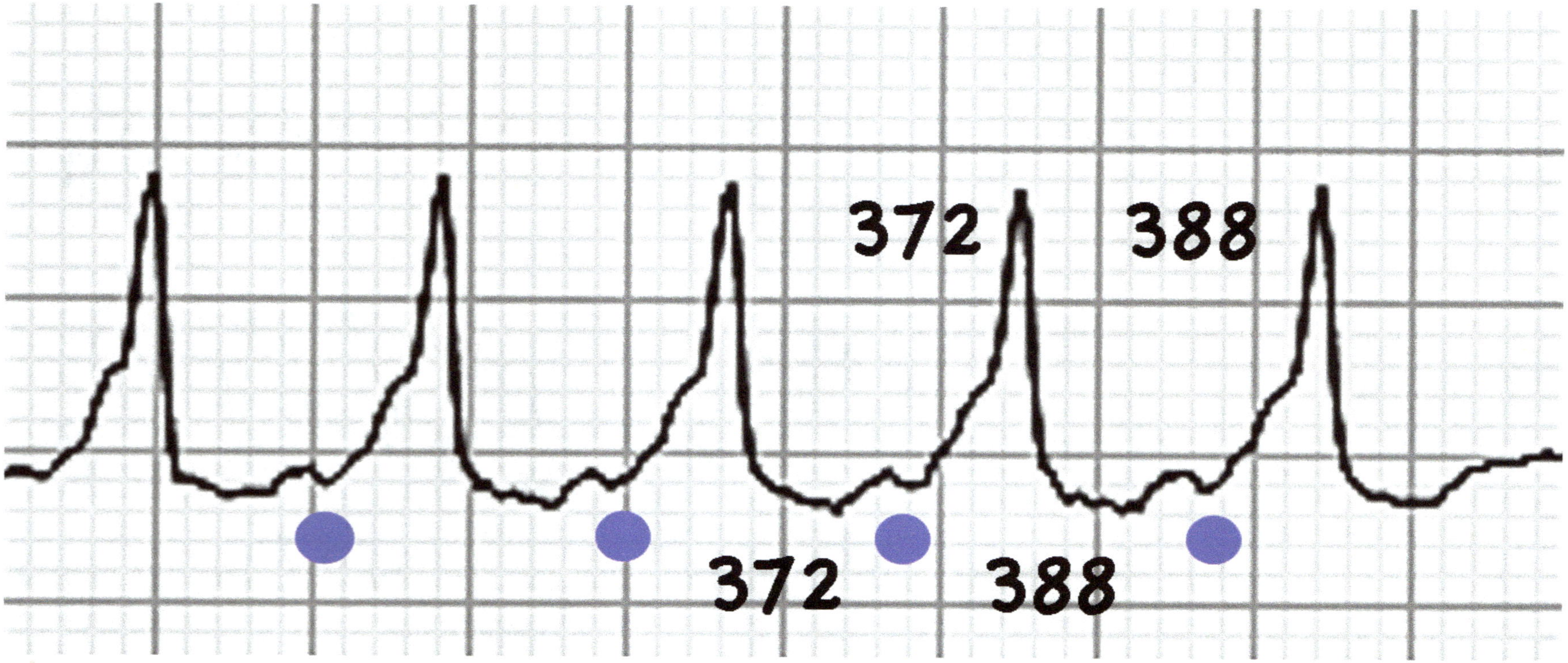

# Index

## A

## P



## Q



## R



## S

## T



## V



## W



## Z

www.ingramcontent.com/pod-product-compliance
Lightning Source LLC
Chambersburg PA
CBHW080716220326
41598CB00033B/5435
* 9 7 8 1 9 4 2 9 0 9 2 4 8 *